ONCOLOGY MCQS FOR NEET-SS

Volume 4: hematology

Dr. Bhratri Bhushan
MBBS, MD, DM

Dedicated to Varchasv
My shining light

CONTENTS

INTRODUCTION

When I was preparing for DM entrance, I experienced a dearth of books on the subject of hematology entrance and the books that were available were either not updated or were lacking in depth, that was when I conceived the idea of writing such a book myself.

I have written this book purely from the perspective of a hemat-oncologist and by relying on the highest quality material. The standard textbooks, NCCN guidelines and high impact journals were referenced for every question. The result is this book, which will serve the purpose of equipping the exam going (NEET-SS and board review, along with any other entrance exam where questions about hematology are asked) doctors with the right tool to test and build their knowledge.

As the knowledge in the field of hematology is unfolding at an unprecedented scale and new strategies are being devised at a prolific pace, it is not possible to provide all of the updated information, all at once. I will be updating this book periodically for this purpose. In case of any queries and suggestions regarding this book, kindly send to: bhratri@gmail.com

ACUTE MYELOID LEUKEMIA

Q. Which of the following comes under the intermediate risk AML category according to the 2017 ELN risk stratification:
1. Biallelic mutated CEBPA
2. t(6;9)
3. t(9;11)
4. Wild type NPM1 and FLT3-ITD*high*

Answer: t(9;11)

Please memorise this table of 2017 European LeukemiaNet risk stratification of acute myeloid leukemia by genetics:

Favorable risk category:
1. t(8;21)(q22;q22.1); RUNX1-RUNX1T1
2. inv(16)(p13.1;q22) or t(16;16)(p13.1;q22); CBFB-MYH11
3. Mutated NPM1 without FLT3-ITD or with FLT3-IT-Dlow
4. Biallelic mutated CEBPA

Intermediate risk category:
1. Mutated *NPM1* and *FLT3-ITD*high
2. Wild type *NPM1* without *FLT3-ITD* or with *FLT3-IT-*

*D*low (without adverse-risk genetic lesions)
3. t(9;11)(p21.3;q23.3); *MLLT3-KMT2A*
4. Cytogenetic abnormalities not classified as favorable or adverse

Adverse risk category:
1. t(6;9)(p23;q34.1); *DEK-NUP214*
2. t(v;11q23.3); *KMT2A* rearranged
3. t(9;22)(q34.1;q11.2); *BCR-ABL1*
4. inv(3)(q21.3q26.2) or t(3;3) (q21.3;q26.2); *GATA2,MECOM(EVI1)*
5. −5 or del(5q); −7; −17/abn(17p)
6. Complex karyotype, monosomal karyotype
7. Wild type *NPM1* and *FLT3-ITD*high
8. Mutated *RUNX1*
9. Mutated *ASXL1*
10. Mutated *TP53*

Q. Which of the following is the definition of complex karyotype according to the ELN 2017 risk classification of AML:
1. Three or more unrelated chromosome abnormalities in the absence of one of the World Health Organisation designated recurring translocations or inversions, ie, t(8;21), inv(16) or t(16;16), t(9;11), t(v;11)(v;q23.3), t(6;9), inv(3) or t(3;3); AML with *BCR-ABL1*
2. Two or more unrelated chromosome abnormalities in the absence of one of the World Health Organization designated recurring translocations or inversions, ie, t(8;21), inv(16) or t(16;16), t(9;11), t(v;11)(v;q23.3), t(6;9), inv(3) or t(3;3); AML with *BCR-ABL1*
3. Four or more unrelated chromosome abnormalities

      in the absence of one of the World Health Organiza-
tion designated recurring translocations or inversions, ie, t(8;21), inv(16) or t(16;16), t(9;11), t(v;11)
(v;q23.3), t(6;9), inv(3) or t(3;3); AML with *BCR-ABL1*

4. Five or more unrelated chromosome abnormalities
in the absence of one of the World Health Organization designated recurring translocations or inversions, ie, t(8;21), inv(16) or t(16;16), t(9;11), t(v;11)
(v;q23.3), t(6;9), inv(3) or t(3;3); AML with *BCR-ABL1*

Answer: Three or more unrelated chromosome abnormalities in the absence of one of the World Health Organization designated recurring translocations or inversions, ie,
t(8;21), inv(16) or t(16;16), t(9;11), t(v;11)(v;q23.3), t(6;9),
inv(3) or t(3;3); AML with *BCR-ABL1*

Q. Which of the following is the most common chromosomal abnormality in children with AML:
1. t(8;21)
2. inv(16)
3. t(12;21)
4. t(9;11)

Answer: t(8;21)

Please memorise the WHO classification category of "AML
with recurrent genetic abnormalities":
1. AML with t(8;21); *RUNX1-RUNX1T1*
2. AML with inv(16) or t(16;16); *CBFB-MYH11*
3. APL with *PML-RARA*
4. AML with t(9;11); *MLLT3-KMT2A*

5. AML with t(6;9); *DEK-NUP214*
6. AML with inv(3) or t(3;3); *GATA2, MECOM*
7. AML (megakaryoblastic) with t(1;22); *RBM15-MKL1*
8. AML with mutated *NPM1*
9. AML with biallelic mutations of *CEBPA*

(So, there are a total of 9 AML with "recurrent genetic abnormality" types).

Please memorise the FAB classification of AML (while is also included under the heading of "AML NOS" in the WHO classification):
1. AML-M0: AML with minimal differentiation
2. AML-M1: AML without maturation
3. AML-M2: AML with maturation
4. AML-M3: acute promyelocytic leukemia
5. AML-M4: Acute myelomonocytic leukemia
6. AML-M5: Acute monoblastic/monocytic leukemia
7. AML-M6: Pure erythroid leukemia
8. AML-M7: Acute megakaryoblastic leukemia

Q. In the current World Health Organization classification system, to make a diagnosis of AML, the blast count must account for at least what percent of the total cellularity of bone marrow:
1. 20
2. >20
3. 25
4. >25

Answer: 20

Remember, the blast count must account for **20% or more** of total cellularity of the bone marrow (at least 500 cells must be counted before giving a blast percentage). Also remember that a blast count **20% or more** in the peripheral blood is also diagnostic of AML.

Note, that if the following genetic abnormalities are present, they are considered diagnostic of AML **regardless of** the blast count:
1. AML with t(8;21)(q22;q22); *RUNX1-RUNX1T1* (previously *AML1-ETO*)
2. AML with inv(16)(p13.1q22) or t(16;16) (p13.1;q22); *CBFB-MYH11*
3. APL with t(15;17)(q24.1;q21.1); *PML-RARA*

If myeloid sarcoma is present, then also we don't require the blast percent to make a diagnosis of AML.

Q. Which of the following statement is true:
1. Therapy related myeloid neoplasms typically present five to seven years after initial treatment with alkylating agents
2. Therapy related myeloid neoplasms typically present five to seven years after initial treatment with RT
3. Therapy related myeloid neoplasms typically present one to three years after initial treatment with topoisomerase II inhibitors
4. All of the above

Answer: all of the above

Please remember all these facts.

The typical abnormalities associated with topoisomerase II inhibitors related myeloid neoplasms involve 11q23, for example t(9;11).

Remember that while alkylating agents and RT are associated with many types of myeloid neoplasms (AML, MDS, MPN etc.); topoisomerase II inhibitors are almost exclusively associated with AML.

Q. Myeloid sarcoma is more common in paediatric AML with all of the following features except:
  1. Older age
  2. High white blood cell count at diagnosis
  3. t(8;21)
  4. FAB M4 and M5 AML

Answer: older age

Myeloid sarcomas are more common in younger paediatric patients.

Q. Children with Down syndrome have:
  1. 2 to 5 times increased risk of developing AML
  2. 2 to 5 times increased risk of developing ALL

3. 10 to 20 times increased risk of developing AML
4. 10 to 20 times increased risk of developing ALL

Answer: 10 to 20 times increased risk of developing AML

Q. Up to what percent of infants with Down syndrome may develop transient abnormal myelopoiesis (TAM):
　　1. <5
　　2. 10
　　3. 20
　　4. 30-43

Answer: 10%

Q. Which of the following is not true:
　　1. Children with Down syndrome with AML have superior overall survival when compared with children with AML who do not have Down syndrome
　　2. AML-M7 is associated with Down syndrome
　　3. The leukemic cells of Down syndrome associated AML show increased sensitivity to cytarabine
　　4. Children with Down syndrome associated AML have lower rates of cardiotoxicity from daunorubicin

Answer: Children with Down syndrome associated AML have lower rates of cardiotoxicity from daunorubicin

In fact, children with Down syndrome associated AML have

higher rates of cardiotoxicity from daunorubicin. This is an important point, because it has clinical implications. Studies have shown that DS related AML patients can not tolerate intensive chemo regimens used in paediatric AML.

Q. Children with Down syndrome related AML who relapse after chemotherapy have:
1. Higher cure rates with allogeneic HCT compared with relapsed AML patients without Down syndrome
2. Lower cure rates with allogeneic HCT compared with relapsed AML patients without Down syndrome
3. Similar cure rates with allogeneic HCT compared with relapsed AML patients without Down syndrome
4. They are not treated with allogeneic HCT at all

Answer: Lower cure rates with allogeneic HCT compared with relapsed AML patients without Down syndrome

Q. What is the preferred approach for remission induction in a young and medically fit patient of AML, without any targetable mutation:
1. A 7-day continuous infusion of cytarabine and 3 days of anthracycline
2. A 7-day continuous infusion of anthracycline and 3 days of cytarabine
3. A 7-day course of cytarabine and 3 days continuous infusion of anthracycline
4. A 7-day course of anthracycline and 3 days continu-

ous infusion of cytarabine

Answer: A 7-day continuous infusion of cytarabine and 3 days of anthracycline

This is more commonly known as the "7 + 3 regimen".

The dosages are as follows:
1. Cytarabine = 100 to 200 mg/m2 daily as a continuous infusion for 7 days
2. Daunorubicin = 60 to 90 mg/m2 on days 1 to 3

We may use idarubicin in place of daunorubicin. The dose of idarubicin is 12 mg/m2 on days 1 to 3 (this recommendation is based on the ALFA 9801 study, in which survival outcomes and toxicities were similar between the daunorubicin arm and the idarubicin arm).

Q. As a part of the 7 + 3 regimen for induction in AML, higher dose (60 to 90 mg/m2) daunorubicin results in all of the following compared with lower dose (45 mg/m2) daunorubicin, except:
1. Superior complete response rates
2. Superior median relapse free survival
3. Superior overall survival
4. Increased incidence of grade 3 adverse events

Answer: Increased incidence of grade 3 adverse events

When we talk about low dose versus high dose daunorubicin in the induction of AML, it means that we are comparing 45 mg/m2 with 60-90 mg/m2 (not comparing 60 mg/2 with 90 mg/m2).

The 60-90 mg/m2 dose resulted in higher CR rates, higher RFS and higher OS but a similar rate of grade 3 or more adverse events compared with the 45 mg/m2 dose.

These results are based on the ECOG 1900 and other phase III trials.

Q. Which of the following statement is wrong:
1. A high mutation fraction of *FLT3*-ITD is associated with adverse outcomes in AML
2. In *FLT3* mutant AML midostaurin should be added to 7+3 induction therapy
3. In the RATIFY trial the majority of AML patients had FLT3-TKD mutation
4. In the RATIFY trial the midostaurin arm resulted in higher median overall survival

Answer: In the RATIFY trial the majority of AML patients had FLT3-TKD mutation

There are two types of FLT3 mutations in AML:
1. FLT3-ITD
2. FLT3-TKD

The FLT3-ITD mutations are more important and have been clearly shown to be adverse risk factors. The FLT3-ITD mutations are further classified as high and low.

Notes on the RATIFY trial:
1. It was a phase III trial
2. Included <60 years old adults with AML, who had FLT3 mutations. The patients had: *FLT3*-ITD (77 percent) or *FLT3*-TKD (23 percent).
3. Patients were randomly assigned to 7+3 chemotherapy plus midostaurin versus 7+3 chemotherapy plus placebo.
4. Midostaurin achieved superior median OS (75 versus 26 months), four-year OS (51 versus 44 percent), median EFS (8 versus 3 months), and four-year EFS (28 versus 21 percent). The two arms had similar rates of CR, time to recovery of neutrophils and platelets, severe (grade 3/4) toxicity, and treatment-related deaths.

Q. Gemtuzumab ozogamicin is an antibody directed towards:
1. CD33
2. CD31
3. CD32
4. CD34

Answer: CD33

Q. When should the bone marrow examination be done in an

AML patient:

1. Before staring treatment, on day 14 of induction chemo and four to five weeks after starting induction chemo
2. Before staring treatment and four to five weeks after starting induction chemo
3. Before staring treatment, on day 7 and 14 of induction chemo and four to five weeks after starting induction chemo
4. Before staring treatment, on day 14 and 21 of induction chemo and four to five weeks after starting induction chemo

Answer: Before staring treatment, on day 14 of induction chemo and four to five weeks after starting induction chemo

Bone marrow examination is performed on three occasions:

1. Before starting treatment.
2. On day 14, counting from the day of initiation of induction: the bone marrow done on day 14 tells us about the initial response, which has implication on further management. Three types of results may be obtained on day 14:
    1. Hypoplastic bone marrow: bone marrow cellularity <5 to 20% and <5% blasts. These patients are observed for 2 to 4 weeks and then bone marrow biopsy is repeated.
    2. Indeterminate bone marrow: bone marrow cellularity <5 to 20% with ≥5% blasts. These patients are observed for 1 to 2 weeks and then bone marrow examination is performed again.
    3. Persistent leukemia: bone arrow cellularity >20% and persistence of blasts or only min-

imal response. These patients are treated with either the same 7 + 3 regimen used before or with a more intensive chemo protocol.

3. When bone marrow recovers from the induction chemo: this bone marrow examination, performed four to five weeks after starting induction chemo, tells us whether or not patient has achieved complete remission. This timeline of four to five weeks is based on general observation. Most of the centres perform the bone marrow examination when absolute neutrophil count (ANC) is >1000/microL and platelet count >100,000/microL, which generally coincides with four to five weeks since the initiation of induction.

Q. Routine evaluation of the CNS is recommended in which of the following patients of AML:
1. Less than one year old infants
2. Adults with acute promyelocytic leukaemia in the first remission
3. Adults with AML M4
4. All of the above

Answer: less than one year old infants

Remember that routine evaluation of CNS is not indicated in all patients of AML because it is uncommon for a patient of AML to have CNS involvement at the time of presentation.

There are two indications for routine evaluation of CNS in AML:

1. All infants (≤1 year old)
2. Adults with acute promyelocytic leukemia in second remission

These two patient populations have higher chance of CNS involvement.

If a patient is showing any CNS related symptoms, then we obviously have to do a full workup.

Q. What is the initial treatment of choice for a patient of AML with confirmed CNS involvement:
1. IT chemotherapy
2. Cranial radiation
3. High dose systemic chemo
4. Any of the above

Answer: IT chemo

CNS irradiation is reserved for those patients who don't fully respond to IT (intrathecal) chemo.

Q. In young and medically fit patients with favourable risk AML, which of the following is the consolidation therapy of choice:
1. High dose cytarabine
2. Standard dose cytarabine
3. Myeloablative conditioning followed by allogeneic HCT

4. Nonmyeloablative conditioning followed by allogeneic HCT

Answer: high dose cytarabine

Generally, in these patients, three courses of cytarabine 3 g/m2, IV over 3 hours, twice per day, on days 1, 3, and 5 are used.

If a patient is older than 60 years and younger than 70 years then the dose is 2 g/m2 and in those older than 70 years the dose is 1.5 g/m2.

Remember these important points:
1. Consolidation high dose cytarabine (HiDAC) is begun after confirmation of complete remission and resolution of all toxicities from induction therapy.
2. It is given for three cycles (usually).
3. The minimum duration between two cycles is 28 days.
4. It is extremely important to use saline or steroid eye drops in both eyes, four times daily until 24 hours after completion of the HiDAC infusion. This is done to prevent chemical conjunctivitis.

Q. Which of the following is the preferred consolidation treatment option for a young, medially fit AML patient having intermediate risk disease:
1. High dose cytarabine (HiDAC)

2. HiDAC followed by autologous HCT
3. Allogeneic HCT
4. Any of the above

Answer: any of the above

In intermediate risk AML patients, who are medically fit, the optimal consolidation treatment in not known. The above mentioned are the three strategies that may be used and the choice depends on individual factors.

Q. Which of the following is the preferred consolidation treatment option for a young, medially fit AML patient having adverse risk disease:
1. High dose cytarabine (HiDAC)
2. HiDAC followed by autologous HCT
3. Allogeneic HCT
4. Any of the above

Answer: allogeneic HCT

Experts differ in their opinion about using myeloablative versus reduced intensity conditioning regimens before allogeneic HCT. Most experts, however, use myeloablative conditioning regimens.

Q. Which of the following is not a favorable prognostic factor for AML patients:

1. t(8;21)
2. inv(16)
3. t(6;9)
4. t(15;17)

Answer: t(6;9)

Q. Which of the following is a favorable prognostic factor for AML patients:
1. FLT3/ITD mutation
2. MLL partial tandem duplication
3. BAALC overexpression
4. CEBPA mutation

Answer: CEBPA mutation

Q. Ivosidenib is useful for:
1. IDH1 mutant AML
2. IDH2 mutant AML
3. IDH1 mutant ALL
4. IDH2 mutant ALL

Answer: IDH1 mutant AML

Q. For a medically fit patient, who is 65 years old with favorable risk AML, what will be the induction regimen of choice:
1. 7 + 3 regimen

   2. Liposomal daunorubicin-cytarabine
   3. Azacitidine plus venetoclax
   4. Decitabine alone

Answer: 7 + 3 regimen

Please carefully go through these important points:
   1. Treatment of elderly AML patients is different from young AML patients. Generally the age cutoff is 60 years.
   2. Not all elderly AML patients are treated in the same way. They are divided in three groups based on fitness: medically fit, intermediate fitness and medically frail.
   3. The treatment selection in these three groups is further based on the risk stratification of AML: favorable, intermediate and adverse.
   4. If an elderly patient is medically fit and has favorable risk or intermediate risk AML then he should be treated with the 7 + 3 regimen (cytarabine by continuous infusion daily for seven days together with daunorubicin for three days); which is the same regimen used in younger patients.
   5. If an elderly patient is medially fit and has adverse risk AML, then liposomal daunorubicin-cytarabine may be used. This combination of drugs in also known as CPX-351. Another choice for these patients is decitabine plus venetoclax or azacitidine plus venetoclax. In these patients, 7 + 3 regimen is not preferred.
   6. If an elderly patient has intermediate medical fitness and has favorable or intermediate risk AML, the options are 7 + 3 regimen, CPX-351 or azacitidine/ decitabine plus venetoclax. If the patient is IDH1 or

IDH2 positive then ivosidenib or enasidenib are also options, respectively.

7. If an elderly patient has intermediate medical fitness and has adverse risk AML, the options are azacitidine or decitabine. If the patient is IDH1 or IDH2 mutation positive then ivosidenib or enasidenib are also options, respectively.

8. In an elderly patient, who is medically frail, the primary goal is not complete cure but it is relief of symptoms and improving quality of life. The options include azacitidine or decitabine. If the patient is IDH1 or IDH2 positive then ivosidenib or enasidenib are also options, respectively.

Q. Venetoclax is approved by the FDA for use in combination with all of the following agents in newly diagnosed AML in patients ≥75 years old, except:
1. Cytarabine
2. Glasdegib
3. Azacitidine
4. Decitabine

Answer: glasdegib

Q. Which of the following is not true about glasdegib:
1. It is an oral inhibitor of the hedgehog pathway
2. It is used as a single agent in relapsed AML
3. It is FDA approved for AML patients of 75 years of age or more who are unable to tolerate intensive therapies
4. It was studied in the BRIGHT AML 1003 trial

Answer: It is used as a single agent in relapsed AML

Remember these important point about glasdegib:
1. It is FDA approved for use in patients who are more than or equal to 75 years of age and are unable to tolerate intensive chemo.
2. It is approved for use in first line therapy (newly diagnosed AML).
3. It is never used as a single agent. It is used in combination with low dose cytarabine.

Q. For medically fit elderly patients of AML, who have intermediate risk AML, which of the following is the most appropriate consolidation therapy:
1. Intermediate dose cytarabine
2. Allogeneic HCT
3. High dose cytarabine
4. Low dose cytarabine

Answer: intermediate dose cytarabine

Remember these points:
1. For medically fit elderly patients of AML, who have favorable or intermediate risk AML; intermediate dose cytarabine is the consolidation therapy of choice.
2. For medically fit elderly patients of AML, who have adverse risk AML; nonmyeloablative or reduced intensity conditioning HCT is the consolidation ther-

apy of choice (myeloablative conditioning is not used in this population).
3. For medically frail patients, generally no consolidation therapy is chosen. Best supportive care is the most appropriate option in them. Although it depends on the protocol being followed.

Definition of complete response (remission) in AML:

All of the following criteria should be met:
1. Less than 5 percent blast cells are present in the bone marrow, and none can have a leukemic phenotype (eg, Auer rods).
2. Absolute neutrophil count >1000/microL, platelet count >100,000/microL and independence from red cell transfusion.
3. Extramedullary leukemia (eg, central nervous system or soft tissue involvement) must be absent.

There are some other criteria as well, like all lineages should show normal maturation and bone marrow biopsy should not show any clusters of blasts.

Q. Gilteritinib is a:
1. FLT3 inhibitor
2. NPM1 inhibitor
3. CEBPA inhibitor
4. RUNX1 inhibitor

Answer: FLT3 inhibitor

Q. Ivosidenib is an:
1. IDH1 inhibitor
2. IDH2 inhibitor
3. IDH3 inhibitor
4. IDH4 inhibitor

Answer: IDH1 inhibitor

Q. Enasidenib is an:
1. IDH1 inhibitor
2. IDH2 inhibitor
3. IDH3 inhibitor
4. IDH4 inhibitor

Answer: IDH2 inhibitor

Q. Which of the following is the treatment of choice for a patient of relapsed AML:
1. Allogeneic HCT
2. Salvage chemo followed by autologous HCT
3. Intensive chemotherapy alone
4. Any of the above

Answer: allogeneic HCT

Note that the question is about "treatment of choice"; not

"treatment options". The other two are also sometimes used in relapsed AML but they are not the preferred treatment options.

When allogeneic HCT is planned for treatment of relapsed AML, most experts recommend using myeloablative conditioning regimens instead of nonmyeloablative/reduced intensity regimens.

Acute promyelocytic leukemia

Q. Which of the following statement is not right:

1. APL was classified as AML-M3 in the older French-American-British (FAB) classification system
2. APL is associated with a high rate of early mortality, often due to haemorrhage from a characteristic coagulopathy
3. Treatment should be started with a differentiation agent but only after definitive cytogenetic or molecular confirmation of the diagnosis has been made
4. APL accounts for 5 to 20 percent of cases of acute myeloid leukemia (AML)

Answer: Treatment should be started with a differentiation agent but only after definitive cytogenetic or molecular confirmation of the diagnosis has been made

APL is a medical emergency and treatment with a differentiation agent, like ATRA, **must be started as soon as there is clinical and cytological suspicion**. We have to send cytogenetic and molecular tests also, and their results may lead to change in treatment plans but the results of these tests are **not needed** for beginning the therapy directed towards APL.

Q. Which of the following drugs are associated with development of APL:

1. Etoposide
2. Doxorubicin
3. Mitoxantrone
4. All of the above

Answer: all of the above

The topoisomerase-II inhibitors are most frequently associated with APL, particularly when they are used in the treatment of breast cancer. Radiation therapy is also associated with APL.

Q. Coagulopathy associated with APL involves:

1. Disseminated intravascular coagulation (DIC)
2. Primary hyperfibrinolysis
3. Both of the above
4. None of the above

Answer: both of the above

The coagulopathy of APL is a unique disorder. This coagu-lopathy develops over time but it is diagnosed only when clinical manifestations are there and at that time, the mor-tality rates are very high. If left untreated, it results in pul-monary or cerebrovascular hemorrhage in up to 40 percent of patients and a 10 to 20 percent incidence of early hemor-rhagic deaths.

Interestingly, thrombosis may also be seen in a minority of patients.

Q. Which of the following is not true about the mechanism of coagulopathy in APL:

1. The rearranged *RARA* in APL activates the tissue factor (TF) promoter and increases its expression in the leukemic cells
2. Death of APL cells by ETosis releases extracellular chromatin and phosphatidylserine, which lead to a hypercoagulable state
3. Primary hyperfibrinolysis is a result of expression of annexin I
4. None of the above

Answer: Primary hyperfibrinolysis is a result of expression of annexin I

If fact primary hyperfibrinolysis is a result of expression of:
   1. Annexin II
   2. Tissue and urokinase plasminogen activator
   3. An acquired deficiency of alpha-2 antiplasmin
   4. An acquired deficiency of plasminogen activator inhibitor-1

Q. Which of the following is not true about promyelocytes in APL:

   1. They are usually >20 microns in diameter
   2. High nucleus to cytoplasmic ratio
   3. Coarse chromatin
   4. Prominent nucleoli

Answer: coarse chromatin

Note that chromatin is **fine** in these cells.

Q. Promyelocytes in APL are larger than normal promyelocytes and typically have "folded" nuclei. They are characterised by presence of granules of which color:

   1. Violet
   2. Purple
   3. Magenta
   4. Lilac

Answer: violet

The presence of violet colored granules in the cytoplasm is a cardinal feature of promyelocytes in APL.

Q. Which of the following types of APL is associated with a high WBC count:

1. Usual APL
2. Hypergranular APL
3. Microgranular APL
4. None of the above

Answer: microgranular APL

APL can present with low WBC counts and many times, no abnormal cells are visualised in the peripheral blood.

Note that the hypergranular form of APL is the "typical" form of APL.

Q. Which of the following is not true about the microgranular variant of APL:

1. It accounts for approximately 25 percent of cases

2. The cells of this variant have a unilobed nucleus
3. There are no apparent granules on light microscopy
4. The myeloperoxidase reaction is strongly positive, and the non-specific esterase reaction is negative or only weakly positive

Answer: The cells of this variant have a unilobed nucleus

In fact, the cells of this variant have a bilobed nucleus.

Q. The APL cells have all of the following features except:

1. The hypergranular variants have a low side scatter
2. They express bright cytoplasmic myeloperoxidase
3. They show bright positivity for CD13, CD33 and CD34
4. HLA-DR and CD11b are only dimly expressed

Answer: there are two correct options here: "the hyper-granular variants have a low side scatter" and "they show bright positivity for CD13, CD33 and CD34".

The facts are that the hypergranular variants have a **high** side scatter. And while it's true that promyelocytes of APL brightly express **CD13 and CD33** but they either don't stain or stain only weakly for CD34.

It should be noted here that the above mentioned pattern

is also expressed by normal promyelocytes, to differentiate the cells of APL from normal promyelocytes, there are two markers, CD15 and CD117. Normal promyelocytes express these markers but malignant promyelocytes express only very low levels of these markers.

Hypogranular variant of APL may express two additional markers: CD2 and CD56.

Q. Which of the following is not true about the classical genetic abnormality in APL:

1. The characteristic translocation is t(15;17) (q24.1;q21.2)
2. *PML-RARA* is defined by the presence of a reciprocal translocation between the long arm of chromosomes 15 and short arm of chromosome 17
3. The retinoic acid receptor alpha (*RARA*) gene is found on chromosome 17
4. The promyelocytic leukemia (*PML*) gene is found on chromosome 15

Answer: *PML-RARA* is defined by the presence of a reciprocal translocation between the long arm of chromosomes 15 and short arm of chromosome 17

If we read the first option carefully then it becomes apparent then one of the first two options must be wrong (there are two "q"s in the first option).

In fact, *PML-RARA* is defined by the presence of a reciprocal translocation between the long arm of chromosomes 15 and **long** arm of chromosome 17 (the long arms of both chromosomes are involved).

Q. The diagnosis of APL can be confirmed by using various methods. Which of the following methods is currently the gold standard method of diagnosing APL:

    1. Conventional karyotype
    2. Light microscopy
    3. FISH
    4. RT-PCR

Answer: RT-PCR

Q. APL is characterized by t(15;17), but there can be variant translocations. Which of the following will lead to PLZF-RARA fusion:

    1. t(11;17)
    2. t(5;17)
    3. t(15;17)
    4. t(17;17)

Answer: t(11;17)

The most important variants are:

1. t(11;17) which leads to *PLZF-RARA*
2. t(5;17) which leads to *NPM1-RARA*
3. t(11;17) which leads to *NuMA-RARA* [the break-point are different than the PLZF-RARA producing t(11;17)]
4. t(17;17) which leads to *STAT5b-RARA*

Q. According to the data of patients of APL treated in the Italian GIMEMA and the Spanish PETHEMA trials, which of the following will constitute an intermediate risk group:

1. WBC 12000/microL and platelets 40000/microL
2. WBC 12000/microL and platelets 80000/microL
3. WBC 8000/microL and platelets 40000/microL
4. WBC 12000/microL and platelets 140000/microL

Answer: WBC 8000/microL and platelets 40000/microL

This question seems difficult for two reasons: one, that now-adays APL is divided into two groups, low risk and high risk. There is no intermediate risk group in most of the guide-lines. And the second reason is the numbers in the options seem closely linked.

The explanation however is very simple: if WBC are more

than 10000/microL then the patient is always **high risk** regardless of platelet counts, that's why the three options having WBC count of 12000/microL (which is more than 10000/microL) are ruled out.

In the GIMEMA and PETHEMA trials the risk categories were:

1. Low risk – WBC ≤10,000/microL and platelets >40,000/microL associated with a relapse free survival (RFS) of 98 percent
2. Intermediate – WBC ≤10,000/microL and platelets ≤40,000/microL associated with an RFS of 89 percent
3. High risk – WBC >10,000/microL associated with an RFS of 70 percent

Presently, in most of the guidelines worldwide, there are only two risk groups. WBC count alone is used for risk stratification, and platelet count **is not considered** in risk stratification:

1. Low-risk: WBC count ≤10,000/microL at diagnosis
2. High-risk: WBC count >10,000/microL at diagnosis

Q. What percent patients of APL have chromosomal abnormalities in addition to t(15;17):

1. 10
2. 20
3. 30
4. 40

Answer: 40%

But there is no evidence that these additional abnormalities have any impact on prognosis (unlike other types of AML, where such abnormalities play a significant role).

It is important to remember that FLT3 mutations are identified in many patients of APL and they may be associated with certain unique clinical features but their presence **does not have any impact on prognosis or treatment selection.**

Q. ATRA must be promptly started once the diagnosis of APL is suspected. But it must be combined with other agents since remissions induced by ATRA therapy alone are usually only about what median duration:

    1. 11 months
    2. 4 months
    3. 14-23 months
    4. Less than 2 months

Answer: 4 months

Q. The therapy of choice for low risk APL is:

1. ATRA plus anthracycline-based chemotherapy
2. ATO plus anthracycline-based chemotherapy
3. ATRA plus ATO
4. Anthracycline-based chemotherapy alone

Answer: ATRA plus ATO

Q. The preferred initial therapy for high-risk APL patients is:

1. ATRA plus ATO
2. ATO plus anthracycline based chemo
3. ATRA plus anthracycline based chemo
4. ATRA plus gemtuzumab ozogamicin

Answer: ATRA plus anthracycline based chemo

Q. In low risk APL patients, ATO plus ATRA is the preferred initial therapy. There are various schedules available but generally this combination therapy should be continued until:

1. There is marrow remission, but should not exceed 60 days
2. There is marrow remission, but should not exceed 90 days
3. There is molecular remission regardless of number of days
4. There is molecular remission but it should not ex-

ceed 90 days

Answer: There is marrow remission, but should not exceed 60 days

This is an important point to remember that only marrow remission is our target for the induction phase of APL by ATRA plus ATO. Molecular remission is **not** our target in the induction phase.

Notes on the APL0406 trial:

1. The Intergroup APL0406 trial is a very important trial in APL
2. In this trial patients with newly diagnosed low- or intermediate-risk APL were included
3. These patients were randomized to ATRA plus ATO versus ATRA plus chemotherapy
4. In the ATRA plus ATO arm, the dose of ATRA was 45 mg/m2 and ATO was 0.15 mg/kg daily. This combination was administered daily until complete remission (CR), followed by consolidation with intermittent ATRA and ATO for seven and four courses, respectively.
5. In the ATRA-chemotherapy arm, patients received ATRA and idarubicin induction therapy, followed by three cycles of consolidation therapy with ATRA plus chemotherapy, and maintenance therapy with low dose chemotherapy and ATRA.
6. The results of this trial suggested that for patients with low/intermediate-risk APL, ATO plus ATRA is not inferior compared with ATRA-chemotherapy

and may even be superior. In summary, ATRA-ATO is associated with less toxicity, fewer deaths during induction therapy, and fewer short- and long-term relapses compared with ATRA-chemotherapy.

Notes on AML17 trial:

1. The United Kingdom's AML17 trial included patients of APL of all risk groups.
2. Patients were randomly assigned to receive ATRA plus ATO versus ATRA plus idarubicin (AIDA).
3. In some high-risk patients an initial dose of gemtuzumab ozogamicin (GO, 6 mg/m2) was offered.
4. At 30 months of median follow up, ATRA plus ATO resulted in similar rates of CR (94 versus 89 percent), similar mortality, similar estimated rates of survival at four years (93 versus 89 percent), superior estimated EFS at four years (91 versus 70 percent), the rates of molecular remission were higher and toxicity was lower.
5. Even after more than 60 months of follow up ATRA plus ATO showed superior outcomes.
6. Note that in this trial **all** risk groups were included.

So, the above mentioned trials compared ATRA plus ATO to ATRA plus chemo. There are many trials comparing ATRA plus chemo to chemo alone in APL and in all of them the use of ATRA was associated with favorable outcomes.

Q. APL is especially susceptible to anthracycline therapy because of:

1. Low expression of MDR-1 on the cell membrane of the leukemic cells
2. Low expression of MDR-2 on the cell membrane of the leukemic cells
3. Low expression of MDR-1 on the cell membrane of the normal promyelocytes
4. Low expression of MDR-2 on the cell membrane of the normal promyelocytes

Answer: Low expression of MDR-1 on the cell membrane of the leukemic cells

There are three chemo molecules that are most commonly used in APL: daunorubicin or idarubicin and cytarabine.

Q. In patients of APL, receiving ATRA plus anthracycline, the use of cytarabine is associated with:

1. Similar CR rates
2. Fewer relapses
3. Improved overall survival
4. All of the above

Answer: all of the above

Notes on the APML4 trial:
1. In the Australian APML4 trial, newly diagnosed pa-

tients of APL received ATRA, idarubicin, and intravenous ATO as induction therapy and 95 percent attained a hematologic CR.

2. Following two cycles of consolidation with ATRA and intravenous ATO, all patients achieved a molecular CR and received two years of maintenance therapy with ATRA, oral methotrexate, and mercaptopurine.

3. DFS at two years was 98 percent.

Q. When using ATRA plus chemotherapy in patients with APL, chemo can be given simultaneously or sequentially with ATRA. Which of the following is not true in this context:

1. When given simultaneously chemo is started from third day of ATRA
2. When given sequentially, chemotherapy is postponed until after achievement of CR
3. Rates of CR are higher in the simultaneous administration but overall survival is the same
4. Simultaneous ATRA-chemo is associated with lower rates of differentiation syndrome

Answer: Rates of CR are higher in the simultaneous administration but overall survival is the same

In fact, the rates of CR are the same whether chemo is given simultaneously or sequentially with ATRA.

However, relapse free survival at 2 years is higher with simultaneous administration.

An important point to remember is that the rates of differentiation syndrome are **lower** when chemo is given **simultaneously** with ATRA. It makes sense because chemo will lead to reduced number of myeloid cells, leading to reduced numbers of malignant promyelocytes that may undergo differentiation with ATRA.

Q. The North American Intergroup study C9710 used which of the following protocol in patients of APL:
1. Daily ATRA (45 mg/m2/day orally divided into two doses), starting on day 0, followed by seven days of cytarabine by continuous infusion (200 mg/m2 per day) and four days of daunorubicin (50 mg/m2 per day), both starting on day 3
2. Daily ATRA (25 mg/m2/day orally divided into two doses), starting on day 0, followed by seven days of cytarabine by continuous infusion (200 mg/m2 per day) and three days of daunorubicin (50 mg/m2 per day), both starting on day 3
3. Daily ATRA (45 mg/m2/day orally divided into two doses), starting on day 0, followed by seven days of cytarabine by continuous infusion (200 mg/m2 per day) and three days of daunorubicin (50 mg/m2 per day), both starting on day 3
4. Daily ATRA (45 mg/m2/day orally divided into two doses), starting on day 0, followed by seven days of cytarabine by continuous infusion (100 mg/m2 per day) and four days of daunorubicin (50 mg/m2 per day), both starting on day 3

Answer: Daily ATRA (45 mg/m2/day orally divided into two doses), starting on day 0, followed by seven days of cytarabine by continuous infusion (200 mg/m2 per day) and four days of daunorubicin (50 mg/m2 per day), both starting on day 3

But note that some other combinations were also used in this important trial.

The dose of ATRA in children is 25 mg/m2.

Q. What is the goal of induction therapy in APL:
1. Attainment of morphological CR
2. Attainment of molecular CR
3. Attainment of two log reduction in PML-RARA
4. Attainment of deep molecular remission

Answer: Attainment of morphological CR

This point should be remembered by heart that the goal of **induction** is **morphological CR.**

Q. The most appropriate time for evaluation of bone marrow in a patient undergoing induction therapy for APL is:
1. 14 to 16 days
2. 30 to 35 days
3. 22 to 26 days
4. After 60 days

Answer: 30 to 35 days

This timing is unique to APL among myeloid leukemias. All other AMLs, except AML-M3 (APL), are evaluated for treatment response on day 14 of induction by doing a bone marrow examination. But in cases of APL, the bone marrow on day 14 is **not examined**, because it is not much informative. In cases of APL, bone marrow is usually examined around day 30 to 35 of induction.

Q. Which of the following statement is not true about patients of APL treated with ATRA and ATO in induction:
  1. For patients treated with ATRA and ATO induction, it is important to incorporate chemotherapy in combination with ATO in the consolidation phase
  2. In the APL0406 trial, consolidation therapy consisted of intermittent ATRA and ATO for seven and four courses, respectively
  3. In the AML17 trial, consolidation consisted of intermittent ATRA and ATO, administered over three months
  4. Anthracycline based chemo should be incorporated in consolidation but cytarabine may be omitted

Answer: 1 and 4

This concept should be clear that patients of APL have various treatment options and protocols available. So there is no single treatment that is superior to every other treatment. But adherence to the protocol chosen is a must. What I mean to say is that whatever protocol you chose, you must stick to **that** protocol, then only optimal results can be expected. So, while there are many protocols that use chemo in the consolidation phase but if the patient has been treated with ATRA and ATO in induction (the induction didn't include an anthracycline based chemo regimen) then in consolidation too, ATRA and ATO are to be used and chemo should not be used; as most of the protocols have been designed this way.

On the other hand, standard consolidation after chemotherapy-based induction consists of two cycles of an anthracycline plus ATRA. In this setting, many experts recommend two cycles of consolidation therapy with ATO followed by two cycles of daunorubicin plus ATRA.

Q. What is the goal of consolidation therapy in APL:
    1. Achievement of molecular CR
    2. Achievement of cytological CR
    3. Achievement of morphological CR
    4. Achievement of flow negative CR

Answer: Achievement of molecular CR

This is defined by the absence of the *PML-RARA* fusion transcript using RT-PCR methods.

Notes on post consolidation therapy in APL:

1. Assessment of molecular response by RT-PCR is done **after the completion of consolidation.** The reason for doing it so late is that it takes time for a patient of APL to achieve molecular remission and doing it before completion of consolidation will lead to confounding results.

2. Patients who achieve molecular CR should proceed directly to maintenance therapy.

3. Patients who have a positive RT-PCR test at the conclusion of the planned consolidation sequence should have a second bone marrow aspirate and biopsy with RT-PCR testing repeated in four weeks. If this second test is negative, the patient may proceed to maintenance therapy. If the second RT-PCR is still positive, the patient should proceed to treatment for resistant disease.

Q. Which of the following statement is not true about maintenance therapy in APL:

1. Patients who receive ATO as part of their induction and/or consolidation do not need maintenance after a molecular CR is achieved

2. Observation is preferred for patients with low-risk APL who achieve a molecular CR with a regimen that includes both ATRA and ATO

3. In the APL0406 trial, patients who were treated with ATRA plus ATO were randomized to receive ATRA based maintenance versus no maintenance and in this trial maintenance did not result in superior outcomes

4. Maintenance therapy is recommended rather than observation alone after induction with ATRA plus anthracycline-based chemotherapy without ATO

43

Answer: In the APL0406 trial, patients who were treated with ATRA plus ATO were randomized to receive ATRA based maintenance versus no maintenance and in this trial maintenance did not result in superior outcomes

In this trial, maintenance therapy was **not** offered to patients who were treated with ATRA plus ATO.

Notes on maintenance therapy:

There are two basic options for maintenance therapy:

1. Single agent ATRA 45 mg/m2 orally for seven days repeated every other week for one year.
2. A combination of ATRA 45 mg/m2 orally daily for 15 days every three months plus 6-mercaptopurine (MP) 60 mg/m2 orally daily plus methotrexate 20 mg/m2 orally per week. This regimen is followed for a total duration of one year.

The choice between these two depends on many clinical factors and the protocol being used but most of the times single agent ATRA is chosen due to lesser toxicity and ease of administration.

Q. In patients of APL who are receiving maintenance, what is the preferred modality for monitoring of the disease:

1. RT-PCR on bone marrow every three months for the first year of CR
2. RT-PCR on bone marrow every six months for the first year of CR
3. RT-PCR on peripheral blood every three months for the first year of CR
4. RT-PCR on peripheral blood every six months for the first year of CR

Answer: RT-PCR on bone marrow every three months for the first year of CR

It is a fact that bone marrow RT-PCR outperforms peripheral blood RT-PCR in APL monitoring, but it's also true that performing these tests from peripheral blood is easy and allows for more frequent monitoring. So the best option is RT-PCR on bone marrow every three months for the first year of CR but doing it from peripheral blood every three months is also an **acceptable** alternative.

If at any time during monitoring, molecular CR is lost then bone marrow evaluation is done for confirmation and the patient will proceed to therapy for relapsed disease.

Q. The concentration of plasma fibrinogen in patients with APL undergoing treatment should be maintained at what level:

1. Above 150 mg/dL

2. Below 150 mg/dL
3. Above 450 mg/dL
4. Below 450 mg/dL

Answer: above 150 mg/dL

The platelet count should be maintained above 20,000 to 30,000/microL and the plasma fibrinogen concentration above 150 mg/dL.

Notes on differentiation syndrome:

1. It occurs in approximately 25 percent of APL patients.
2. It usually occurs within 2 to 21 days after initiation of treatment.
3. It is more frequent in high-risk APL cases, i.e., those with more than 10000 WBCs/microL.
4. ATRA is the most commonly implicated drug (another name for this syndrome is retinoic acid syndrome).
5. But it can occur without ATRA too. Arsenic trioxide may also cause it. And it can also occur spontaneously.
6. It is characterized by fever, peripheral edema, pulmonary infiltrates, hypoxemia, respiratory distress, hypotension, renal and hepatic dysfunction, and serositis resulting in pleural and pericardial effusions.
7. Hyperleukocytosis is often associated with it but it is not necessarily always there.

Q. Once differentiation syndrome is identified in a patient of APL being treated with ATRA, what is the drug and its schedule of choice:

1. Dexamethasone 10 mg intravenously every 12 hours for at least three days
2. Dexamethasone 12 mg intravenously every 12 hours for at least three days
3. Dexamethasone 10 mg intravenously every 24 hours for at least seven days
4. Dexamethasone 20 mg intravenously every 12 hours for at least three to seven

Answer: Dexamethasone 10 mg intravenously every 12 hours for at least three days

Q. Once differentiation syndrome in a patient of APL reaches the stage of respiratory distress, which of the following intervention may prove to be effective:

1. Dexamethasone
2. Cessation of ATRA
3. Cytotoxic chemotherapy
4. Leukapheresis

Answer: dexamethasone

Other interventions listed above are not effective once respiratory distress sets in.

Q. Hyperleukocytosis is seen in up to 50 percent of patients of APL treated with ATRA alone at induction. Which of the following is usually not used for its management:

1. Leukapheresis
2. Cytarabine
3. Daunorubicin
4. Corticosteroids

Answer: leukapheresis

Generally leukapheresis is not used for this indication because leukapheresis has the potential to exacerbate the underlying coagulopathy of APL.

Q. Which of the following is not true about idiopathic intracranial hypertension in APL:

1. Idiopathic intracranial hypertension is more common in children and adolescents treated with ATRA
2. Lower doses of ATRA are associated with reduced incidence of pseudotumor cerebri in APL
3. The diagnosis of IIH in APL is confirmed in patients with increased intracranial pressure, normal cerebrospinal fluid, and positive cerebral imaging stud-

ies

4. Steroids and acetazolamide are therapeutic options for treatment of pseudotumor cerebri induced by ATRA in APL

Answer: The diagnosis of IIH in APL is confirmed in patients with increased intracranial pressure, normal cerebrospinal fluid, and positive cerebral imaging studies

While it's true that intracranial pressure is increased and CSF examination is normal but imaging studied (like CT, MRI) are **negative** in IIH.

Q. If APL is diagnosed in a woman during first trimester of pregnancy, which of the following is a treatment option:

1. ATRA
2. ATO
3. Anthracycline
4. All of the above

Answer: anthracycline

Note that both ATRA and ATO are highly teratogenic and **must not** be used in the first trimester.

It goes without saying that if the woman is willing for termination of pregnancy then the usual treatment protocols of APL are to be instituted.

If the examiner specifically asks about which chemo is to be used in the first trimester then the answer will be daunorubicin.

If a patient undergoes remission with chemo alone then we should wait and once the patient's pregnancy reaches the second or third trimester, then ATRA may be added.

If APL is diagnosed in second or third trimester then ATRA alone or ATRA plus chemo are good options.

Q. Patients with treatment related APL have:

    1. A similar prognosis as de novo APL
    2. Better prognosis than de novo APL
    3. Worse prognosis than de novo APL
    4. None of the above

Answer: a similar prognosis as de novo APL

Q. Which of the following variant translocations in APL is not ATRA-sensitive:

    1. *NuMA-RARA* and t(11;17)
    2. *NPM1-RARA* and t(5;17)
    3. *FIP1L1-RARA*
    4. *STAT5B-RARA*

Answer: *STAT5B-RARA*

The other three are ATRA sensitive.

The *STAT5B-RARA* and interstitial chromosome 17 deletion variant is considered resistant to ATRA.

The *PLZF/RARA* and t(11;17) variant is considered relatively resistant and the sensitivity of *PRKAR1A/RARA* variant to ATRA is unknown.

Note again that patients of FLT3 mutation positive APL **do not** have a worse prognosis than those without this mutation. And additional chromosomal abnormalities **do not** impart a poorer prognosis.

Q. Approximately what percentage of high risk APL cases relapse:
    1. 20 to 30
    2. 5 to 10
    3. 30 to 40
    4. Less than 5

Answer: 20 to 30 percent

Q. In patients with relapsed APL, who achieve a second molecular complete remission, the preferred therapy is:
1. Autologous HCT
2. Allogeneic HCT
3. Observation
4. Continuation of second line with intense surveillance

Answer: autologous HCT

In all other AML subtypes, allogeneic HCT is the preferred therapy in case of relapse but in APL, autologous HCT is preferred.

The point to be understood here is that autologous HCT can only be performed in those relapsed APL patients who **achieve a molecular CR with second line therapy.** In relapsed APL patients who fail to achieve molecular CR, autologous HCT is not done and **allogeneic HCT is preferred.**

Q. Which of the following is not true:

1. Up to 10 percent of patients with relapsed APL will demonstrate involvement of the CNS
2. Arsenic trioxide does not penetrate into CSF, hence it is not used in patients of relapsed APL having CNS involvement

   3. Gemtuzumab ozogamicin can effectively control disease in patients with APL who have had a molecular relapse

   4. None of the above

Answer: Arsenic trioxide does not penetrate into CSF, hence it is not used in patients of relapsed APL having CNS involvement

In fact, ATO **penetrates** into CSF.

Q. Differentiation syndrome can be seen in:

   1. Acute promyelocytic leukemia patients treated with ATRA

   2. Treatment of AML with enasidenib or ivosidenib

   3. Treatment of AML with gilteritinib

   4. All of the above

Answer: all of the above

Enasidenib is an IDH2 inhibitor, ivosidenib is an IDH1 inhibitor and gilteritinib is FLT3 inhibitor.

Q. Differentiation syndrome is reported in approximately what percent of patients of APL treated with ATRA:

1. 25
2. 10
3. 50
4. 66

Answer: 25%

Q. Differentiation syndrome associated with APL generally occurs after how many days of starting ATRA:

1. 2-3
2. 7-14
3. 14-28
4. Within 48 hours

Answer: 7-14 days

But this is a generalisation. This syndrome may manifest within 24 hours as well.

Notes:

There are no formal diagnostic criteria for differentiation syndrome and that is the cause of discrepancies in reporting of this diagnosis among studies. Most experts agree that the presence of three or more of the following features is sufficient for a confident clinical diagnosis of DS (other reasons that may lead to these manifestations must be excluded):

1. Fever ≥ 38° C
2. Weight gain > 5 kg
3. Hypotension
4. Dyspnea
5. Radiographic opacities
6. Pleural or pericardial effusion
7. Acute renal failure

Q. What is the optimal schedule for administration of dexamethasone in a case of differentiation syndrome:

1. 10 mg 12 hourly for at least three days and then taper by 50% every two to three days
2. 12 mg 12 hourly for at least three days and then taper by 50% every two to three days
3. 10 mg 12 hourly for at least seven days and then taper by 50% every two to three days
4. 10 mg 12 hourly for at least three days and then stopped without taper

Answer: 10 mg 12 hourly for at least three days and then taper by 50% every two to three days

The minimum duration is three days but if the symptoms don't resolve then it may be continued beyond three days. And if the clinical picture deteriorates despite this schedule then dexamethasone may be administered on a more frequent basis.

In children and adolescents the dose of dexamethasone is 0.25 mg/kg/dose (maximum dose: 10 mg) IV or orally every 12 hours for 3 days followed by a taper.

Notes on highlights of differentiation syndrome management:

1. Prompt initiation of glucocorticoids.
2. Empiric antibiotics should be started.
3. Diuretics may be started depending on the clinical presentation
4. For treatment of coagulopathy, cryoprecipitate, fibrinogen or fresh-frozen plasma are used. Fresh frozen plasma is the **least** preferred option.

Q. ATRA should preferably be taken:

1. With a meal
2. On empty stomach
3. Four hours after meal
4. At any time, regardless of the last meal

Answer: with a meal

Notes on ATRA and pregnancy issues:

1. It is extremely teratogenic
2. If it must be given to a woman of childbearing potential then two reliable forms of contraception must be used simultaneously during therapy and for 1 month following discontinuation of therapy.

3. Within 1 week prior to ATRA therapy, serum or urine pregnancy test is a must

Q. Which of the following is a "boxed warning" of arsenic trioxide:

1. Differentiation syndrome
2. QTc interval prolongation
3. Encephalopathy
4. All of the above

Answer: all of the above

Q. When arsenic is used for the induction phase of low-risk APL, which of the following is the maximum duration of its use:

1. 30 days
2. 60 days
3. 90 days
4. 120 days

Answer: 60 days

The trials done on this subject, like that conducted by Lo-Coco, reached to a conclusion that ATO should be continued until bone marrow remission but not exceeding 60 days.

The dose in induction is 0.15 mg/kg once daily in combination with ATRA.

When used in consolidation, it is given at 0.15 mg/kg once daily for 5 days each week during weeks 1 to 4 of each 8-week consolidation cycle (in combination with tretinoin) for a total of 4 consolidation cycles.

Notes:

While ATRA acts on the underlying mechanism of APL development and leads to the removal of "maturation block", arsenic trioxide has a different mechanism of action. Arsenic trioxide induces apoptosis in APL cells via morphological changes and DNA fragmentation. It also acts by damaging the PML-RARA fusion protein.

ACUTE LYMPHOBLASTIC LEUKEMIA

Q. The t(9;22) is present in what percentage of children and adults with ALL, respectively:
   1. 2-5% and 25-30%
   2. 25-30% and 2-5%
   3. 10-30% and 60-70%
   4. 60-70% and 10-30%

Answer: 2-5% and 25-30%

Notes: WHO classification of B lymphoblastic leukemia/lymphoma (L/L):
   1. B-L/L, NOS
   2. B-L/L with t(9;22); BCR-ABL1
   3. B-L/L with t(v;11q23.3); KMT2A rearranged
   4. B-L/L with t(12;21); ETV6-RUNX1
   5. B-L/L with hyperdiploidy
   6. B-L/L with hypodiploidy
   7. B-L/L with t(5;14); IL3-IGH
   8. B-L/L with t(1;19); TCF3-PBX1
   9. B-L/L, BCR-ABL1-like
   10. B-L/L with iAMP21

Q. The t(12;21) is present in what percentage of children and adults with ALL, respectively:
   1. 25% and 3%
   2. 3% and 25%
   3. 10% and 30-40%
   4. 30-40% and 10%

Answer: 25% and 3%

So, as we can see here, the distribution of t(9;22) and t(12;21) is just vice versa (this is just to remember these facts).

Q. The t(4;11) is present most frequently in which population of ALL patients:
   1. Infants
   2. Adolescents
   3. Adults
   4. Elderly

Answer: infants

The t(4;11) is present in up to 60 percent of infants younger than 12 months, but is rarely observed in adult ALL patients.

Q. Which is the most common genetic lesion in childhood ALL:

1. t(9;22)
2. t(12;21)
3. t(4;11)
4. Hyperdiploidy

Answer: t(12;21)

The t(12;21) is found in 15-25% of children with B-ALL. It is far less common in adults, where is it present in around 3-4%.

The t(12;21) results in fusion of *ETV6* with *RUNX1*.

Remember that this transaction is associated with **favorable prognosis.**

Q. The t(8;14) is most frequently present in which type of ALL:
1. FAB-L1
2. FAB-L2
3. FAB-L3
4. It is not found in ALL

Answer: FAB-L3

The t(8;14) is most frequently found in patients of Burkitt's lymphoma. It is a fact that Burkitt's lymphoma and FAB-L3 ALL are different manifestations of the same disease.

Q. Which of the following results in fusion of the *KMT2A* gene to the *AFF1* (AF4) gene:
1. t(4;11)
2. t(11;14)
3. t(9;22)
4. t(11;19)

Answer: t(4;11)

The KMT2A gene was previously known as the MLL gene. It is found on chromosome 11.

The AFF1 gene is found on chromosome 4.

This translocation is present in about 5% of ALL patients and it carries a poor prognosis.

On the other hand, 60 to 80 percent of infants with ALL have translocations involving 11q (*KMT2A* gene) and in this population, it carriers an even worse prognosis.

Q. Which is the most frequent rearrangement in adult ALL:
1. t(4;11)
2. t(9;22)
3. t(12;21)
4. t(8;14)

Answer: t(9;22)

Read the question carefully. The "most frequent" facts and figures are different for different patient populations. Here the question is about **adult ALL.**

This rearrangement carries a worse prognosis.

Q. Which of the following is not true about pre-B cell ALL:
1. There is absence of cytoplasmic immunoglobulin mu-chain expression
2. The t(1;19) occurs in approximately 30 percent of patients
3. The immunophenotype shows CD19+, CD10+ (CALLA+), CD22+, CD34-, and CD20+/-
4. Unbalanced translocations of t(1;19) are more common than reciprocal translocations

Answer: there is absence of cytoplasmic immunoglobulin mu-chain expression

In fact, expression of the cytoplasmic immunoglobulin mu-chain is **characteristically present**.

The t(1;19) is associated with a favourable prognosis.

Although the list is long, but remember that following three

chromosomal abnormalities are associated with good prognosis in ALL patients:
1. t(1;19)
2. t(12;21)
3. Hyperdiploidy

Q. Which of the following is not true about acute lymphoblastic leukemia:
1. iAMP21 is associated with poor prognosis
2. Chromosome 9p deletion is associated with a worse outcome
3. Hyperdiploidy is associated with a good outcome and chromosome 10 is gained most frequently
4. Near haploidy is exclusively observed in children and imparts a poorer prognosis

Answer: Hyperdiploidy is associated with a good outcome and chromosome 10 is gained most frequently

This statement is half right and half wrong. While it's true that hyperdiploid state is associated with **good** outcomes but the most frequently "gained" chromosome in these patients is chromosome 21 (which is gained in 100% of patients having hyperdiploid karyotype).

On the other hand, hypodiploidy is associated with bad prognosis. There are three types of hypodiploidy: near-haploidy (23 to 29 chromosomes), low hypodiploidy (33 to 39 chromosomes) and high hypodiploidy (42 to 45 chromosomes).

Out of these, near-haploidy is exclusively observed in children. If we compare these three types of hypodiploidy, the "high hypodiploidy" type is associated with better outcomes compared with the other two.

Q. On which chromosome is *IKZF1* located:
1. 7p
2. 7q
3. 17p
4. 17q

Answer: 7p

Q. Which of the following is true about BCR-ABL1-like B cell ALL:
1. It shares a similar gene expression profile with B cell ALL with the t(9;22), but lacks the *BCR-ABL1* fusion
2. It is more commonly found in adults
3. It is mutually exclusive of t(12;21), t(4;11) and a hyperdiploid karyotype
4. Event free survival at 5 years is lower in this type of ALL but overall survival at 5 years is no different than normal karyotype ALL

Answer: options 1, 2 and 3 are true but option 4 is false

In fact, EFS and OS, **both** are lower compared with normal karyotype ALL.

Q. In T cell ALL, the most common rearrangements involve the TCR genes. On which chromosome is TCR beta chain gene located:
1. 14q
2. 7q
3. 7p
4. 14p

Answer: 7q

There are four TCR chain genes of interest in ALL: TCR alpha/delta chain is located at 14q, TCR beta chain located at 7q and TCR gamma chain located at 7p.

Note here that T cell ALL has a worse prognosis, compared with B cell ALL in general. There are some features that are more commonly associated with T cell ALL, like a higher WBC count and presence of a mediastinal mass.

Q. Which is the most common childhood cancer:
1. ALL
2. AML
3. Retinoblastoma
4. Wilms tumor

Answer: ALL

ALL accounts for about 25% of all childhood cancers.

Q. Which of the following genetic syndrome is associated with ALL:
1. Down syndrome
2. Neurofibromatosis type 1
3. Bloom syndrome
4. Ataxia-telangiectasia

Answer: all of the above

All of the above are associated with increased incidence of ALL.

Q. In children with ALL, which of the following clinical finding is most commonly found at the time of presentation:
1. Hepatomegaly
2. Fever
3. Bleeding manifestations
4. Musculoskeletal pain

Answer: hepatomegaly

This may surprise you, if you haven't gone through standard textbooks carefully. The most common clinical finding in childhood leukemia is **organomegaly.** Organomegaly is most commonly in the form of hepatomegaly (64 percent) and/or splenomegaly (61 percent).

Fever, musculoskeletal pain, bleeding manifestations or lymphadenopathy are found in nearly half of the children.
On the other hand, children may present rarely with headache, testicular enlargement or a mediastinal mass. Note that mediastinal mass is more frequently found in T cell leukemia/lymphoma.

Q. Which of the following statement is true:
1. In children an epitrochlear node is considered normal if it's less than 10 mm in size
2. Any lymph node in a child is considered enlarged if it's more than 10 mm in size
3. A cervical lymph node is considered abnormal in a child, only if it is more than 20 mm in size
4. If an inguinal lymph node is more than 10 mm in size in a child, it will be considered abnormal

Answer: A cervical lymph node is considered abnormal in a child, only if it is more than 20 mm in size

As we all know, a multiple choice question sometimes has no "absolutely correct answer"; sometimes we have to choose what is best among the choices given. Now, this topic of size of lymph nodes is a very confusing one as there are differing views on this and also, the cutoffs are different in different age groups.

As far as this question is concerned, I would like you to go through the following facts (remember that we are talking about lymph node size cutoff values, above which they will be considered abnormal, **in children**):

1. A lymph node is generally considered enlarged when it is >10 mm
2. But there are some exceptions:
   a. The cutoff for epitrochlear nodes is >5 mm
   b. The cutoff value for inguinal nodes is >15 mm
   c. The cutoff value for cervical nodes is >20 mm

Q. The lymphoblasts of acute lymphoblastic leukemia stain positively with which of the following:

1. Periodic acid-Schiff
2. Nonspecific esterase
3. Myeloperoxidase
4. None of the above

Answer: periodic acid-Schiff

But note that PAS staining is **not specific** to the lymphoblast lineage. On the other hand, myeloperoxidase is a lineage defining marker for the myeloid lineage. **By definition, MPO staining is absent in lymphoblasts.**

Notes on immunophenotyping:
It is important to understand that the topic of immunophenotyping is not an easy one; entire books have been written on this subject. So any level of knowledge in this regard may prove to be insufficient at some point. We will just try to go over some very basic facts and in my opinion, most

of the questions can be answered if we apply this limited amount of knowledge carefully.

1. B cell antigens are: CD19, CD20, CD22, CD79a, PAX5
2. T cell antigens are: CD1a, CD3, CD4, CD5, CD7, CD8
3. NK cell antigen: CD56
4. Immature lymphoid cells markers: CD10, terminal deoxyribonucleotide transferase [TdT]
5. Marker of intermediate pre-B cell maturation: CD10
6. Marker of late pre-B cell maturation: CD20
7. Myeloid antigens are: CD13, CD33, CD11b, CD64

These "markers" have to demonstrate a certain level of staining in the cells present, to be called "positive". Generally, if a marker stains more than 20% of cells, it is labelled as positive.

There are some exceptions to this but we don't need to memorise them all.

Q. In children having ALL, before initiation of therapy a lumbar puncture has to be done. If the CSF shows 4 blasts/microL, which of the following will be the correct categorisation of such a patient:

1. CNS-1
2. CNS-2
3. CNS-3
4. CNS-4

Answer: CNS-2

There are three categories in the classification of CSF in pa-

tients of ALL:
1. CNS-1: No lymphoblasts in cerebrospinal fluid (CSF) regardless of the white blood cell count
2. CNS-2: < 5 WBCs/microL in CSF with the presence of lymphoblasts
3. CNS-3: ≥ 5 WBCs/microL in CSF with the presence of lymphoblasts

There is no such category as CNS-4.

Notes on initial treatment of acute lymphoblastic leukemia/lymphoma in adults:
1. The goal of induction therapy traditionally has been to reduce the leukemia cell burden to 5 percent or less blasts in the bone marrow. Nowadays measurable residual disease (MRD) is being frequently used, the aim of which is to provide a measure of reduction of tumor cell burden beyond microscopic levels.
2. Extensive pretreatment evaluation and preparations have to be made, discussion of which is provided in excellent detail in the standard textbooks.
3. It is beyond the scope of this book to provide a detailed analysis of all the different protocols being used today in the treatment of ALL. Some general principles are as follows:
    A. Most induction chemo regimens contain vincristine, anthracycline (like daunorubicin) and prednisone (or dexamethasone).
    B. CNS prophylaxis is included in the induction regimens, like intrathecal methotrexate.
    C. Using these protocols, around 80% of adults with B cell ALL are expected to achieve a com-

plete response.

D. Paediatric protocols contain agents like cyclophosphamide, cytarabine, high-dose methotrexate etc. While these protocols may be used in adults, their role is less clear.

4. Some commonly used protocols are: CALGB study 8811, CALGB study 9111, CALGB study 10403, DFCI ALL/LBL Consortium study, Berlin-Frankfurt-Munster (BFM), Hyper-CVAD alternating with high dose methotrexate and cytarabine, French GRAALL 2003 and French GRAALL 2005 etc.

5. Note that the above mentioned regimens are for **adults.** Some of these protocols are specifically designed for a particular age group, so it must be taken into account before starting a protocol. That being said, the differences among these protocols are not very substantial.

Q. What is the dose of asparaginase in the CALGB protocols:
1. 5000 mg/m2
2. 6000 mg/m2
3. 10000 mg/m2
4. 20000 mg fixed dose

Answer: 6000 mg/m2

I must admit that this question is difficult and it's not at all necessary to remember all the doses used in all the protocols.

Some notes on asparaginase:

1. Asparaginase is an essential component of many adult protocols for ALL and almost all pediatric protocols for ALL.
2. It leads to depletion of asparagine in the plasma. The leukemic cells are not capable of producing this essential amino acid, and they depend on the supply of asparagine from the plasma; so they die due to lack of asparagine.
3. There are following types of asparaginase preparations available in the market:
   a. Native *Escherichia coli* asparaginase (half-life approximately one day)
   b. *Erwinia* asparaginase (half-life approximately 14 hours)
   c. Pegylated *Escherichia coli* asparaginase, also known as pegasparaginase (half-life approximately six days)
   d. Calaspargase pegol is an asparagine specific enzyme
4. Asparaginase preparations are associated with many toxicities like, allergic reactions, coagulopathies, acute pancreatitis, and increased liver transaminases.
5. Pegylated asparaginase is the preferred option because it is less immunogenic and has a greater efficacy. The dose schedules may be different in different protocols. The most commonly used schedule is 2000 to 2500 units/m2 every 14 days.

Q. Which of the following steroid used in acute lymphoblastic leukemia protocols more efficiently crosses the blood brain barrier:
1. Dexamethasone
2. Prednisone

3. Both cross the BBB with equal efficacy
4. None of the above cross the blood brain barrier

Answer: dexamethasone

In many protocols, however, prednisone is used. One important thing to consider is that use of dexamethasone is not associated with improvement in overall survival.

Q. The use of rituximab is recommended in patients of B cell ALL who are Philadelphia chromosome negative and are less than 60 years of age:
1. True
2. False

Answer: true

Although the studies have shown mixed results. Based on the prospective and retrospective data, expert consensus is in favour of giving rituximab in this patient population.

Q. Which of the following is not a method of CNS prophylaxis in the commonly used treatment protocols for acute lymphoblastic leukemia:
1. High dose methotrexate
2. Intrathecal methotrexate
3. Cranial irradiation
4. Pulse vincristine plus high dose steroids

Answer: pulse vincristine plus high dose steroids

It is important to follow one protocol in its entirety. We should not mix the drugs, doses and schedules of various protocols together.

Q. If a patient of ALL presents with CNS involvement, what is the standard minimum therapy required:
1. 2400 cGy of radiation is given to the entire cranium over 12 doses and at least six doses of intrathecal methotrexate
2. 1200 cGy of radiation is given to the entire cranium over 12 doses and at least twelve doses of intrathecal methotrexate
3. 2400 cGy of radiation is given to the entire cranium over 10 doses and at least sixteen doses of intrathecal methotrexate
4. 2400 cGy of radiation is given to the entire cranium over 12 doses and at least sixteen doses of intrathecal methotrexate

Answer: 2400 cGy of radiation is given to the entire cranium over 12 doses and at least six doses of intrathecal methotrexate

Q. Which of the following is not true about ALL and Down syndrome:
1. Patients with Down syndrome who develop ALL/

LBL have more treatment-related complications
2. These patients have increased chances of developing more serious adverse events with methotrexate
3. Patients with Down syndrome have higher incidence of hyperglycaemia when treated with corticosteroids
4. There is no increased risk of developing cardiotoxicity with anthracyclines

Answer: There is no increased risk of developing cardiotoxicity with anthracyclines

In fact, the risk is **increased.**

Q. Which of the following is the preferred TKI in patients with Philadelphia chromosome positive ALL:
1. Imatinib
2. Dasatinib
3. Nilotinib
4. Bosutinib

Answer: dasatinib

Notes on overview of treatment of ALL in children and adolescents:
1. There are basically four phases of treatment of ALL: induction, consolidation, delayed intensification and maintenance. Note that sometimes intensification may be started early, just after induction.
2. **Induction therapy** is the initial phase of treatment.

The goal of induction therapy is achieving complete remission (defined as less than 5 percent blasts in the bone marrow) and restoration of normal hematopoiesis.

3. The drugs used during induction phase depend on the risk stratification and the protocol being followed. Vincristine, a steroid and asparaginase are always used (unless there are contraindications) and an anthracycline may be added in high risk patients.

4. There are many indicators of good outcomes, during the induction phase. In some protocols these indicators are routinely incorporated and they may guide further treatment. The **good indicators** are: early clearance of lymphoblasts from peripheral blood during the first week of therapy, clearance of blasts from the bone marrow by the end of induction, and the absence of MRD at the end of induction therapy.

5. If a patient has t(9;22) then a BCR-ABL1 tyrosine kinase inhibitor is added to the regimen.

6. CNS prophylaxis is a must. If CNS prophylaxis is not given then 80% of patients, who achieve complete remission in the bone marrow, will develop leukaemic involvement of CNS. There are three ways to give CNS prophylaxis: intrathecal methotrexate (some protocols may use more drugs), high dose methotrexate and cranial or craniospinal irradiation. Many studies have been done on this subject and most studies conclude that radiation may be avoided. But it depends on the clinical context and the protocol, the drug doses and intensity/density being used.

7. Once induction therapy is over, **consolidation therapy**, is begun. Consolidation is important because it's a fact that induction chemotherapy can not eliminate all tumor cells and the cells that are not killed go under clonal evolution and ultimately a

new population of tumor cells will take over, which will be resistant to the previous chemotherapy molecules; if consolidation is not given.

8. Consolidation is usually 4 to 8 months long and different trials use different drugs, e.g., cytarabine, methotrexate, anthracyclines, cyclophosphamide/ifosfamide and epipodophyllotoxins.

9. Consolidation may be given as **intensification**, especially in those patients who do not achieve MRD negativity at the end of induction (UKALL 2003 trial). Alternatively, intensification may be given after the consolidation phase is over, which is known as **delayed intensification,** in which pulses of high dose combination therapy are given for 4 to 8 weeks (sometimes more), which are similar to induction therapy.

10. After the induction, consolidation and intensification phases are over, the final phase is begun; which is known as the **maintenance** phase. The overall duration is variable, it primarily depends on gender (males are given a longer duration maintenance compared with females) and the protocol. The overall treatment duration for most children is 30 to 42 months. Different protocols use different drug combinations and the doses are also different, e.g., oral 6-mercaptopurine (6-MP), weekly methotrexate, periodic vincristine, prednisone and intrathecal therapy.

11. Note that in some patients, allogeneic HCT is performed. The strict criteria for selection of patients are not entirely clear (refer to the section of risk stratification of ALL. The treatment of patients belonging to the "very high risk group" involves allogeneic HCT).

Q. What percent of patients with acute lymphoblastic leukemia develop silent inactivation of asparaginase:

    1. 2-8
    2. 1-4
    3. 8-16
    4. 16-32

Answer: 2-8%

This inactivation occurs due to production of neutralizing anti-asparaginase antibodies.

Q. Which of the following is a predictor of development of tumor lysis syndrome in children with ALL being treated with chemotherapy:

    1. Age > 10 years
    2. Splenomegaly
    3. Mediastinal mass
    4. Initial white blood cell count > 20,000/microL

Answer: all of the above are correct

These four factors are the most commonly used and validated predictors. If all of these four are absent then the patient will be categorised as low risk for development of tumor lysis syndrome, with a negative predictive value of 98 percent.

Q. Which of the following is not true about childhood ALL patients being treated with vincristine containing regimens:

1. 25 to 30 percent of children treated will develop clinically significant peripheral neuropathy
2. The rate of neuropathy is lower in children with single nucleotide polymorphism in the promoter region of CEP72
3. The neuropathy involves both sensory and motor fibers
4. Vincristine induced neuropathy is usually reversible

Answer: The rate of neuropathy is lower in children with single nucleotide polymorphism in the promoter region of CEP72

In fact, the rate is very high in children with this SNP.

Q. Which of the following therapy is not used in relapsed B cell ALL:

1. Nelarabine
2. Blinatumomab
3. CAR-T cells therapy
4. Tisagenlecleucel

Answer: nelarabine

Nelarabine is used in **relapsed T cell ALL,** not in B cell ALL.

Another drug used in these patients is liposomal vincristine.

Some notes on therapies used in relapsed B cell ALL:
1. Blinatumomab is a bispecific T cell engager (BiTE) monoclonal antibody directed at both CD19 on precursor B cell ALL tumor cells and CD3 on cytotoxic T cells.
2. Inotuzumab is an anti-CD22 directed monoclonal antibody, with a calicheamicin component.
3. CAR-T cells are genetically modified cells that target the tumor cells of B-ALL. They are a "customised" treatment option, in which the patient's own T cells are generally modified to encode a chimeric antigen receptor which targets the leukemic cells.
4. Tisagenlecleucel is a CD19-directed genetically modified autologous T cell immunotherapy.
5. Clofarabine is also used in the relapsed setting.

Q. In medically fit patients with Philadelphia chromosome positive B cell ALL, who attain complete response with chemotherapy plus TKI (BCR-ABL1 tyrosine kinase inhibitor); which of the following is the most appropriate treatment option:
1. Allogeneic hematopoietic cell transplantation
2. Autologous HCT plus TKI
3. Chemotherapy plus TKI
4. Observation alone

Answer: allogeneic hematopoietic cell transplantation

There is one exception to this approach: autologous HCT or

TKI plus consolidation chemotherapy are acceptable alternatives for patients who achieve a deep molecular remission, i.e., MRD <0.01 percent.

Q. For patients with Ph+ ALL, what is the most appropriate maintenance therapy after the chemotherapy protocol has been finished:
1. TKI alone
2. Chemotherapy with a TKI
3. Chemotherapy without a TKI
4. TKI at the time of molecular relapse

Answer: TKI alone

Note here, that there are no absolutely right or wrong answers to this question. My answer is based on what most institutes follow. The duration of maintenance therapy with a TKI:
1. It is determined by the status of MRD in bone marrow after completing HCT or consolidation chemotherapy.
2. If a patients has MRD <0.01% after HCT or completion of chemotherapy, TKI is continued for 12 more months in patients who received HCT and 24 more months in patients who were treated with chemotherapy.
3. On the other hand if a patient has MRD of 0.01% or more at the end the treatment (either HCT or chemo), further treatment in guided by MRD status:
   a. In those patients who continue to show MRD 0.01% or more, TKI is continued indefinitely until the MRD becomes <0.01%

b. If in a patient, two consecutive MRD results are <0.01%, TKI are continued for at least 12 more months.

c. After the maintenance therapy is over, bone marrow MRD is evaluated every 2 to 3 months for a period of 5 years, along with peripheral blood counts. Although, the data in this regard are still evolving and in the future we may see this change.

Notes on immunophenotype and markers used to diagnose "biphenotypic leukemia":

1. B lineage markers: CD79a, cytoplasmic IgM, cytoplasmic CD22, CD19, CD20, CD10, TdT, CD24

2. T lineage markers: CD3 (cytoplasmic or membrane), anti-TCR alpha/beta/gamma/delta, CD2, CD5, CD8, CD10, TdT, CD7, CD1a

3. Myeloid lineage markers: anti-MPO, CD13, CD33, CDw65, CD117, CD14, CD15, CD64

There is a scoring system assigned to these markers. The diagnosis of biphenotypic leukemia is made when the scores are 3 or more for the myeloid lineage and 1 for the lymphoid lineage.

Also note that a marker is considered positive only if >20% cells stain positive with a monoclonal antibody. There are four exceptions to this rule: CD79a, TdT, MPO and CD3; they are considered positive if >10% cells stain positive.

Notes on diagnosis of "mixed phenotype acute leukemia (MPAL)":

The WHO 2008 criteria are used to defined MPAL. Follow the following steps:

1. If a leukemia fulfils criteria for both myeloid and lymphoid lineages according to the WHO 2008 criteria but does not meet any WHO AML category then it is diagnosed as MPAL.

2. Once this diagnosis is made then sequentially the following tests are done: t(9;22) or BCR-ABL1 rearrangement and t(v;11q23). If the leukemia tests positive for either of these then it is designated as MPAL with that particular mutation.

3. If both of these mutations are absent then it is searched that whether the leukemia shows both B cell and myeloid lineage markers, if so then it is diagnosed as MPAL, B/Myeloid, NOS.

4. If both of these mutations are absent then it is searched that whether the leukemia shows both T cell and myeloid lineage markers, if so then it is diagnosed as MPAL, T/Myeloid, NOS.

5. If none of these definitions are met then the leukemia is diagnosed as MPAL, NOS, rarer types.

Notes on risk stratification of ALL patients:
I would suggest that the reader must go through the following text thoroughly. Remember that many institutes have formulated their own risk stratification systems, so the answer of a particular question will depend on the clinical context and the best option must be chosen.

This risk stratification scheme is primarily for childhood ALL.

Low risk ALL patients must fulfil **all** of the following criteria. A low risk ALL patient has >95% five-year EFS. The treatment of such patients is conventional antimetabolite based therapy.

    a. NCI standard risk group (WBC <50,000/microL **AND** age one to <10 years)

    b. Lesser risk cytogenetics: Trisomies 4 and 10 **or** ETV-RUNX1 (United States) **or** Hyperdiploid (Europe)

    c. Rapid response to therapy (MRD negative at days 8 and 29)

Average risk ALL patients have **either** of the following two sets of criteria. The 5-year EFS in these patients is 90-95% and the treatment is intensified antimetabolite therapy.

    a. NCI standard risk group **and** Rapid response to therapy

    b. NCI standard risk group **and** Lesser risk cytogenetics **and** Slow response to therapy

The "slow response to therapy" means: MRD positive at day 8 and negative at day 29.

High risk ALL patients have **any** of the following sets of criteria. The 5-year EFS is 88-90% and the treatment is intensive multiagent chemotherapy.

    a. NCI high risk group (WBC ≥50,000 microL **OR** age ≥10 years [up to 13 years if treated on a COG protocol]) **and** Rapid response to therapy

    b. NCI standard risk group **and** Slow response to therapy

    c. CNS-positive leukemia

    d. Testicular leukemia

Very high risk ALL patients have **any** of the following sets of criteria. The 5-year EFS is <80%. The treatment is intensive multiagent chemotherapy followed by allogeneic HCT in the first remission.

    a. MRD+ at day 29 (there may be some exceptions to this particular criterion)

    b. Induction failures

    c. MLL rearrangements **or** iAMP21 amplification

    d. Age <1 year (or >13 years if treated on a COG protocol)

Special groups of ALL patients are the following:

1. T cell ALL: here the 5-year EFS is 66-80% and the treatment is multiagent chemotherapy

2. Philadelphia chromosome positive ALL: here the 5-year EFS is 70% and the treatment is multiagent chemotherapy containing a BCR-ABL1 tyrosine kinase inhibitor.

Q. What does the term "rapid response to therapy" means in adult patients of ALL receiving induction chemotherapy:

1. Disappearance of bone marrow blasts at days 8

2. Disappearance of bone marrow blasts at days 14

3. Disappearance of bone marrow blasts at days 29

4. Disappearance of bone marrow blasts at days 36

Answer: Disappearance of bone marrow blasts at days 14

They key word here is "adult". The definitions of responses to therapy are different for adults and children. In children, "rapid response to therapy" means disappearance of bone marrow blasts at day 8 and in adults it means disappearance of bone marrow blasts at day 14.

A "slow response to therapy" means that bone marrow blasts haven't disappeared at day 8 in children and day 14 in adults but by day 29 bone marrow has become negative.

If the bone marrow is positive for blasts even on day 29 then the disease is said to be unresponsive.

As we can infer from the above mentioned discussion, these criteria are based on morphology alone. Many modern day protocols now routinely include assessment of MRD at various time points in the treatment schedule, which gives a more in-depth assessment of the response.

Q. Which of the following statement is not true about MRD in ALL:
  1. Children with detectable MRD have decreased disease-free survival (DFS) and overall survival (OS)
  2. In children the level of detectable MRD correlates with relapse
  3. Semi-quantitative PCR in currently the only way to clinically assess MRD
  4. MRD studies have demonstrated prognostic value when measured before and after allogeneic hematopoietic cell transplantation in ALL

Answer: Semi-quantitative PCR in currently the only way to clinically assess MRD

There are two accepted methods for assessment of MRD: semi-quantitative PCR and flow cytometry.

Q. Approximately what percent of patients with Philadelphia-chromosome positive ALL have the p210 subtype:
  1. 25
  2. 70
  3. >90
  4. <10

Answer: 25

Approximately 70 percent of Ph+ve ALL patients have the p190 subtype and the p210 subtype accounts for 25 to 30 percent of Ph+ve ALL cases.

Note that the p210 subtype is present in the overwhelming majority of CML patients.

Notes on HCT in ALL:
  1. Allogeneic transplant is performed in first or second complete remission.
  2. The preferred donor is a human leukocyte antigen (HLA)-matched sibling or a matched unrelated donor (MUD).

3. The most commonly used conditioning regimen is total body irradiation (TBI) plus cyclophosphamide.
4. Graft versus leukemia effect **does not** play a major role in ALL.

HODGKIN LYMPHOMA

Q. B symptoms are present in approximately what percent of
classical HL cases:
1. 10
2. <5
3. 40
4. >70

Answer: 40

Q. HL has a bimodal age distribution. The two peaks in incidence are seen in:
1. Late adolescence and older adults
2. Infancy and late adolescence
3. Infancy and older adults
4. Early adolescence and older adults

Answer: late adolescence and older adults

Roughly, the two peaks occur at 20 years and 65 years of age.

Q. EBV is most commonly associated with which type of HL:
1. Mixed cellularity
2. Lymphocyte depleted
3. Nodular sclerosis
4. NLPHL

Answer: lymphocyte depleted

EBV is most commonly associated with mixed cellularity and lymphocyte depleted types of HL. But in lymphocyte depleted type of HL, nearly 100% patients show EBV positivity, thus the association is more strong between these two.

Q. Which of the following is not true about lymphadenopathy in classical HL:
1. It is present in more than 60% patients at presentation
2. It is nontender
3. Neck is the most common site of involvement
4. Infradiaphragmatic lymphadenopathy is common

Answer: infradiaphragmatic lymphadenopathy is common

In fact, infradiaphragmatic lymphadenopathy is quite rare. It is found in less than 10% of cases.

On the other hand, mediastinal lymphadenopathy is quite common; it is found in around 50% of cases.

Remember that in HL, the spread of lymphadenopathy is **contiguous.** Contiguous means that HL spreads from one lymph node region to another "adjacent" lymph node region via lymphatics. Sometimes HL may spread to distant regions without involving adjacent regions, but such cases are rare.

Q. Which of the following is not considered a B symptoms in HL:
1. Fever
2. Night sweats
3. Weight loss
4. Alcohol associated pain

Answer: alcohol associated pain

The B symptoms are:
1. Persistent temperature $>38°C$ ($>100.4°F$)

2. Drenching night sweats
3. Unexplained loss of >10 percent of body weight over the past **six** months

The characteristic fever of HL is Pel-Ebstein fever, but is not common.

Q. Alcohol associated pain is highly specific for HL:
   1. True
   2. False

Answer: true

It is very specific to HL. Its mechanism of development is not known.

Q. Which of the following is not a laboratory feature of HL:
   1. Hypocalcemia
   2. Anemia
   3. Eosinophilia
   4. Lymphopenia

Answer: hypocalcemia

In fact, **hypercalcemia** is a lab feature of HL.

Q. Generally Reed-Sternberg cells constitute what percent of involved tissue in HL:
1. <10
2. 20-30
3. 30-60
4. >60

Answer: <10%

Remember that while RS cells are the hallmark of HL, they constitute only a small proportion of cells of tissues involved by HL.

Q. The characteristic RS cells of HL have an "owl eyes" appearance on microscopy. Which of the following variant of RS cells is mononuclear:
1. Hodgkin cell
2. Lacunar cell
3. Popcorn cell
4. L and H cell

Answer: Hodgkin cell

Q. Which of the following is not expressed by neoplastic cells of classical HL:

1. CD15
2. CD30
3. PAX5
4. CD79a

Answer: CD79a

Remember the immunophenotype features of classical HL: CD15+, CD30+, PAX5+, CD45-, CD20-, CD19-, CD79a-, BOB1-, OCT2-.

The most commonly expressed antigen is CD30, which is expressed in nearly 100% cases. PAX5 is expressed but only very weakly.

Q. Clonal immunoglobulin gene rearrangements can be detected in what percent of classical HL patients:

1. <10
2. 20-30
3. 50-70
4. >90

Answer: >90%

Clonal Ig gene rearrangements play a very important role in the pathogenesis of classical HL.

Q. Which of the following is the most common gene mutation in classical HL:
1. Beta-2 microglobulin
2. *STAT6*
3. *SOCS1*
4. *PTPN1*

Answer: Beta-2 microglobulin

Q. Which of the following is the least common subtype of classical HL:
1. Nodular sclerosis
2. Mixed cellularity
3. Lymphocyte rich
4. Lymphocyte depleted

Answer: lymphocyte depleted

Remember that the most common subtype HL in the western world is NS but the most common subtype of HL in India is MC.

Q. What percent of patients initially diagnosed with HL have NLPHL:
1. <1%
2. 5%
3. 10-20%
4. Nearly 30%

Answer: 5%

Q. L and H Reed-Sternberg cells are the neoplastic cells of NLPHL. These cells arise from which of the following:
1. Germinal center B cells
2. Activated B cells
3. Primordial B cells
4. Undifferentiated bone marrow stromal cells

Answer: germinal center B cells

Q. B symptoms are least common in:
1. Mixed cellularity HL
2. NLPHL
3. Lymphocyte rich HL
4. Lymphocyte depleted HL

Answer: NLPHL

Q. Lymphadenopathy is present in nearly all patients of NLPHL. Which of the following site is most commonly involved with lymphadenopathy:
1. Central lymph nodes above diaphragm
2. Peripheral lymph nodes
3. Mediastinal lymph nodes
4. Central lymph nodes below diaphragm

Answer: peripheral lymph nodes

Mediastinal lymph nodes are rarely involved by NLPHL.

Q. Popcorn cells are characteristic of:
1. Mixed cellularity HL
2. Nodular sclerosis HL
3. Lymphocyte depleted HL

4. NLPHL

Answer: NLPHL

Although these cells are not pathognomonic for NLPHL.

Q. All of the following are characteristics of NLPHL immunophenotype except:
1. CD45+
2. BCL6-
3. CD20+
4. CD15-

Answer: BCL6-

Remember these important facts:
1. Classical HL: CD15+, CD30+, CD45-, CD20-
2. NLPHL: CD45+, BCL6+, CD19+, CD20+, CD22+, CD79a+, BCL6+, and CD15- and usually CD30-

This data has implications on selection of treatment. Like in case of NLPHL, rituximab plays an important role because NLPHL is CD20+. And in case of classical HL, brentuximab is an important drug because it targets CD30 and classical HL is CD30+.

Q. EBV in the neoplastic cells is found more commonly in:
1. Classical HL
2. NLPHL
3. Both of the above
4. None of the above

Answer: classical HL

Q. All of the following are features of NLPHL and not of classical HL, except:
1. EMA positivity
2. Presence of CD57+ T cells
3. Fibrosis
4. Abundance of B cells in the background

Answer: fibrosis

Fibrosis is more commonly found in classical HL and not in NLPHL. Note that in classical HL, T cells are more common in background than B cells, while the opposite is true for NLPHL.

Notes on staging of lymphoma:

I would request you to go through the below mentioned points and remember them by heart. So many questions are asked out of these:

1. The most commonly used staging system for lymphomas worldwide is the Lugano classification, which is derived from the Ann Arbor staging system with Cotswolds modifications.

2. Stage I: involvement of a single lymph node region (there are fine rules about what constitutes a lymph node region) or lymphoid structure (such as the spleen, thymus, or Waldeyer's ring)

3. Stage II: involvement of two or more lymph node regions or lymph node structures on the same side of the diaphragm.

4. Stage III: involvement of lymph node regions or lymphoid structures on both sides of the diaphragm.

5. Stage IV: diffuse or disseminated involvement of one or more extranodal organs or tissues beyond that designated E, with or without associated lymph node involvement.

6. All cases are subclassified to indicate the absence (A) or presence (B) of the systemic symptoms of significant unexplained fever, night sweats, or unexplained weight loss exceeding 10% of body weight during the six months prior to diagnosis.

7. The designation "E" refers to extranodal contiguous extension that can be encompassed within an irradiation field appropriate for nodal disease of the same

anatomic extent. More extensive extranodal disease is designated stage IV.

8. Bulky disease: A single nodal mass, in contrast to multiple smaller nodes, of 10 cm or more than or equal to 1/3 of the transthoracic diameter at any level of thoracic vertebrae as determined by CT

9. The term "X" (used in the Ann Arbor staging system) is no longer necessary.

10. The subscript "RS" is used to designate the stage at the time of relapse.

Q. Which of the following was not an arm of the GHSG HD10 trial done in favourable prognosis early stage HL:

1. Four cycles of ABVD followed by 30 Gy IFRT
2. Four cycles of ABVD followed by 20 Gy IFRT
3. Three cycles of ABVD followed by 30 Gy IFRT
4. Two cycles of ABVD followed by 20 Gy IFRT

Answer: Three cycles of ABVD followed by 30 Gy IFRT

The fourth arm was two cycles of ABVD followed by 30 Gy IFRT.

The inclusion criteria of this trial were:

1. No more than two sites of disease
2. No extranodal extension

3. No mediastinal mass greater than or equal to one-third the maximum thoracic diameter
4. ESR less than 50 (less than 30 if B symptoms present).

Please remember that this trial was done in **early stage, favorable risk group** patients. In such patients, the survival outcomes were not different in the four treatment arms described above and the toxicities were markedly less in the lower chemo cycles and lower radiation dose arms. So if a patient fits these criteria then 2 cycles of ABVD followed by 20 Gy IFRT can be used without compromising the survival outcomes.

Q. Which of the following radiation therapy techniques involves the least amount of healthy tissue:
1. EFRT
2. IFRT
3. INRT
4. ISRT

Answer: INRT

The problem with INRT is that we need a pretreatment PET scan, to which contouring of lymph nodes is done post completion of chemo. This PET scan is not adequately available in many patients, that's why ISRT is the most commonly used technique worldwide.

Memorise these important facts about treatment of early stage (I or II) HL:

1. First of all, we have to decide whether or not the patient belongs to the unfavourable category.
2. In the patient belongs to unfavorable category then the minimum adequate treatment is 4 cycles of ABVD followed by 30 Gy radiation.
3. If the patient belongs to the favorable group **and** meets the eligibility criteria of GHSG HD10 trial, 2 cycles of ABVD and 20 Gy radiation is adequate.
4. If the patient belongs to the favorable group **but** does not meet the eligibility criteria of GHSG HD10 trial, then 3 to 4 cycles of ABVD and 30 Gy of radiation is appropriate.
5. Radiation therapy is an integral part of treatment of early stage HL. In some patients, however, radiation therapy may not be chosen. In them, six cycles of ABVD may be appropriate. If such patients show complete response after 2 cycles of ABVD, then 4 cycles of ABVD may suffice in selected patients.

Q. Which of the following is not true about treatment of stage III/IV HL:

1. ABVD is the preferred therapy in the majority of pa-

tients
2. The full course of ABVD in this setting is 8 cycles
3. Response evaluation by PET is done after two cycles of chemotherapy
4. In younger patients having IPS 4 or more, BEACOPP is more suitable choice

Answer: The full course of ABVD in this setting is 8 cycles

Remember, the full course of ABVD in this setting is **6** cycles. It is very important to remember this fact.

ABVD is administered every 14 days and 2 such courses constitute one cycle. So six cycles mean total twelve courses of ABVD. But we never describe them as courses. In summary, if ever a question is asked then the answer will be: for advanced stage (III/IV) HL, **six cycles of ABVD** are the standard of care.

Please memorise the doses and schedule of ABVD:
1. Doxorubicin (A)= 25 mg/m2 (on days 1 and 15 of every 28 days cycle)
2. Bleomycin (B)= 10 units/m2 (on days 1 and 15 of every 28 days cycle)
3. Vinblastine (V)= 6 mg/m2 (on days 1 and 15 of every 28 days cycle)

4. Dacarbazine (D)= 375 mg/m2 (on days 1 and 15 of every 28 days cycle)

BEACOPP is of two types, fixed dose and escalated. BEACOPP is used by European centres for younger patients, having good performance status and with IPS 4 or more. It is much more toxic than ABVD, thus its use is mostly limited to young and fit individuals with advanced HL.

Q. One unit of bleomycin is equal to:
1. 1 mg of bleomycin
2. 10 mg of bleomycin
3. 0.1 mg of bleomycin
4. 0.01 mg of bleomycin

Answer: 1 mg of bleomycin

Q. In the Stanford V regimen used for advanced HL, chemo-therapy is given for:
1. 12 weeks
2. 8 weeks
3. 16 weeks
4. 24 weeks

Answer: 12 weeks

Radiation therapy is an integral part of Stanford V and it is given 1 to 3 weeks after completion of chemotherapy.

Q. Which of the following is not true about the RATHL trial done in HL:
1. In it PET scan was done after first two cycles of ABVD
2. It was done in limited stage HL
3. If PET was negative after two cycles, then therapy was de-escalated in the experimental arm
4. The PFS and OS was same for the arms containing ABVD and AVD

Answer: It was done in limited stage HL

In fact, it was done in advanced stage HL.

The main purpose of this trial was to study the feasibility of omitting bleomycin in patients of advanced stage HL who achieved a negative PET scan after 2 cycles of ABVD. This trial showed that in such patients omitting bleomycin resulted in reduced toxicity and equal survival outcomes.

Q. Which of the following was a finding of the German Hodgkin Study Group HD18 trial done in HL:

1. The five-year PFS with four cycles of escalated BEACOPP was equal versus either six or eight cycles of escalated BEACOPP in patients with advanced stage HL who achieved PET negativity after two cycles of escalated BEACOPP

2. The five-year PFS with four cycles of escalated BEACOPP was equal versus either six or eight cycles of BEACOPP in patients with advanced stage HL who achieved PET negativity after two cycles of escalated BEACOPP

3. The five-year OS with four cycles of escalated BEACOPP was equal versus either six or eight cycles of escalated BEACOPP in patients with advanced stage HL who achieved PET negativity after two cycles of escalated BEACOPP

4. The five-year OS with four cycles of escalated BEACOPP was equal versus either six or eight cycles of BEACOPP in patients with advanced stage HL who achieved PET negativity after two cycles of escalated BEACOPP

Answer: The five-year PFS with four cycles of escalated BEACOPP was equal versus either six or eight cycles of escalated BEACOPP in patients with advanced stage HL who achieved PET negativity after two cycles of escalated BEACOPP

The four cycles arm was associated with fewer toxicities.

Q. Which of the following trial done in HL studied using escalated BEACOPP for two cycle and then de-escalation to ABVD if PET scan was negative after 2 cycles of escalated BEACOPP:

1. AHL2011
2. GHSG HD18
3. RATHL
4. GITIL HD0607

Answer: AHL2011

In the GITIL/FIL HD0607 trial, a different strategy was tried. The other three trials (options 1, 2 and 3) were trials of "de-escalation", but in the GITIL trial "escalation" was done. In this trial, if the patient had a positive PET scan after two cycles of ABVD then he was assigned to escalated BEACOPP.

Another trial using escalation strategy was SWOG S0816.

Q. What percent of patients with advanced HL are expected to achieve complete response after 6 cycles of ABVD:

1. 50-60
2. 20-30

3. 70-80
4. Nearly 100

Answer: 70-80%

Q. All are true about the ECHELON-1 trial except:
1. Patients of stage III or IV HL were included, not of stage I or II
2. Patients randomised to the brentuximab plus AVD arm showed equivalent modified PFS compared with the bleomycin plus AVD arm
3. OS did not differ significantly between the two arms of the trial
4. Growth factor support was needed with the brentuximab plus AVD arm

Answer: Patients randomised to the brentuximab plus AVD arm showed equivalent modified PFS compared with the bleomycin plus AVD arm

In this trial, the modified PFS was superior with the brentuxiamb plus AVD arm (not equivalent).

Q. Which of the following is an indication for RT in patients

with advanced HL:
1. Initial bulky mediastinal disease
2. Partial response after completion of chemotherapy
3. Both of the above
4. None of the above

Answer: both of the above

Usually, these two are the only two indications of RT in advanced HL. RT is contemplated in initial bulky mediastinal disease, even if the patient achieves complete response with chemotherapy.

Remember that these two are not absolute indications.

Q. In treatment of advanced HL, when can autologous hematopoietic transplant be used:
1. In the first remission
2. In the second remission
3. In chemotherapy refractory disease
4. All of the above

Answer: options 2 and 3 are correct

But option 1 is not correct. HCT has no place in the treatment of HL in the first remission.

Q. All of the following are factors in the International Prognostic Score for Hodgkin lymphoma except:
1. Serum albumin
2. LDH
3. Hemoglobin
4. Absolute lymphocyte count

Answer: LDH

There are **seven** factors in the IPS for HL:
1. Serum albumin <4 g/dL
2. Hemoglobin <10.5 g/dL
3. Male gender
4. Age >45 years
5. Stage IV disease
6. White blood cell count ≥15,000/microL
7. Absolute lymphocyte count <600/microL and/or <8 percent of the total white blood cell count

If any of these is present then one point is given to the total score. So, the total score ranges from zero to seven. There are six score group (0, 1, 2, 3, 4 and 5 or more). These scores give estimates of 5-year freedom from progression rate and

5-year overall survival.

It is very important to note that IPS is used only for **advanced HL** (not for early stage HL).

Q. Which of the following is true about bone marrow examination in HL:

1. Bone marrow aspirate and biopsy is generally-not required
2. Bone marrow examination is indicated only in patients showing bone marrow uptake in PET scan to confirm the findings
3. If PET scan is negative, bone marrow examination is not necessary
4. All of the above

Answer: Bone marrow aspirate and biopsy is generally-not required

This is a very important question. Read these facts about bone marrow examination in HL carefully:

1. Bone marrow aspirate and biopsy is generally-not required.
2. Bone marrow examination is indicated only when unexplained cytopenias are present in the setting of a PET that is **negative** for bone marrow involve-

ment.

Q. Early stage (I and II) HL is further classified into favorable and unfavourable groups according to a variety of systems. Which of the following is not an unfavourable characteristic according to the EORTC definition:

1. Age >50
2. Large mediastinal adenopathy
3. Erythrocyte sedimentation rate (ESR) ≥50 mm/h and no B symptoms
4. ≥3 sites of involvement

Answer: ≥3 sites of involvement

In fact, in the EORTC system the criterion for belonging to unfavourable group is involvement of ≥**4 sites.**

Remember that favorable and unfavourable groupings are only for early stage HL patients (stage I and II); **not for advanced stages (stage III and IV).** If any one or more of the following is present then the patient will belong to the unfavourable group according to the EORTC:

1. Age >50
2. Large mediastinal adenopathy (it is defined as mediastinal mass width measuring >1/3 of the thoracic width at the T5-6 level)

3. ESR ≥ 50 mm/h and no B symptoms or ESR ≥ 30 mm/h in those with B symptoms
4. ≥**4** sites of involvement

Another commonly used system is the GHSG system:

If any one or more of the following is present then the patient will belong to the unfavourable group according to the GHSG:

1. Large mediastinal adenopathy (defined as mediastinal mass measuring >1/3 of the maximum thoracic diameter)
2. ESR ≥ 50 mm/h and no B symptoms or (ESR ≥ 30 mm/h in those with B symptoms)
3. ≥3 sites of involvement

Note that the number of "sites of involvement" is different in EORTC and GHSG systems.

Another system used for this stratification is the NCIC/ECOG system. If any one or more of the following is present then the patient will belong to the unfavourable group:

1. Large mediastinal adenopathy (>1/3 maximum transverse thoracic diameter)
2. Involvement of four or more sites
3. Age ≥40 years at diagnosis
4. ESR > 50 mm/hour
5. Mixed cellularity histology

Q. What will be the Deauville score of a lesion in FDG-PET showing uptake more than mediastinal blood pool but equal to liver:

1. 2
2. 3
3. 4
4. 5

Answer: 3

Please memorise the Deauville score for interpreting FDG-PET in lymphoma:

Deauville score 1 = no uptake

Deauville score 2 = Uptake ≤ mediastinal blood pool

Deauville score 3 = Uptake > mediastinal blood pool but ≤ liver

Deauville score 4 = Uptake moderately more than liver uptake, at any site

Deauville score 5 = Uptake markedly higher than liver (ie, two to three times the maximum SUV in the liver) and/or new lesions

X = New areas of uptake unlikely to be related to lymphoma

Q. For autologous hematopoietic cell transplant in HL, which is the conditioning regimen of choice and which is the preferred source of stem cells, respectively:
1. BEAM and peripheral blood
2. BuCy and bone marrow
3. BEAM and bone marrow
4. BuCy and peripheral blood

Answer: BEAM and peripheral blood

BEAM is the conditioning regimen of choice for autologous HCT in HL, it consists of BCNU, etoposide, cytarabine and melphalan.

Remember that BEAM is a myeloablative regimen.

Q. Which of the following is not an indication of brentuximab maintenance after autologous HCT in HL:
1. Primary refractory disease
2. Relapse within 12 months after initial therapy
3. Relapse with extranodal disease

4. Relapse after four or more lines of chemo

Answer: relapse after four or more lines of chemo

There are three indications of brentuximab maintenance after auto-HCT in HL (options 1, 2 and 3).

Notes on treatment of NLPHL:
Remember that NLPHL is a very different kind of disease than classical HL. The principles of its management are quite different from classical HL.

NLPHL patients are divided in the following groups:
1. Non-bulky early stage NLPHL: <10 cm stage IA **or** non-bulky, *contiguous* stage IIA disease. The patients must not have any significant symptoms or threat of organ compromise
2. Bulky early stage NLPHL: stage I or II with ≥10 cm mass
3. Non contiguous early stage NLPHL: stage II with non contiguous disease
4. Early stage NLPHL threatening organ function or causing significant symptoms
5. Advanced NLPHL: Stage III or stage IV NLPHL

The treatment of these patients is as follows:

1. Non-bulky early stage NLPHL: involved-site radiation therapy (ISRT) **or** active surveillance (AS)
2. Bulky or non-contiguous early stage NLPHL: RCHOP (or other combinations) alone **or** ISRT alone
3. Advanced NLPHL: stage III and IV patients of NLPHL are known as advanced NLPHL. They can be further divided into two categories:
   a. Patients with significant symptoms: they are best treated with RCHOP (or other such combinations)
   b. Patients with minimal symptoms or asymptomatic patients: they may be treated with RCHOP like regimens or single agent rituximab. In these patients, we may choose to just do active surveillance without any treatment.

Q. Which of the following is true about brentuximab vedotin:

1. It is a conjugate of anti-CD30 antibody linked to the anti-tubulin agent, monomethyl auristatin E
2. It is approved for the treatment of patients with HL after failure of autologous HCT
3. It is approved for treatment of patients with HL after failure of at least two prior multi-agent chemotherapy regimens who are not candidates for HCT
4. All of the above

Answer: all of the above

Q. Which of the following is true about HL:
1. PD-L1 and PD-L2 are overexpressed by Reed-Sternberg cells
2. Nivolumab is approved for patients with classic HL that relapse or progress after autologous HCT and post transplantation brentuximab
3. Pembrolizumab is approved by the FDA for patients whose disease is refractory or has relapsed after three or more lines of therapy
4. Pembrolizumab is approved in Europe for patients with progression after autologous HCT and brentuximab

Answer: all of the above are true. Please remember these facts.

NON-HODGKIN LYMPHOMA

Diffuse large B cell lymphoma

Q. Which of the following is the most common lymphoma:
1. Burkitt lymphoma
2. DLBCL
3. Mantle cell lymphoma
4. Hodgkin lymphoma

Answer: DLBCL

Note that DLBCL is not a single disease and there are many entities, which are classified by WHO in separate diagnostic categories:
1. T cell/histiocyte-rich large B cell lymphoma
2. Primary DLBCL of the mediastinum
3. Intravascular large B cell lymphoma
4. Lymphomatoid granulomatosis
5. Primary DLBCL of the central nervous system
6. Primary cutaneous DLBCL, leg type
7. DLBCL associated with chronic inflammation

Q. The BCL6 gene is located on which chromosome:
1. 3
2. 11

    3. 4
    4. 18

Answer: 3

Note that there is no "characteristic" translocation or genetic abnormality that defines DLBCL. Instead, a collection of features is used to make its diagnosis.

Q. Which of the following is not a characteristic of International Prognostic Index (IPI) for non-Hodgkin lymphoma:
    1. Age
    2. Serum LDH
    3. ECOG PS
    4. Number of involved nodal areas

Answer: Number of involved nodal areas

In fact, the IPI for NHL requires the number of involved **extranodal** sites (not nodal).

You must read the question very very carefully. There are many types of "IPI". One IPI is generally applicable to NHL as a whole; but there are specific IPIs for many lymphomas, for example, there is an IPI for follicular lymphoma (FLIPI) and another for mantle cell lymphoma (MIPI), among many others. There are also different IPIs for organ involvement, like for CNS. Thus, I would like to repeat that you must read the question carefully.

Notes of the IPI for NHL:
There are five characteristics in it, each is given one point if present and the final score ranges from 0 to 5:
1. Age >60
2. Serum lactate dehydrogenase concentration above normal
3. ECOG performance status ≥2
4. Ann Arbor stage III or IV
5. Number of extranodal disease sites >1

The final score determines the risk group:
1. Low risk = 0 to 1
2. Low intermediate risk = 2
3. High intermediate risk = 3
4. High risk = 4 to 5

The 5 year overall survival in the low risk group is around 75%, whereas it is only around 25% in the high risk group.

Notes on the revised staging system for primary nodal lymphomas (Lugano classification):
Lugano classification divides stages in to limited and advanced. Limited stage disease is stage I and stage II. Advanced stage is stage III and IV.

Read the following text carefully:

Limited stage:
Stage I: one node or a group of adjacent nodes **OR** single ex-

tranodal lesion without nodal involvement

Stage II: two or more nodal groups on the same side of the diaphragm **OR** stage I or II by nodal extent with limited **contiguous** extranodal involvement
Stage II bulky: same as stage II but with **bulky** disease

Advanced stage:

Stage III: nodes on both sides of the diaphragm OR nodes above the diaphragm with spleen involvement

Stage IV: additional **noncontiguous** extralymphatic involvement

Q. Which of the following is not a factor in the Follicular lymphoma international prognostic index (FLIPI):
1. Age
2. Serum LDH
3. Hemoglobin
4. ECOG PS

Answer: ECOG PS

Note here that the question is not about IPI for NHL but about FLIPI, which is different from the former. There are five characteristics in it, each is given one point if present and the final score ranges from 0 to 5:
1. Age >60
2. Serum lactate dehydrogenase concentration above

normal
3. Hemoglobin <12 g/dL
4. Ann Arbor stage III or IV
5. Number of involved nodal areas >4

The final score determines the risk group:
1. Low risk = 0 to 1
2. intermediate risk = 2
3. High risk = 3 or more

The 2 year overall survival in the low risk group is around 98%, whereas it is around 87% in the high risk group. These figures are based on recent data, in which the patients were treated with rituximab.

Q. Which of the following is not a factor in the Mantle cell lymphoma international prognostic index (MIPI):
1. Age
2. ECOG PS
3. Serum LDH
4. Ann Arbor stage

Answer: Ann Arbor stage

The MIPI has four factors:
1. Age
2. ECOG PS
3. Serum LDH
4. WBC count

Q. CNS-IPI, which is used in DLBCL, includes all of the following except:
1. Age
2. Stage
3. Kidney involvement
4. Number of nodal sites

Answer: number of nodal sites

There are six factors in CNS-IPI:
1. Kidney and/or adrenal glands involved
2. Age >60 years
3. LDH above normal
4. ECOG PS >1
5. Stage III/IV disease
6. Extranodal involvement of ≥2 sites

Q. What is the recommendation about the number of cycles of R-CHOP in a patient of limited stage DLBCL, with no bulky disease, normal LDH, ECOG PS <2:
1. 4
2. 6
3. 3
4. 3-6

Answer: 4

Note that this question is about the number of cycles of "R-CHOP"; not "total number of cycles of any therapy".

Six cycles of R-CHOP have been standard therapy for many subsets of lymphomas. This notion was challenged by the results of the FLYER study, which included patients of ≤60 years with stage I-II DLBCL and no adverse risk factors. It showed that four cycles of R-CHOP followed by two additional treatments of rituximab was not inferior to six cycles of R-CHOP, and was associated with less toxicity.

This is my take on the question, although choosing 6 cycles of R-CHOP as the answer will also not be entirely wrong.

Q. What is the treatment of choice for limited stage DLBCL with bulky disease:
1. 6 cycles of R-CHOP plus RT
2. 6 cycles of R-CHOP alone
3. 4 cycles of R-CHOP plus RT
4. 4 cycles of R-(DA)EPOCH with RT

Answer: 6 cycles of R-CHOP plus RT

There is no universal definition of bulky disease in NHL and even within a subset like DLBCL, varying definitions have been used. Most commonly DLBCL is said to be bulky if a tumor mass is ≥10 cm in diameter. That being said, sometimes 7.5 cm may be taken as the cutoff for defining bulky disease.

The dose of RT may be fixed, depending on the protocol being used or it may be modulated depending on the results of the PET scan performed after 6 cycles of R-CHOP.

Q. MInT trial studied addition of which of the following to the backbone of CHOP chemotherapy:
1. Obinutuzumab
2. Ofatumumab
3. Rituximab
4. Venetoclax

Answer: rituximab

Notes on the MabThera International trial (MInT Trial) in DLBCL:
1. Patients with DLBCL were randomised between CHOP-like chemotherapy with or without rituximab.
2. Radiation therapy (RT) was given to patients with bulky or extra nodal disease
3. 6 year OS, EFS and PFS were superior with the R-CHOP arm compared with the CHOP arm.
4. Another important finding of this study was that 6 cycles of R-CHOP were non inferior to 8 cycles of R-CHOP regarding the survival outcomes and that 6 cycles resulted in significantly lesser toxicities.

Q. The treatment of limited stage germinal center DLBCL is less aggressive than treatment of limited stage activated B cell DLBCL:
1. True
2. False

Answer: false

While the cell of origin (germinal centre B cell versus activated B cell) play a role in deciding the management of advanced stage DLBCL; this differentiation plays no role in treatment decision making in limited stage DLBCL.

Q. Which of the following post remission therapy has shown benefit in patients with DLBCL:
1. Rituximab
2. Pulse administration of chemoimmunotherapy
3. Hematopoietic cell transplantation (HCT)
4. All of the above

Answer: this is a trick question and the goal is to test the depth of knowledge of the student. In fact, none of these maintenance therapies has shown benefit

A study, ReMARC, has shown increased PFS with two years of maintenance lenalidomide in DLBCL patients older than 60 years who achieved CR or PR with 6 to 8 cycles of R-CHOP.

Remember the dosing and schedule of R-CHOP:
1. Rituximab: 375 mg/m2 IV on day 1
2. Cyclophosphamide: 750 mg/m2 IV on day 1
3. Doxorubicin: 50 mg/m2 IV on day 1
4. Vincristine: 1.4 mg/m2 IV on day 1
5. Prednisone: 100 mg orally daily on days 1 to 5

The cycle is repeated every 21 days.

Q. Which of the following in not a risk factor for CNS involvement by non-Hodgkin lymphoma:
1. Stage III disease
2. Testicular involvement
3. Bone marrow involvement
4. Low hemoglobin level

Answer: low hemoglobin level

Q. Which of the following is not a stage in the Lugano classification of gastrointestinal lymphomas:
1. I
2. IIE
3. II2
4. III

Answer: III

Remember that there is **no stage III** in gastrointestinal lymphomas. The staging of GI lymphomas is different than other sites:
a. Stage I: The tumor is confined to the gastrointestinal tract. It can be a single primary lesion or multiple, noncontiguous lesions.
b. Stage II - The tumor extends into the abdomen. This is further subdivided based upon the location of nodal involvement:

a. Stage II$_1$: Involvement of local nodes (paragastric nodes for gastric lymphoma or para-intestinal nodes for intestinal lymphoma)

b. Stage II$_2$: Involvement of distant nodes (para-aortic, para-caval, pelvic, or inguinal nodes for most tumors; mesenteric nodes in the case of intestinal lymphoma)

c. Stage IV - There is disseminated extranodal involvement or concomitant supra-diaphragmatic nodal involvement.

Q. Which of the following statement is not true about advanced stage DLBCL:

1. For germinal center B cell DLBCL, 6 cycles of R-CHOP is the preferred therapy

2. R-CHOP for 6 cycles is not considered sufficient for activated B cell DLBCL

3. Maintenance rituximab improves outcomes in patients with activated B cell advanced stage DLBCL

4. High-dose chemotherapy with autologous hematopoietic cell rescue in first complete remission in not recommended in patients with activated B cell advanced stage DLBCL

Answer: Maintenance rituximab improves outcomes in patients with activated B cell advanced stage DLBCL

As we have noted before, the differentiation between germinal center B cell and activated B cell DLBCL plays no role in limited stage DLBCL treatment decision making but it does play a role in treatment selection of advanced stage DLBCL.

The best treatment strategy for advanced stage activated B cell DLBCL is unknown but it is agreed upon that 6 cycles of R-CHOP is not enough. The best place for treatment of such patients is in a clinical trial. Many strategies have been developed, like adding lenalidomide etc.

Q. Polatuzumab vedotin is:
1. An anti-CD79b antibody-drug immunoconjugate
2. Active against B cell lymphomas
3. Approved by the US Food and Drug Administration
4. Approved for multiply relapsed DLBCL

Answer: all of the above are correct

Q. What is the meaning of "double hit DLBCL":
1. *MYC* translocation plus rearrangement of *BCL2*, *BCL6*, or both
2. *BCL2* translocation plus rearrangement of *MYC*, *BCL6*, or both
3. *BCL6* translocation plus rearrangement of *MYC*, *BCL2*, or both
4. None of the above

Answer: *MYC* translocation plus rearrangement of *BCL2*, *BCL6*, or both

It is a very important concept. Double hit lymphomas have

worse prognosis.

Q. Which of the following is the preferred treatment for first relapse of DLBCL:
1. Salvage therapy followed by autologous HCT
2. Salvage therapy followed by allogeneic HCT
3. Chemoimmunotherapy alone, followed by HCT in the second relapse
4. CAR-T cell therapy

Answer: Salvage therapy followed by autologous HCT

R-GDP is the most commonly used salvage chemoimmuno-therapy regimen before autologous HCT.

Q. For patients of relapsed DLBCL who have chemoresistant disease, what is the most appropriate treatment:
1. Autologous HCT
2. Allogeneic HCT
3. CAR-T cell therapy
4. Any of the above

Answer: options 2 and 3 are correct. Option 1 is not correct.

If we have to choose between options 2 and 3 then option 2 will be a better choice. But both allogeneic HCT and CAR-T cell therapy are equally acceptable treatment options for relapsed DLBCL patients who are:

1. Chemoresistant
2. Who relapse after autologous HCT

Mantle cell lymphoma

Q. Which of the following forms of MCL develops from B cells expressing SOX11:
  1. Classical MCL
  2. Leukemic MCL
  3. Both of the above
  4. None of the above

Answer: classical MCL

There are two major forms of MCL, classical and leukemic.
  1. Classical MCL arises from SOX11 expressing naive B cells.
  2. Leukemic MCL arises from SOX11-negative B cells.

Q. MCL is associated with which the following translocations:
  1. t(11;14)
  2. t(8;14)
  3. t(14;18)
  4. t(9;22)

Answer: t(11;14)

This translocation dysregulates the cyclin D1 gene.

Q. All of the following are expressed by MCL cells except:
1. CD20
2. CD23
3. CD5
4. FMC7

Answer: CD23

Remember:
1. MCL cells are CD5+, CD23-
2. CLL cells are CD5+, CD23+

Q. Which of the following statements is not true:
1. Nuclear staining for cyclin D1 is present in almost all MCL cases
2. Cyclin D1 is not produced if MCL cells lack t(11;14)
3. The t(11;14) is a translocation between the *C-CND1* locus and the immunoglobulin heavy chain locus
4. t(11;14) is not specific for MCL

Answer: Cyclin D1 is not produced if MCL cells lack t(11;14)

Studies have shown that cyclin D1 is produced even by cells lacking t(11;14).

Q. Which of the following is the preferred therapy for most of the patients of MCL:
1. BR
2. R-CHOP
3. R-DHAP
4. Hyper-CVAD

Answer: BR

This question is inherently controversial because different institutes have different protocols for treatment of MCL, which according to them are the best. The point of this question is that the data available till date shows equal outcomes with more intense therapies than BR but BR is far less toxic. That's why many experts prefer it in most of the patients.

Hyper-CVAD alternating with high dose methotrexate and cytarabine is reserved for young and very fit patients.

Q. For young and fit patients with newly diagnosed MCL who achieve partial response with chemoimmunotherapy, what is the most appropriate next step:
1. Observation
2. Maintenance rituximab
3. Autologous HCT

    4.   Allogeneic HCT

Answer: autologous HCT

Maintenance rituximab is an option for patients who achieve CR or PR with chemoimmunotherapy but are not candidates for autologous HCT for any reason.

Remember that even after autologous HCT, many experts recommend maintenance rituximab for a total of three years.

Q. Which of the following is true about treatment options in patients with relapsed MCL:
    1.   Ibrutinib is approved by the FDA for the treatment of patients with MCL who have received at least one prior therapy
    2.   Acalabrutinib has received accelerated approval by the FDA treatment of adults who have received at least one prior therapy for MCL
    3.   Zanubrutinib has received accelerated approval by the FDA for treatment of adults with MCL who have received at least one prior treatment
    4.   All of the above

Answer: all of the above

All these "brutinib" drugs are BTK inhibitors. The recommended dose of ibrutinib is 560 mg orally once daily in relapsed MCL.

The dose in relapsed CLL is different: 420 mg orally once daily.

Burkitt lymphoma

Q. Which of the following types of BL occurs at the median age of 30 years:
1. Endemic
2. Sporadic
3. Immunodeficiency-associated
4. All of the above

Answer: sporadic

The endemic variety presents at the median age of 4 to 7 years.

Note that BL disproportionately affects males.

Q. The development of BL is dependent on the MYC gene. The MYC gene is a:
1. Proto-oncogene located on chromosome 8q
2. Tumor suppressor gene located on chromosome 8q
3. Proto-oncogene located on chromosome 8p

4. Tumor suppressor gene located on chromosome 8p

Answer: Proto-oncogene located on chromosome 8q

Q. Epstein-Barr virus is associated most strongly with which of the following types of BL:
1. Endemic
2. Sporadic
3. Immunodeficiency associated
4. EBV is equally strongly associated with all types of BL

Answer: endemic

The endemic for of BL, which is also known as the African BL, is almost always associated with EBV.

Q. Which of the following form of BL generally presents as facial bone tumors:
1. Endemic
2. Sporadic
3. Immunodeficiency associated
4. All of the above

Answer: endemic

Remember:

1. The endemic (African) form presents as a jaw or facial bone tumors.
2. The non-endemic (sporadic) form presents as abdominal mass.

Q. A "starry-sky" pattern is present in the tumor biopsy of which of the following;.
1. Burkitt lymphoma
2. DLBCL
3. NK/T cell lymphoma
4. Mantle cell lymphoma

Answer: BL

BL is a very rapidly dividing malignancy. The fraction of Ki-67+ (MIB-1+) cells is nearly 100 percent.

Q. Which of the following antigen is not expressed by BL cells:
1. CD20
2. CD23
3. CD10
4. BCL6

Answer: CD23

Notes:
1. BL cells express: surface IgM, CD19, CD20, CD22,

CD79a, CD10, BCL6, HLA-DR and CD43.
2. BL cells **don't** express: CD5, BCL2, TdT and CD23.

Remember that BL arises from germinal centre B cells, that's why BL cells express CD10 and BCL6.

Q. Which of the following translocation is found in BL:
1. t(8;14)
2. t(2;8)
3. t(8;22)
4. All of the above

Answer: all of the above

Notes:
1. The MYC gene is responsible for development of BL. It is a proto-oncogene located on chromosome 8q.
2. MYC gene translocation most common occurs as t(8;14). On chromosome 14, the Ig heavy chain gene is present.
3. Some patients may have t(2;8). On chromosome 2, kappa light chain gene is present.
4. Very few patients may have t(8;22). On chromosome 22, lambda light chain gene is present.

Q. For young and fit adults with BL, which of the following is the treatment of choice:
1. R-CODOX-M/IVAC

2. Dose-adjusted EPOCH-R
3. R-CHOP
4. BR

Answer: R-CODOX-M/IVAC

Follicular lymphoma

Q. Which of the following is not a characteristic of pediat-ric-type follicular lymphoma:
1. They are generally stage I/II
2. They usually have abdominal disease
3. There is absence of *BCL2* rearrangements
4. There are activating mutations involving MAP2K1 and TNFRSF14

Answer: they usually have abdominal disease

In fact, paediatric type FL generally present in the head and neck region.

Q. Which of the following are the predominant cell popula-tion in FL:
1. Centrocytes
2. Centroblasts
3. Both of the above are present in almost equal num-

bers
4. None of the above

Answer: centrocytes

Q. If, in a case of FL, 10 centroblasts are present per high power field, what will be the grade:
1. 1
2. 2
3. 3a
4. 3b

Answer: 2

Notes on grading of FL:
1. Grade 1: 0 to 5 centroblasts/high power field
2. Grade 2: 6 to 15 centroblasts/hpf
3. Grade 3: More than 15 centroblasts/hpf
    1. Grade 3a: centrocytes are still present
    2. Grade 3b: solid sheets of centroblasts are present

Notes on immunophenotype of FL:
1. Surface immunoglobulin+
2. Either kappa or lambda light chains present (not both)
3. HLA-DR+
4. CD19+, CD20+, CD79a+, CD10+, CD21+
5. CD5-, CD43-, CD11c-
6. BCL2 is positive in the majority but many types of FL

don't express BCL2

Q. Which of the following is the characteristic molecular and cytogenetic feature of FL:
1. An IgH/BCL1 fusion gene produced by t(14;18)
2. An IgH/BCL1 fusion gene produced by t(11;18)
3. An IgH/BCL2 fusion gene produced by t(14;18)
4. An IgH/BCL2 fusion gene produced by t(11;18)

Answer: An IgH/BCL2 fusion gene produced by t(14;18)

There are many other variant translocations as well.

Q. Which of the following is not a criterion in the Follicular Lymphoma International Prognostic Index 2 (FLIPI2):
1. Age
2. LDH
3. Bone marrow involvement
4. Serum beta-2 microglobulin

Answer: LDH

Note that FLIPI2 is different from FLIPI1. There are five factors in FLIPI2:
1. Age >60 years
2. Bone marrow involvement
3. Hemoglobin level <12.0 g/dL
4. Greatest diameter of the largest involved node more

than 6 cm
5. Serum beta-2 microglobulin level greater than the upper limit of normal

The final score ranges from 0 to 5; dividing patients in low (zero factors), intermediate (1 to 2 factors), or high (3 to 5 factors) FLIPI2 groups.

Q. A bone marrow biopsy is indicated in all patients of advanced stage FL, regardless of imaging results:
1. True
2. False

Answer: false

Note:
1. Bone marrow biopsy is indicated in early stage FL, as its results will impact the treatment strategy.
2. On the other hand, bone marrow biopsy is not indicated in advanced stage FL, as confirmed by imaging.

Q. The treatment of choice for stage I FL is:
1. Radiation therapy
2. Chemoimmunotherapy
3. Immunotherapy alone
4. Observation

Answer: radiation therapy

Q. Initial RT is the treatment of choice for stage II FL:
1. True
2. False

Answer: false

While RT is the TOC for stage I FL, it is not the case with stage II FL. Stage II is FL is more often treated on the lines of advanced stage FL.

Q. Which of the following is true about results of the PRIMA study in advanced stage FL:
1. Two years of rituximab maintenance was associated with PFS benefit relative to observation
2. Two years of rituximab maintenance was associated with OS benefit relative to observation
3. Adverse events were similar between the rituximab maintenance arm and observation arm
4. All of the above

Answer: Two years of rituximab maintenance was associated with PFS benefit

Only PFS benefit was there in this study. That's why experts are divided on the subject of maintenance rituximab in advanced FL. Some recommend for it because of PFS benefit while others recommend against it because of adverse effects and no OS benefit.

Very important notes:
1. TOC in stage I FL is RT.
2. TOC in stage II FL is not well defined.
3. Treatment is **not** indicated in **all** patients of stage II to IV FL:
    1. Patients are generally treated only when they are symptomatic or organ function is threatened.
    2. GELF and FLIPI criteria are used for deciding whether or not a patient with stage II to IV should be treated.
    3. If treatment is indicated, then rituximab plus chemo is the therapy of choice. Bendamustine is the most commonly used chemo in this setting.
    4. In some patients obinutuzumab may be used instead of rituximab.

Q. What is the ideal schedule of rituximab maintenance in patients of advanced stage FL:
1. Every month for a total of two years
2. Every two months for a total of two years
3. Every month for a total of three years
4. Every two months for a total of three years

Answer: Every two months for a total of two years

This recommendation is based on the GALLIUM and PRIMA studies.

Q. The combination of lenalidomide plus rituximab was studied in which of the following trials and in which setting:
1. AUGMENT in relapsed or refractory FL
2. AUGMENT in newly diagnosed FL
3. LEORY in relapsed or refractory FL
4. LEORY in newly diagnosed FL

Answer: AUGMENT in relapsed or refractory FL

Q. Which fo the following is true:
1. Idelalisib is approved by the FDA as a single agent for the treatment of patients with relapsed FL who have received at least two prior systemic therapies
2. Copanlisib is approved by the FDA as a single agent for the treatment of patients with relapsed FL who have received at least two prior systemic therapies
3. Duvelisib is approved by the FDA as a single agent for the treatment of patients with relapsed FL who have received at least two prior systemic therapies
4. **Ibritumomab tiuxetan** is approved by the FDA for the treatment of patients with relapsed or refractory FL

Answer: all of the above are true

Idelalisib, copanlisib and duvelisib are phosphoinositide 3-

kinase inhibitors (PI3K inhibitors).

Ibritumomab is a murine monoclonal antibody against CD20 that has been radiolabeled with yttrium-90.

Miscellaneous

Q. Which of the following is not an AIDS-defining malignancy:
1. Kaposi sarcoma
2. Invasive cervical carcinoma
3. T cell non-Hodgkin lymphomas
4. Primary central nervous system lymphoma

Answer: T cell NHL

High grade B cell lymphomas are AIDS-defining malignancies (not T cell).

Q. Which is the most common systemic NHL subtype in HIV patients:
1. Burkitt lymphoma
2. Diffuse large B cell lymphoma
3. Plasmablastic lymphoma
4. T cell lymphoma

Answer: DLBCL

Approximately 75% of HIV associated lymphomas are DLBCL.

The next most common one is BL.

Q. Approximately what percent of patients with HIV-AIDS develop non-Hodgkin lymphoma:
1. <5
2. 10
3. 20-30
4. 50-70

Answer: 10

Q. What is the usual cutoff of CD4 cell count (per microL), below which rituximab is generally not given, in the treatment of HIV related DLBCL:
1. 50
2. 100
3. 150
4. 200

Answer: 50

Q. Which of the following is the regimen of choice for high risk HIV associated DLBCL:
1. DA-EPOCH plus rituximab
2. Rituximab-CODOX-M/IVAC
3. R-CHOP
4. BR

Answer: DA-EPOCH plus rituximab

On the other hand, for patients with HIV-related Burkitt lymphoma R-CODOX-M/IVAC is the regimen of choice.

HIV is itself a risk factor for CNS involvement in NHL. Remember these sites, which if involved by NHL, impart a higher risk of CNS involvement (even if the patient is not HIV positive):
1. Paranasal sinuses
2. Testes
3. Epidural space
4. Adrenals
5. Kidneys
6. Bone marrow

Q. Which of the following is the most common extranodal site of lymphoma in the western world:
1. Stomach
2. Small intestine
3. Lungs
4. CNS

Answer: stomach

Note that *H. pylori* infection is associated with the development of MALT lymphoma of the stomach.

Q. Which of the following is the characteristic appearance of primary CNS lymphoma on an MRI scan:
1. Isointense to hypointense on T2-weighted MRI images, and enhance homogeneously after contrast administration
2. Isointense to hypointense on T1-weighted MRI images, and enhance homogeneously after contrast administration
3. Isointense to hyperintense on T2-weighted MRI images, and enhance homogeneously after contrast administration
4. Isointense to hyperintense on T1-weighted MRI images, and enhance homogeneously after contrast administration

Answer: Isointense to hypointense on T2-weighted MRI images, and enhance homogeneously after contrast administration

Q. Which is the most common histopathologic subtype of PCNSL:
1. DLBCL
2. BL
3. MCL
4. MALToma

Answer: DLBCL

Notes on treatment of PCNSL:
1. High-dose methotrexate-based multiagent chemo-therapy is the treatment of choice in patients who can tolerate it.
2. Majority of experts recommend including rituximab as first line therapy, in combination with high dose MTX-based multiagent chemotherapy.
3. Consolidation therapy should be given after the above mentioned therapy is finished.
    1. In young and fit patients, further cycles of chemo (different agents) or high dose chemo followed by autologous HCT are appropriate options.
    2. The optimal consolidation therapy is not known in older population. Chemo may be given if they are fit enough, otherwise observation is also an option.

Some patients may not be candidates for cure. In them whole brain RT and glucocorticoids may provide good palliation.

Q. Which of the following is correctly matched with the type of EMZL:
1. *Helicobacter pylori* with gastric EMZL
2. *Chlamydia psittaci* with ocular adnexa EMZL
3. *Campylobacter jejuni* with small intestine EMZL

4. *Borrelia afzelii* with skin EMZL

Answer: all of the above are correct

Achromobacter xylosoxidans is associated with lung EMZL.

Q. EMZLs are negative for which of the following antigen:
1. CD19
2. CD20
3. CD22
4. CD23

Answer: CD23

Usually the EMZLs express B cell markers and don't express T cell markers.

Q. MCD is caused by which of the following virus:
1. HIV
2. EBV
3. HHV-8
4. CMV

Answer: HHV-8

Q. Which of the following is the preferred therapy for patients with HHV-8-associated MCD without evidence of life-threatening organ failure and without Kaposi sarcoma:

1. Observation
2. Rituximab alone
3. Rituximab plus pegylated liposomal doxorubicin
4. Rituximab plus etoposide

Answer: rituximab

Remember:

1. In HHV-8 associated MCD patients who don't have life threatening organ dysfunction or Kaposi sarcoma, rituximab alone is the drug of choice.
2. In HHV-8-associated MCD patients with life-threatening organ failure but without Kaposi sarcoma, rituximab plus pegylated liposomal doxorubicin is the therapy of choice. In some cases etoposide may be used instead of PLD.
3. In HHV-8-associated MCD patients with Kaposi sarcoma, rituximab plus PLD is the therapy of choice.

Q. Which of the following is not considered a post-transplant lymphoproliferative disorder:

1. Follicular lymphomas
2. Small lymphocytic lymphoma
3. Marginal zone lymphomas
4. Classical Hodgkin lymphoma

Answer: options 1, 2 and 3 are correct

Note that the follicular lymphomas, small lymphocytic lymphoma and marginal zone lymphomas are not considered PTLDs.

Q. Which of the following statements is not correct:
1. EBV is the most common pathogen associated with PTLD
2. PTLD accounts for a minority of secondary cancers following allogeneic HCT
3. PTLD accounts for the majority of secondary cancers following solid organ transplant

Q. Which of the following is not an entity of PTLD as per the WHO:
1. Plasmacytic hyperplasia and infectious mononucleosis-like PTLD
2. Polymorphic PTLD
3. Monomorphic PTLD
4. Classical non-Hodgkin lymphoma-like PTLD

Answer: Classical non-Hodgkin lymphoma-like PTLD

In fact, the fourth category is Classical **Hodgkin** lymphoma-like PTLD.

Q. Which of the following is not true about prevention of PTLD:

1. Limiting exposure to immunosuppressive regimens
2. Early and rapid withdrawal immunosuppressants
3. Anti-viral prophylaxis
4. Chronic administration of low dose immunosuppression as opposed to high dose short term immunosuppressants

Answer: Chronic administration of low dose immunosuppression as opposed to high dose short term immunosuppressants

Note that options 1 and 2 are in contradiction with option 4.

Q. Which of the following is considered the cornerstone of therapy of PTLD:
1. Immunosuppression reduction
2. Rituximab
3. Chemotherapy with or without rituximab
4. Chemotherapy with or without radiation

Answer: immunosuppression reduction

Notes on treatment of PTLD:
1. Early lesions: generally reduction in immunosuppression alone is enough.
2. Polymorphic PTLD: reduction in immunosuppression is a must, along with it single agent rituximab is preferred (obviously rituximab can only be given in PTLDs expressing CD20). If the tumor doesn't ex-

press CD20 then chemotherapy is used.

3. Monomorphic PTLD: reduction in immunosuppression is a must, along with it single agent rituximab is preferred (obviously rituximab can only be given in PTLDs expressing CD20). If the tumor doesn't express CD20 then chemotherapy is used.

4. Classic Hodgkin lymphoma-like PTLD: these patients are treated with reduction of immunosuppressive drugs plus chemotherapy regimens used in classical Hodgkin lymphoma.

CLL AND HCL

Q. The most common leukemia in western countries is:
1. CML
2. CLL
3. AML
4. ALL

Answer: CLL

Q. The characteristic immunophenotype of CLL cells is:
1. CD5+, CD20+, CD23+
2. CD5+, CD20-, CD23+
3. CD5+, CD20+, CD23-
4. CD5-, CD20+, CD23+

Answer: CD5+, CD20+, CD23+

There is sometimes confusion between CLL and MCL. We can remember this by using a trick that CLL has two "L" so it is positive for both CD5 and CD23 whereas MCL (mantle cell lymphoma) has only one "L" in it so it is positive for only one of these markers: positive for CD5 and negative for CD23.

CD200 is expressed on CLL cells, but not on mantle cell lymphoma cells, and may be used as a distinguishing marker.

Notes on MBL (monoclonal B lymphocytosis):
1. Around 3.5% of otherwise normal individuals over the age of 40 years may harbor a population of clonal (by light chain analysis) CD5+/CD19+/CD23+ B cells.
2. These asymptomatic individuals **do not** have an absolute lymphocytosis, lymphadenopathy, or other clinical evidence of CLL.

Q. The most common chromosomal abnormality in CLL is:
1. Del(13q)
2. Del(11q)
3. Trisomy 12
4. Del(17p)

Answer: del(13q)

Deletion 13q [del(13q)] is the most common chromosome abnormality in CLL; it is found by FISH as a sole abnormality in 55% of cases, followed by 11q deletion (18%) [del(11q)], 12q trisomy (16%), and 17p deletion (7%) [del(17p)].

The prognosis is worst for del(17p).

The prognosis is best for del 13q.

The survival times associated with these abnormalities are: 32, 79, 114, 111, and 133 months for del(17p), del(11q), 12q trisomy, no abnormalities, and del(13q), respectively.

Notes on diagnostic criteria of CLL:
These criteria are proposed by the International Workshop on Chronic Lymphocytic Leukemia:

1. A blood monoclonal B lymphocyte count >5 × 109/L, with <55% of the cells being atypical (prolymphocytes)
2. B lymphocyte monoclonality should be demonstrated with cells expressing B-cell surface antigens (CD19, CD20, CD23), low density surface Ig (M or D), and CD5

Q. The monoclonal B cell count specified to distinguish CLL from small lymphocytic lymphoma (SLL) in patients with palpable lymph nodes or splenomegaly is:
1. 5000/mm3
2. 10000/mm3
3. 3000/mm3
4. There is no such distinction and it depends on the immunophenotype

Answer: 5000/mm3

Q. Wells syndrome is frequently seen in:
1. CLL
2. CML
3. MDS
4. T-PLL

Answer: CLL

Exaggerated skin reaction to a bee sting or an insect bite (Wells syndrome) is frequent in CLL.

Notes on certain interesting features associated with CLL:
1. Smudge cells are commonly seen in the peripheral smear, reflecting fragility and distortion dur-

ing preparation of the peripheral smear on the glass slide.

2. A positive direct antiglobulin (Coombs) test is seen in approximately 25% of cases, but autoimmune hemolytic anemia (AIHA) of clinical significance is not common.

Q. Which of the following belongs the Rai stage III of CLL:
1. Lymphocytosis with splenomegaly
2. Lymphocytosis with lymphadenopathy and hepatomegaly
3. Anemia with or without lymphocytosis
4. Thrombocytopenia with lymphocytosis

Answer: Anemia with or without lymphocytosis

Following are the Rai stages of CLL:
0 = Lymphocytosis only

I = Lymphocytosis and lymphadenopathy

II = Lymphocytosis and splenomegaly with/without lymphadenopathy

III = Lymphocytosis and anemia (hemoglobin, <11 g/dL)

IV = Lymphocytosis and thrombocytopenia (platelets, <100,000/mm3)

There is also Binet staging for CLL, which divides the patients in three stage groups A, B and C.

Q. Which of the following patients of CLL will **not** require active treatment:

1. A patient with extreme fatigue
2. A patient with fever
3. If a patient develops AIHA responsive to steroids
4. A patient with lymphadenopathy of more than 10 cm longest diameter

Answer: If a patient develops AIHA responsive to steroids

Treatment may be indicated in patients with AIHA **unresponsive** to steroids.

It is an important point to note that not all patients of CLL require treatment and some may be observed without any treatment (as opposed to, for example AML or CML, where all patients have to be treated). For this the IWCLL has proposed criteria for active disease as indications to initiate treatment:

1. Presence of constitutional symptoms attributable to CLL: weight loss (>10% of baseline weight within the preceding 6 months), extreme fatigue (Eastern Cooperative Oncology Group [ECOG] performance status 2 or higher), fever (temperature higher than 38 ° C or 100.5 ° F for at least 2 weeks), or night sweats without evidence of infection.
2. Evidence of progressive bone marrow failure characterized by the development of or worsening of anemia, thrombocytopenia, or both.
3. AIHA or autoimmune thrombocytopenia, or both, poorly responsive to corticosteroid therapy.
4. Massive (>6 cm below the left costal margin) or progressive splenomegaly.
5. Massive (>10 cm in longest diameter) or progressive lymphadenopathy.
6. Progressive lymphocytosis defined as an increase in the absolute lymphocyte count by >50% over a 2-month period, or a doubling time predicted to be <6 months.

The sixth point is especially confusing and should be read very carefully.

If any of these characteristics is present in a patient, then we may initiate treatment.

Q. Which is preferred treatment for a patient aged 55 years, having IGHV-mutated status but without del(17p):
1. Ibrutinib
2. FCR
3. BR
4. Obinutuzumab plus venetoclax

Answer: FCR

Notes on first line therapy of CLL:
1. Tremendous progress has been made in the treatment of CLL, especially over the recent years.
2. The list of approved protocols is too long and one must read a thorough reference book for this purpose, like Devita's oncology (quarterly updates) or the NCCN. I will try to give a brief overview of the treatment here.
3. In young patients (<65 years) who are fit, in young patients (<65 years) who are not fit, in old (65 years or more) patients; **so essentially in all patients having del(17p)**, the Bruton tyrosine kinase inhibitor ibrutinib is the drug of choice.
4. In young fit patients not having del(17p) and having IGHV (immunoglobulin heavy chain) mutated status, FCR is the therapy of choice (combination of fludarabine, cyclophosphamide and rituximab).
5. In older patients and those young patients who are not fit to receive intensive combination FCR

chemo, who don't have del(17p) and have IGHV-mutated status   some less intensive chemo-immunotherapy or ibrutinib should be used.

6. In young fit patients not having del(17p) and having IGHV-**un**mutated status, treatment options are chemoimmunotherapy or ibrutinib. Same is true for old or unfit patients.

7. The term chemoimmunotherapy means use of a anti-CD20 molecule, like rituximab, obinutuzumab, ofatumumab and a chemo molecule like bendamustine, chlorambucil etc.

8. The main clinical implication of choosing ibrutinib over chemoimmunotherapy is that ibrutinib has to be taken lifelong but the chemoimmunotherapy is given for a specific duration of time.

Q. Which of the following drugs used in CLL works on Bcl-2:
1. Ibrutinib
2. Idelalisib
3. Venetoclax
4. Selumetinib

Answer: venetoclax

Idelalisib is a PIK-3 inhibitor.

Selumetinib is not used in CLL.

Q. Which is the most common second neoplasm developing in CLL patients:
1. Skin cancer
2. Lung cancer
3. Myelodysplastic syndrome
4. PNH turning into MDS

Answer: skin cancer

Approximately 25% of patients with CLL develop second neoplasms, the most common benign skin cancer.

Q. CLL may sometimes evolve into a high grade lymphoma, known as Richter transformation, in what percentage of cases:
> 1. 1-5
> 2. 5-10
> 3. <2
> 4. 20

Answer: 1-5%

The exact mentioned percentages are from 2 to 6%.

The prognosis of Richter transformation is poor, with a median survival of only 6 months.

Q. In high risk patients of CLL, not having del(17p), rituximab maintenance is recommended:
> 1. True
> 2. False

Answer: false

A trial was done that randomized patients to receive rituximab every 3 months for up to 2 years versus observation. There was improved PFS with rituximab versus observation; there was no difference in OS. There was also a higher incidence of grade 3/4 neutropenia and infections for patients who received rituximab.

So in conclusion, CD20 MAb maintenance therapy post-CIT improved PFS, but not OS, and is associated with neutropenia and infection. It is **not** recommended.

Q. Which of the following is not true about hairy cell leukemia;

1. Hairy cells may be seen in the peripheral blood which are twice as large as normal lymphocytes
2. Bone marrow has a "fried egg" appearance
3. Immunophenotypic analysis of cHCL cells shows the presence of CD11c, CD23, CD25, CD103, CD123, as well as CD19, CD20, and CD22
4. BRAF V600E gain of function mutation is found in the cells from patients with classical HCL

Answer: Immunophenotypic analysis of cHCL cells shows the presence of CD11c, CD23, CD25, CD103, CD123, as well as CD19, CD20, and CD22

It must be noted that in contrast to CLL, hairy cells are negative for CD5 and CD23 and negative for CD10, CD27, and CD79b.so, the immunophenotypic analysis of cHCL cells shows the presence of CD11c, CD25, CD103, CD123, as well as CD19, CD20, and CD22

Notes:

1. HCL can be of two types: classical and variant.
2. The variant HCL cells are negative for CD25 and CD123.
3. In variant HCL, BRAF V600E mutations are not seen.

Q. Which of the following is curative in cases of HCL:
1. Cladribine
2. Pentostatin
3. Vemurafenib and dabrafenib
4. Vemurafenib plus auto-HSCT

Answer: none of the above

It was a trick question, it should be remembered that in HCL there is no curative therapy for HCL, except perhaps allo-SCT.

Pentostatin (2' deoxycoformycin) and cladribine (2-CdA) are the nucleoside analogs and are the mainstay of treatment of HCL.

Because cladribine is given only for one course and pentostatin for many cycles, cladribine is preferred.

Vemurafenib and other BRAF inhibitors are used in classical HCL, either as monotherapy or in combination with anti-CD20 drugs. It should be noted that variant HCL is devoid of these mutations and not responsive to BRAF inhibitors

Moxetumomab pasudotox is a novel drug which is a CD22 MAb-drug conjugate.

PLASMA CELL DYSCRASIAS

Monoclonal gammopathy of undetermined significance (MGUS)

Q. MGUS occurs in approximately what percentage of general population over the age of 50 years:
1. 0.01
2. 3
3. 5 to 10
4. >10

Answer: 3%

The rate of progression of MGUS to more proliferative plasma cell dycrasias is interesting. To give a broad generalisation, after 25 years of diagnosis around 25% patient of MGUS will progress to smouldering myeloma, multiple myeloma etc. (so, the rate of progression is around 1% per year.)

The important point to note here is that MGUS is usually diagnosed after 65 years of age and because it has such a low probability of progression, and also due to the fact that there are many other competing illnesses that may lead to death, the actual decrement in life expectancy of an individual suffering from MGUS is not much, compared with the age matched healthy population.

Q. IgM MGUS accounts for approximately what percent of MGUS cases:
  1. 1-5%
  2. 10-15%
  3. <1%
  4. >50%

Answer: 10-15%

Non IgM MGUS is the most common type of MGUS. Light chain MGUS (LC-MGUS) is another type.

Q. MGUS has all of the following features except:
  1. Presence of a serum monoclonal protein (M-protein), at a concentration <10 g/dL
  2. Bone marrow with <10 percent monoclonal plasma cells
  3. Absence of end-organ damage
  4. None of the above

Answer: Presence of a serum monoclonal protein (M-protein), at a concentration <10 g/dL

In fact, the M protein is found at a concentration of <3 g/dL

Light chain MGUS (LC-MGUS) is defined by (all of the following must be present):

1. The presence of an abnormal serum FLC ratio (<0.26 or >1.65)
2. Increased level of the involved FLC above the reference range
3. No monoclonal immunoglobulin heavy chain (IgG, IgA, IgD, or IgM)
4. Bone marrow with <10 percent monoclonal plasma cells
5. Absence of end-organ damage

Q. Which of the following is a risk factor useful in predicting the risk of progression of MGUS to multiple myeloma or a related malignancy:
1. Serum M-protein level ≥1.5 g/dL
2. Non-IgG MGUS (ie, IgA, IgM, IgD MGUS)
3. Abnormal serum free light chain (FLC) ratio
4. None of the above

Answer: 1, 2 and 3 are correct

Many risk stratification models have been developed for MGUS, which are useful in predicting the risk of progression. The above mentioned three factors are most commonly used in practice for this purpose.

If all of these 3 factors are present MGUS is high-risk, if 2 are present then it is high-intermediate risk, if 1 risk factor is present then it is low-intermediate risk and if no risk factor is present then it is low-risk MGUS.

Note that (as we have already discussed) the risk of progression of MGUS is around 1% per year; but if all of the above mentioned 3 risk factors are present then the risk becomes almost 3% per year. These data help in formulating an appropriate follow up plan.

Q. MGRS stands for:
1. Monoclonal gammopathy of renal significance
2. Monoclonal gammopathy of robust significance
3. Monoclonal gammopathy of regional significance
4. Monoclonal gammopathy of routine significance

Answer: Monoclonal gammopathy of renal significance

There is another term known as MGCS (monoclonal gammopathy of clinical significance.)

Q. Patients with MGUS have an increased risk of:
1. Axial bone fractures
2. Peripheral bone fractures
3. Both of the above
4. None of the above

Answer: axial bone fractures

The risk of peripheral bone fractures is **NOT** increased in MGUS.

Patients of MGUS also have an increased risk of thromboembolic events and second malignancies.

Q. The International Myeloma Working Group guidelines recommend which of the following imaging studies in patients suffering from MGUS:
    1. Whole body PET-CT
    2. Whole body MRI
    3. Whole body low dose CT
    4. None of the above

Answer: whole body low dose CT

Q. MGUS has been described in approximately what percent of patients with acquired C1 inhibitor deficiency:
    1. 10
    2. 20
    3. 30
    4. 70

Answer: 30%

Q. The M protein may present as a "church spire", in which of the following regions of the densitometer testing:
1. Gamma
2. Beta
3. Alpha-2
4. Any of the above

Answer: any of the above

IgG is the most common type of immunoglobulin heavy chain produced, followed by IgM.

Q. Which of the following is a common artefact affecting the measurements of serum M protein:
1. High value for HDL cholesterol
2. High value for bilirubin
3. Altered level of inorganic phosphate
4. All of the above

Answer: options 2 and 3 are correct but 1 is not correct

In fact, **low** levels of HDL cholesterol are associated with faulty readings of serum M protein.

Q. M protein found in monoclonal gammopathies can:
1. Increase the serum viscosity

2. Decrease the erythrocyte sedimentation rate
3. Decrease the serum viscosity
4. Increase the erythrocyte sedimentation rate

Answer: options 1 and 4 are correct

It seems contradictory but M protein increases serum viscosity as well as ESR.

Notes:

Diagnostic criteria of light chain MGUS (LC-MGUS) are as follows. Note that **all** of these criteria must be met:
1. The presence of an abnormal FLC ratio (ie, ratio of kappa to lambda FLCs <0.26 or >1.65)
2. Increased level of the appropriate involved light chain
3. No monoclonal immunoglobulin heavy chain (IgG, IgA, IgD, or IgM)
4. Fewer than 10 percent clonal lymphoplasmacytic cells in the bone marrow
5. The absence of lytic bone lesions, anemia, hypercalcemia, and renal insufficiency related to the plasma cell proliferative process

Notes:

Although the scope of this chapter does not include smoldering multiple myeloma and multiple myeloma, we should go over their diagnostic criteria right here, so that we can understand the key differences in the diagnostic criteria of MGUS, SMM and MM.

There criteria are the "revised international myeloma working group" criteria:

Definition of multiple myeloma:
Clonal bone marrow plasma cells ≥10% or biopsy-proven bony or extramedullary plasmacytoma is the first and foremost necessary criterion. But just having 10% or more bone marrow plasma cells is not sufficient, because it may also be present in smoldering multiple myeloma. So, remember that a patient having ≥10% bone marrow plasma cells **must fulfil either of the following two criteria** to be diagnosed as multiple myeloma (collectively these two criteria are known as "myeloma defining events"):

1. Evidence of end-organ damage that can be attributed to the underlying plasma cell proliferative disorder.
2. Presence of any one of the three biomarkers of malignancy

The details of these two criteria are as follows:

1. Evidence of end-organ damage that can be attributed to the underlying plasma cell proliferative disorder are:
    a. Hypercalcemia: serum calcium >0.25 mmol/L (>1 mg/dL) higher than the upper limit of normal or >2.75 mmol/L (>11 mg/dL)
    b. Renal insufficiency: creatinine clearance <40 mL per min or serum creatinine >177 μmol/L (>2 mg/dL)
    c. Anemia: hemoglobin value of >20 g/L below the lower limit of normal, or a hemoglobin value <100 g/L

    d. Bone lesions: one or more osteolytic lesions on skeletal radiography, CT, or PET-CT

2. Any one or more of the following biomarkers of malignancy should be:
    a. Clonal bone marrow plasma cell percentage ≥60%
    b. Involved:uninvolved serum free light chain ratio ≥100
    c. >1 focal lesions on MRI studies

Definition of smoldering multiple myeloma:
Both of the following criteria must be present:
    1. Serum monoclonal protein (IgG or IgA) ≥30 g/L or urinary monoclonal protein ≥500 mg per 24 hours and/or clonal bone marrow plasma cells 10 to 60%
    2. Absence of myeloma defining events or amyloidosis

Definition of MGUS:
All of the following three criteria must be met:
    1. Serum monoclonal protein <30 g/L
    2. Bone marrow plasma cells <10%
    3. Absence of myeloma defining events or amyloidosis (or Waldenström macroglobulinemia in the case of IgM MGUS)

There are some finer points that need to be clarified.
    1. We have discussed above that bone marrow plasma cell percentage is important. But the key word in all

the sentences is "clonal". Because there are many dis-orders in which bone marrow plasma cell percent-age may be more than 10% but in those conditions the plasma cells will not be "clonal" rather they will be "polyclonal". Such polyclonal cells can't be used to diagnose multiple myeloma, regardless of their percentage in the bone marrow.

2. Clonality should be established by showing kappa/lambda-light-chain restriction on flow cytometry, immunohistochemistry, or immunofluorescence.

3. Bone marrow plasma cell percentage should prefer-ably be estimated from a core biopsy specimen; in case of a disparity between the aspirate and core bi-opsy, the highest value should be used.

4. In the "biomarker of myeloma" section, we have learned about a criteria: Involved:uninvolved serum free light chain ratio ≥100. But the important thing here is that the involved free light chain must be ≥100 mg/L. So even if the ratio is 100 or more, but the involved light chain is less than 100 mg/L, then it will not count as a biomarker of malignancy.

5. Another criteria in the biomarker of malignancy section is presence of more than 1 focal lesion on MRI. It is important to note that each focal lesion must be 5 mm or more in size.

Plasmacytoma

Q. Which is the most common site involved by solitary extramedullary plasmacytomas (SEP):

1. Oronasopharynx
2. Liver
3. Gastrointestinal tract
4. Central nervous system

Answer: oronasopharynx

45 to 80 percent SEPs involve the upper respiratory tract (ie, oronasopharynx and paranasal sinuses).

Not here that SEPs don't have the CRAB features seen in multiple myeloma.

Notes on diagnostic criteria for SEP (all of the following criteria must be met):
1. Biopsy-proven extramedullary tumor with evidence of clonal plasma cells
2. Imaging studies (preferably 18F-FDG PET/CT) must show no lytic lesions
3. Bone marrow aspirate and biopsy must contain no clonal plasma cells
4. No anemia, hypercalcemia, or renal insufficiency attributable to a plasma cell dyscrasia

Q. What does the diagnostic entity "solitary extramedullary plasmacytoma (SEP) with minimal bone marrow involvement" mean:
1. SEP with upto 1% of clonal plasma cells in the bone marrow
2. SEP with upto 10% of clonal plasma cells in the bone

marrow
3. SEP with upto 5% of clonal plasma cells in the bone marrow
4. SEP with less than 30% of non-clonal plasma cells in the bone marrow

Answer: SEP with upto 10% of clonal plasma cells in the bone marrow

Q. What is the treatment of choice for SEP:
1. Radiation therapy (RT) at a dose of 40 to 50 Gy over a four-week period
2. Complete surgical excision
3. Radiation therapy (RT) at a dose of 40 to 50 Gy over a four-week period followed by adjuvant chemotherapy
4. Radiation therapy (RT) at a dose of 40 to 50 Gy over a four-week period followed bisphosphonates for 2 years

Answer: Radiation therapy (RT) at a dose of 40 to 50 Gy over a four-week period

The treatment of choice is RT. There may be some cases, where the tumor is small and very accessible; in such cases complete surgical resection alone may be used and RT may be omitted.

Q. Which of the following is not true about solitary plasma-

cytoma of bone (SPB):
1. The axial skeleton is more commonly involved than is the appendicular skeleton
2. The lumbar vertebrae are more commonly involved than thoracic, cervical or sacral vertebrae
3. SPB don't have anemia or renal failure by definition
4. The presence of an M band does not exclude the diagnosis of SPB

Answer: The lumbar vertebrae are more commonly involved than thoracic, cervical or sacral vertebrae

In fact, **thoracic** vertebrae are more commonly involved compared with other areas of spine.

As we have already discussed above in a question about SEP, in SPB as well there may be some cases who show upto 10% clonal bone marrow plasma cells; these cases are known as SPB with minimal marrow involvement. The management of such lesions is no different than those without any marrow involvement but prognosis seems to be worse.

Q. Bisphosphonates are not recommended in patient with SPB:
1. True
2. False

Answer: true

Bisphosphonates are not recommended in management of both SPB and SEP.

LABORATORY METHODS

Q. The heavy polypeptide chain IgG has how many sub-classes:
1. Three
2. Two
3. Four
4. Five

Answer: four

IgA has two subclasses.

Q. Which of the following statement is not true about protein electrophoresis in multiple myeloma:
1. Capillary zone electrophoresis is more sensitive method of performing SPEP compared with agarose gel method
2. Using the SPEP techniques, proteins are classified by their final position after electrophoresis is complete into five general regions: albumin, alpha-1, alpha-2, beta, and gamma

3. The various immunoglobulin classes are usually located in the beta or alpha-1 region of the SPEP, but they may also be found in the gamma region
4. The immunoglobulin classes rarely locate to the alpha-2 region

Answer: The various immunoglobulin classes are usually located in the beta or alpha-1 region of the SPEP, but they may also be found in the gamma region

Always remember that the various immunoglobulin classes are usually located in the **gamma** region.

Q. Which of the following statements is not true:
1. Panhypogammaglobulinemia occurs in about 10 percent of patients with multiple myeloma
2. Most of the patients of multiple myeloma who have panhypogammaglobulinemia have a Bence Jones protein
3. Panhypogammaglobulinemia is seen in approximately 20 percent of patients with primary amyloidosis and it is often associated with a nephrotic syndrome like picture
4. None of the above

Answer: none of the above

Note that **options 1,2 and 3 are correct statements.**

Q. Decreased serum albumin and an increased levels of immunoglobulins in alpha-1 and alpha-2 regions may be found in metastatic malignancy:
1. True
2. False

Answer: true

In the disorder of deficiency of alpha-1 antitrypsin, marked reduction of the alpha-1 globulin component is usually seen.

Notes about **false positive M band:** (lab abnormalities which resemble an M protein band on electrophoresis)
1. Fibrinogen is located between the beta and gamma mobility regions.
2. Hemoglobin-haptoglobin complexes may be found in the alpha-2-globulin region.
3. High concentrations of transferrin may produce a localized band in the beta region.
4. Nephrotic syndrome is associated with increased alpha-2 and beta bands
5. Drugs used in the treatment of multiple myeloma, daratumumab and elotuzumab, can be detected on SPEP.

Notes on normal levels of free light chains;
1. Free serum kappa light chains – 3.3 to 19.4 mg/L
2. Free serum lambda light chains – 5.7 to 26.3 mg/L
3. Ratio of kappa to lambda FLCs – 0.26 to 1.65

Multiple myeloma

Q. Which of the following is not true about epidemiology of multiple myeloma:
1. The annual incidence of multiple myeloma is around 4 to 5 per 100,000
2. Multiple myeloma is more frequent in men than in women (approximately 1.4:1)
3. There is no correlation between rising BMI and the incidence of multiple myeloma
4. The risk of developing MM is approximately 4-fold higher for persons with a first degree relative with MM

Answer: There is no correlation between rising BMI and the incidence of multiple myeloma

In fact, higher BMI is a risk factor for development of multiple myeloma.

Q. Anemia is found in approximately what percentage of multiple myeloma patients:
1. 15
2. 25
3. 50
4. 75

Answer: 75%

Anemia in multiple myeloma is normocytic, normo-chromic type. It is defined as hemoglobin ≤12 g/dL and it is found in nearly three fourth patients on presentation.

It is important to note here that the "definitions of anemia" are different for different malignancies. Like in case of CLL, according to the Rai staging classification, if a patient has Hb <11 g/dL then he is said to be anemic. Also in the case of CLL, the Binet classification defines anemia as Hb <10 g/dL.

Bone pain is found in around 60% patients and elevated serum creatinine is found in nearly 50% patients.

Q. In patients of multiple myeloma, *Streptococcus pneumoniae* and gram-negative organisms are the most frequent pathogens leading to infections:
   1. True
   2. False

Answer: true

The primary reason of increased incidence of infections in patients of multiple myeloma is immunodeficiency produced as a result of "functional hypogammaglobulinemia".

Q. What percent of patients with multiple myeloma have no M protein in the serum or urine on immunofixation at the time of diagnosis:
1. <1%
2. 3-5%
3. 5-12%
4. Nearly 30%

Answer: 3-5%

These patients fall into the category of "nonsecretory myeloma". Approximately two thirds of these patients show free light chains in the serum.

There is thus a small subset of patients who not only do not have M protein in the serum or urine on immunofixation but also no serum FLC. They are known as "true nonsecretory myeloma" patients.

Q. Which of the following is not true about the morphological features of plasma cells:
1. Their nucleus is round and eccentrically located with a marked perinuclear hof
2. The nucleus contains "clock-face" or "spoke wheel" chromatin with many nucleoli
3. Their cytoplasms may have grape like cluster, giving the appearance of Morula cells
4. Russell bodies are cherry-red refractive round bodies that may be found in their cytoplasm

Answer: The nucleus contains "clock-face" or "spoke wheel" chromatin with many nucleoli

In fact, the nucleus indeed contains "clock-face" or "spoke wheel" chromatin **but characteristically, there are no nucleoli.**

Q. Which of the following is not true about immunophenotype of plasma cells in multiple myeloma:
1. Lab methods detect either kappa or lambda light chains, but not both, in the cytoplasm of bone marrow plasma cells in patients with myeloma
2. On the surface of plasma cells immunoglobulin (sIg) is found in abundance
3. The normal kappa/lambda ratio in the bone marrow is 2:1
4. If the ratio of kappa/lambda is more than 4:1 or less than 1:2; it defines monoclonality

Answer: On the surface of plasma cells immunoglobulin (sIg) is found in abundance

In fact, surface immunoglobulin is characteristically absent on plasma cells in multiple myeloma.

Please remember options 1, 3 and 4 by heart. They are very important.

Q. Which of the following markers is expressed by normal plasma cells but not by the abnormal plasma cells of multiple myeloma:
1. CD79a
2. CD138
3. CD38
4. CD19

Answer: CD19

Myeloma cells infrequently express CD19.

Two other facts should also be remembered that most myeloma cells don't express CD45 and most myeloma cells express CD56. Note here that CD56 is typically negative in normal plasma cells.

Q. Which of the following is not true about the international staging system (ISS) criteria for multiple myeloma:
1. Stage I is, beta-2-microglobulin <3.5 mg/L and serum albumin ≥3.5 g/dL
2. Stage III is beta-2-microglobulin ≥5.5 mg/L or serum albumin <3.5 g/dL
3. The median overall survival for patients with stage II is 44 months
4. The median overall survival for patients with stage I is 62 months

Answer: stage III is beta-2-microglobulin ≥5.5 mg/L or

serum albumin < 3.5 g/dL

While its true that beta-2-microglobulin ≥ 5.5 mg/L makes a patient of multiple myeloma stage III but serum albumin has no significance when deciding stage III hence the word "OR" in this option is incorrect.

The stage groupings according to the ISS criteria are as follows:

Stage I – B2M < 3.5 mg/L and serum albumin ≥ 3.5 g/dL

Stage II – neither stage I nor stage III

Stage III – B2M ≥ 5.5 mg/L

Median overall survival (OS) for patients:
1. ISS stages I is 62 months
2. ISS stage II is 44 months
3. ISS stage III is 29 months

Notes on the revised ISS (also known as R-ISS):
1. The R-ISS is a revised version of ISS, it includes all the parameters used in ISS along with cytogenetic features and LDH. It gives significantly different survival outcomes at 5 years compared with ISS.
2. R-ISS I is ISS stage I (B2M < 3.5 mg/L and serum albumin ≥ 3.5 g/dL) **and** normal LDH **and** no del(17p), t(4;14), or t(14;16) by FISH. Estimated OS and PFS at five years are 82 and 55 percent, respectively. Median OS is not known as it was not reached in the

original study. Median PFS is 66 months.

3. R-ISS II is neither stage I nor stage III. Estimated OS and PFS at five years are 62 and 36 percent, respectively. Median OS and PFS are 83 and 42 months.

4. R-ISS III is ISS stage III (B2M ≥5.5 mg/L) **plus** LDH above normal limits **and/or** detection of one of the following by FISH: del(17p), t(4;14), or t(14;16). Estimated OS and PFS at five years are 40 and 24 percent, respectively. Median OS and PFS are 43 and 29 months.

Q. Which of the following characteristic will not put a patient of multiple myeloma in the high risk category:

1. t(4;14)
2. t(14;16)
3. Del17q13
4. Gain 1q

Answer: del17q13

In fact, it's the del17**p**13 that puts the patient in high risk myeloma category.

Notes on high risk myeloma:
If any one of the following features in present, the patient will belong to **high risk myeloma** category. Note that there may be minor differences among various national and international guidelines.

1. Presence of t(4;14), t(14;16), t(14;20), del17p13, or gain 1q by FISH (note that around 25% of multiple

       myeloma patients harbour one or more of these abnormalities)
2. Lactate dehydrogenase (LDH) levels ≥2 times the institutional upper limit of normal
3. Features of primary plasma cell leukemia (defined by either ≥2000 plasma cells/microL in peripheral blood or ≥20 percent on a manual differential count)
4. Patients with a high-risk signature on gene expression profiling (GEP)

Patients who do not have the above mentioned features, are classified as "standard risk myeloma". Abnormalities like trisomies, t(11;14), and t(6;14) also fall under this category.

Notes on therapy of multiple myeloma:
The most important question here is: whether or not the patient is transplant eligible?
The next question depends on the answer of the first question. If the answer to the first question is that yes, the patient is eligible then the question is: should we do an early autologous transplant, delayed autologous transplant, tandem autologous transplant or should we rather go for an allogeneic transplant?
If we proceed with any of the above mentioned options, then what should we do next and what is the role of maintenance therapy?
What should we do if a patient relapses after a transplant?
Following text will clarify the above mentioned questions:
    a. High-dose therapy followed by autologous HCT is considered the standard of care. It may be done early (which is done after a fixed number of cycles of chemotherapy) or it may be done in "delayed" fashion (in which chemo is continued till relapse and

once the patient relapses then auto-HCT is done).

b. Note that auto-HCT is **not curative** for multiple myeloma. It improves the survival outcomes compared with standard myeloma directed therapy alone.

c. On the other hand, allogeneic HCT in myeloma may prove to be curative but is associated with substantial transplant related mortality.

d. Induction chemotherapy is administered for approximately four months prior to stem cell collection. Regimens used are many, but the most common ones are VRd (bortezomib, lenalidomide and dexamethasone) and VCd (bortezomib, cyclophosphamide and dexamethasone). It is important to note that melphalan containing regimens should not be used, because melphalan causes stem cell damage. Another important point to remember is that more than four months of initial therapy should also **not** be given, because prolonged initial therapy may also harm stem cells.

e. Both PBPCs and bone marrow may be used for auto-HCT but PBPCs are preferred. Either G-CSF or G-CSF plus cyclophosphamide may be used for mobilising stem cells for collection from peripheral blood. Plerixafor is a reserved agent.

f. Apheresis is begun when the peripheral CD34+ counts reach 10 CD34 cells/microL. The goal of aphaeresis is collecting at least $3 \times 10_6$ CD34+ cells/kg if only one transplant is being considered, or at least $6 \times 10_6$ CD34+ cells/kg if two transplants are being considered. ($2 \times 10_6$ CD34+ cells/kg is considered essential for one transplant).

g. PBPCs are cryopreserved in 5 percent dimethylsulfoxide. They should be thawed at the bedside at the time of infusion.

h. These collected cells are contaminated with tumor

cells. Some experts suggest purging of tumor cells from the collected PBPCs. There are two methods for this: 1. cells can be identified and isolated by CD34+ or CD34+/Thy1+ selection. 2. Tumour cells can be purged by using a combination of monoclonal antibodies. But remember that there is no evidence of a clinical benefit with these methods and thus, most centres don't attempt to purge myeloma cells from PBPC collections.

i. Basically there are two options, once patient has received around 4 months of initial therapy. They can proceed directly with HCT (early transplant) or they can continue induction therapy with transplant being done at the time of relapse (delayed transplant).

j. In many trials, early transplantation resulted in deeper responses and improved progression-free survival (PFS), but no clear overall survival (OS) benefit. This benefit is most apparent in patient with **high-risk** multiple myeloma.

k. Sometimes a second (tandem) preplanned transplant may be done. When it is contemplated, it should be done within 6 to 12 months of the first transplant. Tandem transplantation has not improved outcomes in standard-risk myeloma. In high-risk myeloma some studies have suggested better outcomes compared with single transplant, but the evidence is very flimsy and that's why most centres **do not** perform tandem HCT.

l. The standard conditioning regimen used for HCT in MM is melphalan at a dose of 200 mg/m2. Dose may be reduced depending on the age and comorbidities.

m. Trials have compared 200 mg/m2 melphalan with variants like a) melphalan 140 mg/m2 plus 8 Gy TBI and b) melphalan 100 mg/m2. In both of these trials melphalan 200 mg/m2 resulted in better outcomes.

n. Most experts recommend that the dose of melphalan should be reduced to 140 mg/m2 if creatinine is >2 mg/dL. Melphalan is generally used at dose of 140 mg/m2 in patients more than 70 years of age.

o. After approximately 24 hours after completion of the preparative chemotherapy, peripheral blood progenitor cells (PBPCs) are reinfused in the patient.

p. Neutrophil engraftment usually occurs by day 12 and platelet counts are expected to recover to greater than 20,000/microL by day 16.

q. About 40 percent of patients with multiple myeloma undergoing autologous HCT will experience febrile neutropenia. Prophylactic antibacterial, antifungal and antiviral therapies are indicated in these patients.

r. It is important to understand, once again, that autologous HCT is **not curative** for multiple myeloma. Thus, even after a patient undergoes auto-HCT, some form of therapy should be given as maintenance therapy. Maintenance therapy has consistently shown improved outcomes in studies.

s. Most experts recommend **a minimum of 2 years** of maintenance therapy. For standard-risk patients, lenalidomide is used, whereas for high risk patients, bortezomib is indicated. Ixazomib may be used in patients who are not able to tolerate bortezomib.

t. Monitoring of the disease after transplant must be done. International myeloma working group criteria are used worldwide for this purpose.

u. If a patient of multiple myeloma relapses after autologous HCT, the treatment options are not well defined. Options include a second autologous HCT (experts recommend not performing another auto-HCT in a patient who relapses within 12 to 18 months of first auto-HCT), nonmyeloablative allogeneic HCT, or treatment with salvage chemotherapy.

If, on the other hand, a patient is **ineligible** for HCT; he should receive 8 to 12 cycles of initial therapy with a triplet regimen followed with maintenance therapy until progression unless there is significant toxicity. In patients who are frail and are not felt to be candidates for triplet therapy, doublet therapy with lenalidomide and dexamethasone is preferred.

Q. How was the ALCYONE trial designed:
  1. Newly diagnosed transplant ineligible patients of multiple myeloma were randomised to nine cycles of bortezomib, melphalan and prednisone with or without daratumumab
  2. Newly diagnosed transplant eligible patients of multiple myeloma were randomised to nine cycles of bortezomib, melphalan and prednisone with or without daratumumab
  3. Relapsed/refractory patients of multiple myeloma, who had never underwent transplantation, were randomised to nine cycles of bortezomib, melphalan and prednisone with or without daratumumab
  4. Relapsed/refractory patients of multiple myeloma, who relapsed after an autologous or allogeneic transplant, were randomised to nine cycles of bortezomib, melphalan and prednisone with or without daratumumab

Answer: Newly diagnosed transplant ineligible patients of multiple myeloma were randomised to nine cycles of bortezomib, melphalan and prednisone with or without daratumumab

This trial was done for exploring the idea: is a combination of four drugs superior to a combination of three drugs? As we all know, in fit patients a combination of three drugs, like bortezomib plus lenalidomide plus dexamethasone is preferred. The ALCYONE trial showed improvement in survival outcomes with the use of four drugs compared with three drugs but it was not significant enough to make the four drug regimen the preferred one. Also a very important point of criticism of this trial was the use of a rather nonconventional combination of bortezomib plus melphalan plus prednisone which complicated the application of the results of this study to a wider population.

Notes on important trial data on initial treatment of multiple myeloma:

1. SWOG S0777 phase III study randomised patients with previously untreated MM to receive six months of induction therapy with either VRd (bortezomib, lenalidomide and dexamethasone) or Rd (lenalidomide and dexamethasone), each followed by Rd maintenance until progression or unacceptable toxicity. Median PFS with VRd was 43 months versus 30 months with Rd and median overall survival was 75 months versus 64 months with Rd. This trial established the superiority of VRd over Rd.

2. The phase II EVOLUTION trial studied newly diagnosed patients. They were randomly assigned to receive initial

treatment with twice weekly bortezomib and weekly dexamethasone in combination with lenalidomide (VRd), cyclophosphamide (VCd), or both (VDCR). Corresponding rates of very good partial response (VGPR) or better were 32, 22, and 33 percent.

3. The MAIA trial randomised patients with newly diagnosed multiple myeloma, who were ineligible for HCT, to receive lenalidomide plus dexamethasone with or without daratumumab (Rd versus DRd). DRd resulted in deeper responses, improved PFS and higher toxicity. Overall survival data are not mature. Based on this trial the FDA approved DRd in newly diagnosed autologous HCT ineligible patients of multiple myeloma.

4. Some trials have compared other molecules like cyclophosphamide, thalidomide etc (with a bortezomib and dexamethasone backbone) with many other combinations, which are of historic interest now.

5. The phase III CLARION trial and a few phase II trials have compared carfilzomib combinations with bortezomib combinations in patients with newly diagnosed myeloma, but the results have been mixed.

6. The FIRST trial randomly assigned newly diagnosed, transplant ineligible patients to Rd until progression; Rd for 18 months; or melphalan, prednisone, plus thalidomide (MPT) for 18 months. Rd consistently improved treatment and survival outcomes.

Q. Which of the following statement is not true:
1. Daratumumab containing three drug regimens are preferred combinations for relapsed multiple myeloma pa-

tients

2. The POLLUX trial randomised patients with relapsed/refractory MM to receive lenalidomide plus dexamethasone with or without daratumumab. In this trial daratumumab improved PFS

3. The CASTOR trial randomised patients with relapsed/refractory MM to receive bortezomib plus dexamethasone with or without daratumumab. In this trial daratumumab improved PFS.

4. Elotuzumab is approved by the FDA for use in combination with lenalidomide and dexamethasone (ERd) for the treatment of patients with MM who have received two or more prior therapies

Answer: Elotuzumab is approved by the FDA for use in combination with lenalidomide and dexamethasone (ERd) for the treatment of patients with MM who have received two or more prior therapies

In fact, ERd is approved for the treatment of patients with MM who have received one to three prior therapies.

Q. Which of the following is not true about the drug elotuzumab used in multiple myeloma:
   1. It is a monoclonal antibody directed against SLAMF7
   2. The ELOQUENT-3 trial randomised relapsed or refractory multiple myeloma patients to pomalidomide plus dexamethasone with or without elotuzumab. Elotuzumab led to increased PFS but

    severe toxicities were also higher
3. The ELOQUENT-2 trial demonstrated increased PFS and OS in the elotuzumab containing arm
4. Elotuzumab is not approved in the first-line treatment of multiple myeloma

Answer: **The** ELOQUENT-3 trial randomised relapsed or refractory multiple myeloma patients to pomalidomide plus dexamethasone with or without elotuzumab. Elotuzumab led to increased PFS but severe toxicities were also higher

The above mentioned information is correct, except for one detail. In fact, elotuzumab did increase PFS **but severe toxicities were not increased by addition of elotuzumab.**

Q. Which of the following monoclonal antibody targets CD38:
1. Daratumumab
2. Elotuzumab
3. Isatuximab
4. Siltuximab

Answer: 1 and 3

Both daratumumab and isatuximab are monoclonal antibodies against CD38.

The drug isatuximab was studied in the phase 3 trial ICARIA-MM, in which patients who had received at least two lines of prior therapy, including lenalidomide and a proteasome inhibitor, were randomly assigned to receive pomalidomide plus dexamethasone with or without isatuximab.

In this trial, isatuximab resulted in increased PFS and statistically nonsignificant improvement in OS; whereas toxicities were also higher.

Q. The Tourmaline-MM1 trial studied which of the following drugs:
  1. Siltuximab
  2. Tocilizumab
  3. Ixazomib
  4. Panobinostat

Answer: ixazomib

This trial studied ixazomib in relapsed refractory multiple myeloma.

Q. The trial ASPIRE studied which of the following drugs:
  1. Ixazomib
  2. Carfilzomib
  3. Panobinostat
  4. Pomlidomide

Answer: carfilzomib

This trial was done in relapsed multiple myeloma, in it carfilzomib resulted in improved PFS and OS.

Q. The OPTIMISMM trial studied which of the following drugs:
1. Pomalidomide
2. Ixazomib
3. Isatuximab
4. Carfilzomib

Answer: pomalidomide

Q. Which of the following is not true about panobinostat:
1. It is a histone deacetylase (HDAC) inhibitor
2. It is approved for patients with multiple myeloma who have received at least two prior therapies, including bortezomib and an immunomodulatory drug
3. It is generally used in patients more than 65 years of age with borderline performance status
4. The approval of panobinostat PANORAMA1 trial

Answer: It is generally used in patients more than 65 years of age with borderline performance status

Note that panobinostat is used in a very select population on patients. Since this drug has many life threatening toxicities, it is used in patients less than 65 years of age with good performance status.

Q. Which of the following is not true about selinexor:
1. It was evaluated in the STORM trials
2. It is approved by the FDA for the treatment of adults with relapsed refractory multiple myeloma who have received at least three prior therapies
3. Thrombocytopenia, neutropenia, and hyponatremia are important adverse events with selinexor
4. Selinexor is teratogenic

Answer: It is approved by the FDA for the treatment of adults with relapsed refractory multiple myeloma who have received at least three prior therapies

In fact, it is approved by the FDA for the treatment of adults with relapsed refractory multiple myeloma who have received at least **four** prior therapies. These four prior therapies include two proteasome inhibitors, two immunomodulators and a CD38 directed therapy.

On a different topic, note that the anti-CD38 monoclonal antibody daratumumab is approved as a **single agent** by the US Food and Drug Administration for patients who have received at least **three** prior lines of therapy including a proteasome inhibitor and an immunomodulatory drug or who are double-refractory to a proteasome inhibitor and an immunomodulatory drug.

Q. Which of the following is true:
1. Proteasome inhibitors do not cause fetal harm and can be used in pregnancy
2. Peripheral neuropathy appears to be less common and less severe with bortezomib than with carfilzomib and ixazomib
3. Dose reductions of ixazomib are not needed for patients with hepatic or renal impairment
4. Proteasome inhibitors have been associated with thrombotic microangiopathy (TMA), which can present with Coombs-negative hemolysis

Answer: Proteasome inhibitors have been associated with thrombotic microangiopathy (TMA), which can present with Coombs-negative hemolysis

All other statements are false. The *correct versions* of the above mentioned wrong statements are:
1. Proteasome inhibitors **cause fetal harm.**
2. Peripheral neuropathy is more severe with bortezomib and less severe with carfilzomib and ixazomib.
3. Dose reductions of ixazomib are needed for hepatic or renal impairment.

Notes on adverse effects of some anti myeloma drugs (the percentage values are approximations):
Bortezomib:
1. Thrombocytopenia is seen in 40%. It is generally not severe and there is no evidence that it is cumulative.
2. Peripheral neuropathy develops in 40% of patients who receive bortezomib 1.3 mg/m2 twice weekly

and in 20% of patients who receive bortezomib 1.3 mg/m2 once weekly. Subcutaneous administration is preferred over IV route due to a lower risk of neuropathy.
3. Bortezomib can be used safely in patients with impaired renal function. This was studied in detail in the APEX trial.
4. Dose adjustments are required for liver dysfunction.
5. Antiviral prophylaxis and antimicrobial prophylaxis are generally given.

Carfilzomib:
1. It is associated with less neuropathy compared with bortezomib.
2. It is associated with increased frequency of heart failure, acute renal failure, and hypertension. Cardiovascular toxicity may be seen in 20% of patients or higher.

Immunomodulatory drugs:
1. They are absolutely contraindicated in pregnant and nursing women.
2. Prophylaxis against thromboembolism is required.
3. Dose adjustment is required for lenalidomide and pomalidomide if renal dysfunction is there but no adjustment is required for thalidomide in renal dysfunction.
4. Second primary malignancies are increased with use of lenalidomide based therapies.

Q. Which of the following statement is true about dose re-

ductions of bortezomib in peripheral neuropathy:
1. For grade 1 toxicity (asymptomatic, loss of deep tendon reflexes or paresthesia without pain or loss of function) no dose reduction is needed
2. For grade 2 toxicity (interfering with function but not activities of daily living) or grade 1 toxicity with pain; dose is reduced to 1 mg/m2
3. For grade 3 toxicity (interfering with activities of daily living) or grade 2 toxicity with pain withhold bortezomib until toxicity resolved, and may reinitiate at 0.7 mg/m2 once weekly
4. For grade 4 toxicity (life-threatening, disabling, eg, paralysis) bortezomib should be discontinued

Answer: all of the above are correct

Notes on evaluation of response:
I would sincerely request you to go through the table that summarises the 2016 International myeloma working group uniform response criteria for multiple myeloma. There is no point in writing it all down here and you have to go through that table as many times as you have to, to memorise it. This table is provided in the NCCN guidelines on multiple myeloma as well.

Q. Which of the following is a non-nitrogen containing bisphosphonate:
1. Pamidronate
2. Ibandronate
3. Clodronate
4. Etidronate

Answer: clodronate and etidronate

Pamidronate, zoledronate and ibandronate are nitrogen containing bisphosphonates; whereas clondronate and etidronate are **non**-nitrogen containing bisphosphonates.

Q. Which of the following is not true about osteoclast inhibitors used in multiple myeloma:
1. They repair existing bone damage and also prevent the development of new lesions
2. In patients with multiple myeloma who have no bone lesions and have normal bone density, the routine use of osteoclast inhibitors is not recommended
3. A similar benefit in outcomes is obtained from denosumab when compared with zoledronate
4. Osteonecrosis of jaw is seen in a minority of patients receiving zoledronic acid as well as in patients receiving denosumab

Answer: They repair existing bone damage and also prevent the development of new lesions

Note that osteoclast inhibitors prevent the development of new lesions but they **do not** repair existing bone damage.

Bisphosphonates lead to many kinds of benefits, like reduced rates of vertebral fractures, reduced rate of skeletal related events and reduction in bone pain; all of these lead to a significantly improved quality of life.

A controversial topic is the overall survival benefit obtained with the use of bisphosphonates. Many studies done on this subject demonstrated no OS benefit but in one study OS benefit was seen with zoledronic acid.

Q. The Medical Research Council (Myeloma IX) trial reached to which conclusion:
1. Patients with multiple myeloma without bone disease on skeletal x-rays who were receiving anti-myeloma treatment experienced fewer skeletal related events with monthly zoledronic acid compared with daily oral clodronate
2. Patients with multiple myeloma with bone disease on skeletal x-rays who were receiving anti-myeloma treatment experienced fewer skeletal related events with monthly zoledronic acid compared with daily oral clodronate but those patients who didn't have bone disease own skeletal x-rays, did not experience a reduction in such events
3. Patients with multiple myeloma without bone disease on skeletal x-rays who were receiving anti-myeloma treatment experienced similar rates of skeletal related events with monthly zoledronic acid compared with daily oral clodronate
4. Patients with multiple myeloma without bone disease on skeletal x-rays who were receiving anti-myeloma treatment experienced fewer skeletal related events with daily oral clodronate compared with monthly zoledronic acid

Answer: Patients with multiple myeloma without bone disease on skeletal x-rays who were receiving anti-myeloma treatment experienced fewer skeletal related events with monthly zoledronic acid compared with daily oral clodronate

Q. Reductions in dosage are not required with renal dysfunction, in which of the following drugs:
1. Zoledronate
2. Clodronate
3. Denosumab
4. All of the above

Answer: denosumab

Q. Which of the following statement is wrong:
1. The dose of denosumab 120 mg subcutaneously every four weeks. Its dose is not altered in case there is renal dysfunction.
2. The dose of zoledronate is 4 mg intravenously over 30 to 60 minutes every four weeks. If creatinine clearance is low then many experts recommend a reduced dose.
3. The dose of pamidronate is 90 mg intravenously every four weeks. If creatinine clearance is low then this dose is decreased and the infusion time is shortened.
4. All of the above

Answer: The dose of pamidronate is 90 mg intravenously

every four weeks. If creatinine clearance is low then this dose is decreased and the infusion time is shortened.

In fact, the dose of pamidronate is not reduced if there is renal dysfunction. The infusion time, however, is **increased** in such cases. If the CrCl is ≥30 mL/minute, it is administered over ≥2 hours and if the CrCl is <30 mL/minute, it is administered over over 4 to 6 hours.

Q. In a patient of multiple myeloma, who is receiving anti-myeloma therapy as well as bisphosphonates, what are the recommended dosages of calcium and vitamin D, respectively:
   1. 1000 mg daily and at least 400 IU daily
   2. 500 mg daily and at least 400 IU daily
   3. 1000 mg daily and at least 1200 IU daily
   4. 2000 mg daily and at least 800 IU daily

Answer: 1000 mg daily and at least 400 IU daily

Many experts recommend that the optimal dose of calcium is 1000 mg daily and the dose of vitamin D is at least 400 IU daily.

MISCELLANEOUS TOPICS

Q. Which are the most common abnormalities detected in patients with primary plasma cell leukemia:

1. Deletion of chromosome 13 and monosomy 13
2. Deletion 17p and the consequent loss of TP53
3. Chromosome 1q21 amplification and del(1p21)
4. None of the above

Answer: deletion of chromosome 13 and monosomy 13

"Primary" plasma cell leukemia arises de novo, whereas "secondary" plasma cell leukemia arises in patients already having multiple myeloma.

Notes on the diagnosis of plasma cell leukemia:

1. The diagnosis is confirmed when a monoclonal population of plasma cells is present in the peripheral blood with an absolute plasma cell count exceeding 2000/microL or 20 percent of the peripheral blood white cells.

Q. Which of the following is the most appropriate treatment for a patient of plasma cell leukemia:

1. Induction chemotherapy followed by HCT and maintenance therapy
2. Induction chemotherapy followed by maintenance therapy
3. Single agent lenalidomide maintenance alone
4. Directly proceeding with conditioning regimen followed by allogeneic HCT

Answer: Induction chemotherapy followed by HCT and maintenance therapy

Q. In a patient having high risk smoldering multiple myeloma, as per the Mayo 2018 10/2/2020 criteria, which of the following is the most appropriate management option:
1. Observation alone
2. Single agent lenalidomide
3. Lenalidomide plus dexamethasone
4. Single agent bortezomib with or without dexamethasone

Answer: single agent lenalidomide or lenalidomide plus dexamethasone

This is a very important question. For decades, observation alone had been the modality of choice for management of smoldering multiple myeloma. But now it has changed, and for patients with high-risk SMM by the Mayo 2018 20/2/20 criteria, it is now recommended that treatment with single-agent lenalidomide or lenalidomide and dexamethasone is preferred rather than observation.

Q. Which of the following is a criterion used in stratification of individuals with smoldering multiple myeloma, according to the Mayo 2018 risk stratification system:
1. Bone marrow plasma cells > 10%
2. M protein > 2 g/dL

3. FLC ratio >20
4. All of the above

Answer: options 2 and 3 are correct but option 1 is not correct

An easy way to remember the risk stratification criteria of smouldering multiple myeloma is their alternate name, the 20/2/20 criteria:
1. Bone marrow plasma cells >**20** percent
2. M protein >**2** g/dL
3. Involved/uninvolved free light chain (FLC) ratio >**20**

If 2 or 3 of these factors are present then the patient will belong to the high risk category, if 1 of these factors is present then the patient will belong to the intermediate risk category and if none of these factors is present then the patient will belong to the low risk category.

In the previous question we have noted the recent changes in practice in the management of **high risk** smoldering multiple myeloma, which is defined according to the above mentioned criteria. If, on the other hand, the patient belongs to the low or intermediate risk groups, then observation is the standard of care.

Q. Which of the following is the most common cause of mixed cryoglobulinemia syndrome:
1. HCV infection
2. HBV infection

3. HIV infection
4. Autoimmune diseases and lymphoproliferative disorders

Answer: HCV infection

In up to 90% of MCS patients, chronic HCV infection is the underlying etiology.

Q. Which of the following type of cryoglobulin is abnormally present in the serum of patients of mixed cryoglobulinemia syndrome (MCS):
1. Type I cryoglobulins
2. Type II cryoglobulins
3. Type III cryoglobulins
4. All of the above

Answer: options 2 and 3 are correct. Option 1 is not correct.

Q. MCS is characterised by:
1. A low serum C4 concentration
2. A high serum C4 concentration
3. A low serum C5 concentration
4. A high serum C5 concentration

Answer: A low serum C4 concentration

Q. For most patients with severe mixed cryoglobulinemia syndrome, what is the treatment of choice:

1. High-dose systemic glucocorticoids alone
2. High-dose systemic glucocorticoids plus rituximab
3. Rituximab with or without high-dose systemic glucocorticoids
4. High-dose systemic glucocorticoids plus cyclophosphamide

Answer: High-dose systemic glucocorticoids plus rituximab

Note that there are no uniform, universally accepted criteria classifying MCS in mild, moderate and severe categories. Most clinicians agree that if a patient of MCL has only mild symptoms then treatment of MCS per se is not indicated and the therapy is directed towards the underlying etiology. On the other hand, in patients having moderate or severe MCS, the combination of high-dose systemic glucocorticoids plus rituximab is the preferred option.

In patients with life threatening MCS, plasmapheresis may be used in addition to the above

Notes on POEMS syndrome (**P**olyneuropathy, **O**rganomegaly, **E**ndocrinopathy, **M**onoclonal protein, **S**kin changes):

1. The diagnostic criteria of POEMS syndrome are very extensive and complicated. I would strongly advise you to go through a standard textbook.

2. To summarise, POEMS syndrome is a monoclonal plasma cell disorder. And the most important clinical features is peripheral neuropathy. There are two mandatory criteria, polyneuropathy plus monoclonal plasma cell disorder. These two criteria are absolutely required for this diagnosis.

3. Apart from these two mandatory criteria, at least one major criterion and at least one minor criterion should also be present. The major criteria are **osteosclerotic** bone lesion[s], Castleman disease, or elevated serum or plasma vascular endothelial growth factor [VEGF] levels. Note that the bone lesions in POEMS syndrome are **osteosclerotic.**

4. In patients with one to three isolated bone lesions and no evidence of bone marrow involvement, radiation in a dose of 40 to 50 Gy is the treatment of choice.

5. In patient having widespread disease, systemic therapy is indicated. The most commonly used combination is melphalan plus prednisone, although other combinations used in multiple myeloma management may also be used here. Autologous HCT may be used in young patients and the protocol is similar to multiple myeloma.

Q. Which of the following statement is true:
1. Alpha heavy chain disease is also known as Seligmann disease and it most commonly affects the gastrointestinal system
2. Gamma heavy chain disease is also known as Franklin's disease and it has a lymphoma like presentation
3. Mu HCD resembles chronic lymphocytic leukemia
4. All of the above

Answer: all of the above

Notes on the treatment of heavy chain disease:
1. In patients having alpha-HCD, initial therapy is a trial of antibiotics. If this doesn't work then it is treated like low grade NHL.
2. Gamma-HCD is treated as low grade lymphoma but the treatment is indicated only in those patients who are symptomatic and fit certain other criteria.
3. Mu-HCD is treated like CLL/SLL.

Q. Which of the following is a diagnostic criterion of systemic AL amyloidosis:
1. Presence of an amyloid-related systemic syndrome
2. Positive amyloid staining by Congo red in any tissue
3. Evidence that amyloid is light-chain-related established by direct examination of the amyloid using mass spectrometry-based proteomic analysis, or immunoelectronmicroscopy
4. Evidence of a monoclonal plasma cell proliferative disorder

Answer: all of the above criteria are required for a diagnosis of systemic AL amyloidosis

Abdominal fat pat biopsy is the most preferable method for obtaining a specimen for Congo red staining, the second best is bone marrow sampling. If somehow these two are inadequate then organ biopsy is to be done.

Notes on treatment of systemic AL amyloidosis:
1. In a fit patient, autologous HCT is the treatment of choice. Melphalan is the preferred conditioning chemotherapy for this purpose.
2. In patients who are unfit for autologous HCT, chemo is the only resort. Bortezomib based triplets, e.g. bortezomib plus cyclophosphamide plus dexamethasone (CyBorD) or bortezomib plus melphalan plus dexamethasone are most commonly used.

Q. Which of the following is not true about Waldendstorm macroglobulinemia:
1. Presence of an IgM monoclonal paraprotein on serum immunofixation is must for diagnosis
2. The bone marrow biopsy sample must demonstrate ≥10 percent infiltration by small lymphocytes exhibiting lymphoplasmacytic features
3. The immunophenotype is surface IgM+, CD10-, CD19+, CD20-, CD138+
4. MYD88 L265P mutations can also be seen in over 90 percent of patients with WM

Answer: The immunophenotype is surface IgM+, CD10-, CD19+, CD20-, CD138+

In fact the immunophenotype is surface IgM+, CD10-, CD19+, **CD20+, CD138-**.

Remember that WM is a type of lymphoma and it stains positive for CD20, hence rituximab (anti-CD20 monoclonal antibody) is used in its treatment.

Although MYD88 L265P mutations are seen in >90% of WM patients, this mutation is **not** specific for WM. It may, however, help in doing differential diagnosis in certain situations.

Notes on treatment of WM:

1. Treatment in **not** indicated in every patient of WM. It is indicated only in those who are symptomatic, anemic or thrombocytopenic.
2. For patients who are asymptomatic and have adequate hemoglobin and platelet levels, observation is the standard of care.
3. For patients who require treatment, rituximab plus chemo is the standard of care. Ibrutinib is another treatment option in patients not willing for rituximab based chemo regimens.
4. Bendamustine plus rituximab is the most often used regimen. In some high risk patients a combination containing bortezomib may be used.

MYELODYSPLASTIC SYNDROMES

Q. What percent of MDS patients have one or more driver mutations:
1. 10-20
2. 30-50
3. 50-70
4. >90

Answer: >90%

The most commonly mutated genes are DNMT3A, TET2, ASXL1, TP53, RUNX1 and SF3B1.

Q. Which of the following is not a risk factor for development of MDS:
1. Benzene exposure
2. Trisomy 21
3. Lynch syndrome
4. Congenital neutropenia

Answer: Lynch syndrome

Some important etiologic factors for MDS are:
1. Benzene, radiation and tobacco

2. Exposure to certain chemotherapy drugs
3. Genetic syndromes like trisomy 21, Fanconi anemia, Bloom syndrome, ataxia telangiectasia
4. Benign haematological disorders like paroxysmal nocturnal hemoglobinuria and congenital neutropenia
5. Familial MDS

Q. Which is the most common cytopenia in MDS patients:
   1. Anemia
   2. Neutropenia
   3. Lymphopenia
   4. Thrombocytopenia

Answer: anemia

The most common "symptom" in MDS patients is fatigue, which is found in nearly all patients.

Q. Acquired hemoglobin H disease is found in what percent of MDS cases:
   1. 2
   2. 8
   3. 27
   4. 56

Answer: 8%

Somatic mutations of the ATRX gene are a frequent cause of this disease.

Q. Which of the following is not true about the laboratory findings in anemia caused by MDS:

1. Anemia is nearly universally present in MDS patients and is generally associated with inappropriately high reticulocyte response
2. The mean corpuscular volume (MCV) may be macrocytic or normal but it is only very rarely microcytic
3. The red cell distribution width (RDW) is increased which leads to anisocytosis
4. The mean corpuscular hemoglobin concentration (MCHC) is usually normal

Answer: Anemia is nearly universally present in MDS patients and is generally associated with inappropriately high reticulocyte response

It is true that anemia is almost always present but it is generally associated with **inappropriately low** reticulocyte response.

It is important to pay attention the the second option. While generally, RBCs are either macrocytic or normal but in MDS patients having ring sideroblasts, they may be microcytic.

There are two fundamental findings present in the peripheral blood examination of a patient of MDS:

1. Cytopenia (of which anemia is the most common)
2. Dysplasia (which is most commonly present in red blood cell and white blood cell lines; sometimes platelets may also show morphologic changes)

Q. Which is the most commonly seen abnormality of erythrocytes in MDS patients:
1. Ovalomacrocytosis
2. Elliptocytes
3. Teardrop cells
4. Stomatocytes

Answer: Ovalomacrocytosis

As we all know, red cells may show some other peculiar structural abnormalities in MDS patients like basophilic stippling, Howell-Jolly bodies and spur cells.

Q. In MDS patients granulocytes commonly display:
1. Reduced segmentation
2. Pelger-Huet abnormality
3. Increased granulation
4. All of the above

Answer: reduced segmentation

Memorise some important morphologic features of granulocytes in MDS:

1. Reduced segmentation
2. "Pseudo" Pelger-Huet abnormality
3. Reduced or absent granulation

Q. In MDS, the myeloid:erythroid ratio is most commonly:
1. Increased
2. Decreased
3. Stays the same
4. Infinite

Answer: decreased

But if "variable" was one of the options, that would have been the most correct one.

Please remember that **the blast percentage, by definition, is less than 20 percent.** Because if the blast percentage is more than this, the diagnosis will be acute myeloid leukemia, not MDS. But there are some exceptions to this rule: if a patient has any of the following genetic abnormality, the diagnosis will be AML, **regardless of the blast percentage**:
1. t(8;21)(q22;q22); *RUNX1-RUNX1T1* (previously *AML1-ETO*)
2. inv(16)(p13.1q22) or t(16;16)(p13.1;q22); *CBFB-MYH11*
3. t(15;17)(q22;q21.1); *PML-RARA*

Q. In MDS, the erythroid precursors show a "necklace" like structure around the nuclei with Prussian blue staining.

This gives these cells the name "ring sideroblasts". Which of the following organelles constitutes this so called necklace:
1. Mitochondria
2. Golgi apparatus
3. Endoplasmic reticulum
4. Clumped extranuclear chromatin

Answer: mitochondria

Iron-laden mitochondria surround the nuclei to give the appearance of ring sideroblasts.

Q. The bone marrow in patients of MDS is usually:
1. Hypercellular
2. Hypocellular
3. Normocellular
4. Nearly aplastic

Answer: hypercellular

An important point to remember is that in therapy related MDS, bone marrow is often hypocellular; whereas in all other types of MDS, bone marrow is usually hypercellular. Once again, note these important features of MDS:
1. Bone marrow is hypercellular
2. There is cytopenia in the peripheral blood (despite bone marrow being hypercellular)
3. There is dysplasia in one or more lineages

The reason for cytopenia in patients having hypercellular bone marrow is intramedullary cell apoptosis.

It sometimes happens that there is cytopenia in the peripheral blood, bone marrow is hypercellular but there is no dysplasia. In such patients cytogenetics is of tremendous help. There are many genetic abnormalities, which if present in such patients are considered sufficient for making a presumptive diagnosis of MDS. The list is very long, I would advice the readers to go to a standard textbook to read that list.

Unexplained monocytosis is another very important feature of some of the MDS patients.

Q. In MDS patients, "Pawn ball" changes are seen in which of the following cells:
1. Megakaryocytes
2. Granulocytes
3. Erythroid precursors
4. Bone marrow stromal cells

Answer: megakaryocytes

Multiple dispersed nuclei in the affected megakaryocytes give them this "Pawn ball" look.

Q. In patients of MDS, granulopoiesis may undergo some fundamental changes, one of which is the phenomenon of "ALIP". In this phenomenon, which of the following happens:

1. Granulopoiesis is displaced to paratrabecular location
2. Granulopoiesis is displaced to central marrow spaces
3. Granulopoiesis starts to occur in extramedullary spaces
4. Granulopoiesis halts and abnormally increases in irregular cycles

Answer: Granulopoiesis is displaced to central marrow spaces

Granulopoiesis usually takes place in the paratrabecular locations in marrow, but in MDS patients it may shift to more central marrow spaces. This phenomenon is known as ALIP (abnormal localization of immature precursors).

Q. In MDS patients, myelofibrosis is most commonly found in the therapy related MDS subset:

1. True
2. False

Answer: true

Q. Which of the following is true about laboratory methods

used in MDS:
1. To determine the blast percentage in the peripheral blood, a 200-leukocyte differential is recommended
2. To determine the blast percentage in the bone marrow, a 500-cells differential is recommended
3. Both of the above
4. None of the above

Answer: both of the above

It is important to follow strict protocols in this regard, because a patient may be easily misdiagnosed if standard procedures are not followed.

Notes on diagnosis of MDS (all are required):
1. Presence of cytopenia in the peripheral blood. Cytopenia is defined as one or more of these: hemoglobin <10 g/dL, absolute neutrophil count <1.8 x 10^9/L, platelets <100 x 10^9/L
2. Morphologic evidence of significant dysplasia (ie, ≥10 percent of erythroid precursors, granulocytes, or megakaryocytes) upon visual inspection of the peripheral blood smear, bone marrow aspirate, and bone marrow biopsy in the absence of other causes of dysplasia
3. Blast forms account for less than 20 percent of the total nucleated cells of the bone marrow aspirate and peripheral blood

There are some exceptions to the above mentioned diagnostic criteria:
A. In some patients there may be no or minimal dysp-

lasia, in such patients MDS may still be diagnosed if certain genetic abnormalities are present

B. In some patients blasts may be less then 20% but certain genetic abnormalities may be present and the patients will be diagnosed as having AML, **regardless of the blast percentage**:

1. t(8;21)(q22;q22);   *RUNX1-RUNX1T1*   (previously *AML1-ETO*)
2. inv(16)(p13.1q22) or t(16;16)(p13.1;q22); *CBFB-MYH11*
3. t(15;17)(q22;q21.1); *PML-RARA*

Q. If bone marrow shows loose network of reticulin with many intersections, especially in perivascular areas; what will be WHO grade of such a patient of myelofibrosis;

1. MF-0
2. MF-1
3. MF-2
4. MF-3

Answer: MF-1

Note on WHO grading of myelofibrosis:

1. MF-0: Scattered linear reticulin with no intersections (crossovers) corresponding to normal bone marrow
2. MF-1: Loose network of reticulin with many intersections, especially in perivascular areas
3. MF-2: Diffuse and dense increase in reticulin with extensive intersections, occasionally with focal bundles of thick fibers mostly consistent with collagen, and/or focal osteosclerosis

4. MF-3: Diffuse and dense increase in reticulin with extensive intersections and coarse bundles of thick fibers consistent with collagen, usually associated with osteosclerosis

Note that in MF-2 and MF-3, additional staining with trichrome is recommended.

Q. In which of the following diagnostic category, dysplasia should either be absent or if present then it should be less than 10%:

1. ICUS
2. CCUS
3. CHIP
4. All of the above

Answer: all of the above

Full forms are: idiopathic cytopenia of undetermined significance (ICUS), clonal hematopoiesis of indeterminate potential (CHIP) and clonal cytopenia of undetermined significance (CCUS).

Q. Which of the following is not true about WHO diagnostic criteria for chronic myelomonocytic leukemia:

1. Persistent peripheral blood monocytosis $\geq 1 \times 10^9/$L, with monocytes accounting for at least 20% of the WBC count
2. No evidence of *PDGFRA*, *PDGFRB*, or *FGFR1* re-

    arrangement or *PCM1-JAK2*
3. Dysplasia in 1 or more myeloid lineages
4. Not meeting WHO criteria for *BCR-ABL1*+ CML, PMF, PV, or ET

Answer: Persistent peripheral blood monocytosis ≥1 × 10^9/L, with monocytes accounting for at least 20% of the WBC count

In fact, the diagnostic criteria in this regard are: Persistent peripheral blood monocytosis ≥1 × 10^9/L, with monocytes accounting for **10% or more** of the WBC count.

Notes on WHO diagnostic criteria for CMML (all are required):
1. Persistent peripheral blood monocytosis ≥1 × 10^9/L, with monocytes accounting for ≥10% of the WBC count
2. Not meeting WHO criteria for *BCR-ABL1*+ CML, PMF, PV, or ET
3. No evidence of *PDGFRA*, *PDGFRB*, or *FGFR1* rearrangement or *PCM1-JAK2* (should be specifically excluded in cases with eosinophilia)
4. <20% blasts in the blood and bone marrow
5. Dysplasia in 1 or more myeloid lineages. If myelodysplasia is absent or minimal, the diagnosis of CMML may still be made if the other requirements are met and one of the following is present: An acquired clonal cytogenetic or molecular genetic abnormality is present in hemopoietic cells **or** the monocytosis (as previously defined) has persisted for at least 3 months **and** all other causes of monocytosis have been excluded.

Q. Which of the following is not true about WHO diagnostic criteria for atypical chronic myeloid leukemia, BCR-ABL1 negative:
1. Peripheral blood leukocytosis due to increased numbers of neutrophils and their precursors (pro-myelocytes, myelocytes, metamyelocytes) comprising ≥10% of leukocytes
2. Dysgranulopoiesis, which may include abnormal chromatin clumping
3. No or minimal absolute basophilia; basophils usually >2% of leukocytes
4. Hypercellular bone marrow with granulocytic proliferation and granulocytic dysplasia, with or without dysplasia in the erythroid and megakaryocytic lineages

Answer: No or minimal absolute basophilia; basophils usually >2% of leukocytes

In fact, these diagnostic criteria state that there should be no or minimal absolute basophilia; **basophils usually <2% of leukocytes.**

Notes on WHO diagnostic criteria for atypical chronic myeloid leukemia, BCR-ABL1 negative (all are required):
1. Peripheral blood leukocytosis due to increased numbers of neutrophils and their precursors (pro-myelocytes, myelocytes, metamyelocytes) comprising ≥10% of leukocytes
2. Dysgranulopoiesis, which may include abnormal

chromatin clumping
3. No or minimal absolute basophilia; basophils usually <2% of leukocytes
4. Hypercellular bone marrow with granulocytic proliferation and granulocytic dysplasia, with or without dysplasia in the erythroid and megakaryocytic lineages
5. No or minimal absolute monocytosis; monocytes <10% of leukocytes, <20% blasts in the blood and bone marrow
6. No evidence of *PDGFRA*, *PDGFRB*, or *FGFR1* rearrangement, or *PCM1-JAK2*
7. Not meeting WHO criteria for *BCR-ABL1+* CML, PMF, PV, or ET

Q. Which of the following is not a mandatory diagnostic criterion for juvenile myelomonocytic leukemia according to the WHO:
1. Blast percentage in peripheral blood and bone marrow <20%
2. Splenomegaly
3. Absence of Philadelphia chromosome
4. Germ line *CBL* mutation and loss of heterozygosity of CBL

Answer: Germ line *CBL* mutation and loss of heterozygosity of CBL

The diagnostic criteria for JMML are a little difficult to remember:
There are four mandatory criteria (i.e. all four must be pre-

sent):
1. Blast percentage in peripheral blood and bone marrow <20%
2. Splenomegaly
3. Absence of Philadelphia chromosome
4. Peripheral blood monocyte count $\geq 1 \times 10^9$/L

So, all of these four must be present and along with these four:

Either one of these three genetic abnormalities should be present:
1. Somatic mutation in *PTPN11* or *KRAS* or *NRAS*
2. Clinical diagnosis of NF1 or *NF1* mutation
3. Germ line *CBL* mutation and loss of heterozygosity of CBL

There may be some patients in whom all of the four mandatory criteria are met but who have none of the above mentioned genetic abnormalities present. In these patients, following criteria have to be present if a diagnosis of JMML is to be made:

Monosomy 7 or any other chromosomal abnormality or at least 2 of the following criteria:
a. Hemoglobin F increased for age
b. Myeloid or erythroid precursors on peripheral blood smear
c. GM-CSF hypersensitivity in colony assay
d. Hyperphosphorylation of STAT 5

Q. Which of the following is not a WHO diagnostic criterion for MDS/MPN with ring sideroblasts and thrombocytosis:
1. Anemia associated with erythroid lineage dysplasia with or without multilineage dysplasia, ≥ 15% ring

sideroblasts,* <1% blasts in peripheral blood and <5% blasts in the bone marrow

2. Persistent thrombocytosis with platelet count ≥450 × 10⁹/L

3. Absence of *SF3B1* mutation, *BCR-ABL1* fusion gene, rearrangement of *PDGFRA*, *PDGFRB*, or *FGFR1*

4. No preceding history of MPN, MDS (except MDS-RS), or other type of MDS/MPN

Answer: Absence of *SF3B1* mutation, *BCR-ABL1* fusion gene, rearrangement of *PDGFRA*, *PDGFRB*, or *FGFR1*

The WHO diagnostic criteria for MDS/MPN with ring sideroblasts and thrombocytosis (all are required):

1. Anemia associated with erythroid lineage dysplasia with or without multilineage dysplasia, ≥15% ring sideroblasts, <1% blasts in peripheral blood and <5% blasts in the bone marrow

2. Persistent thrombocytosis with platelet count ≥450 × 10⁹/L

3. Presence of a *SF3B1* mutation or, in the absence of *SF3B1* mutation, no history of recent cytotoxic or growth factor therapy that could explain the myelodysplastic/myeloproliferative features

4. No *BCR-ABL1* fusion gene, no rearrangement of *PDGFRA*, *PDGFRB*, or *FGFR1*; or *PCM1-JAK2*; no (3;3) (q21;q26), inv(3)(q21q26) or del(5q)

5. No preceding history of MPN, MDS (except MDS-RS), or other type of MDS/MPN

Q. Which of the following is not a major diagnostic criterion according to the WHO diagnostic criteria for overt primary

myelofibrosis:
1. Presence of megakaryocytic proliferation and atypia, accompanied by either reticulin and/or collagen fibrosis grades 2 or 3
2. Presence of *JAK2*, *CALR*, or *MPL* mutation or, in the absence of these mutations, presence of another clonal marker, or absence of reactive myelofibrosis
3. Palpable splenomegaly
4. Anemia not attributed to a comorbid condition

Answer: options 3 and 4 are correct (they are **not** the major criteria)

Notes on WHO diagnostic criteria for overt primary myelofibrosis (Diagnosis of overt PMF requires meeting all 3 major criteria, and at least 1 minor criterion):
Major criteria (all three must be present):
1. Presence of megakaryocytic proliferation and atypia, accompanied by either reticulin and/or collagen fibrosis grades 2 or 3
2. Not meeting WHO criteria for ET, PV, *BCR-ABL1*+ CML, myelodysplastic syndromes, or other myeloid neoplasms
3. Presence of *JAK2*, *CALR*, or *MPL* mutation or, in the absence of these mutations, presence of another clonal marker, or absence of reactive myelofibrosis

Minor criteria (at least 1 of the following must be present, confirmed in 2 consecutive determinations):
1. Anemia not attributed to a comorbid condition
2. Leukocytosis $\geq 11 \times 10^9$/L
3. Palpable splenomegaly
4. LDH increased to above upper normal limit of insti-

tutional reference range
5. Leukoerythroblastosis

Notes on WHO diagnostic criteria for pre-primary myelofibrosis:

Major criteria (all three must be present):
1. Megakaryocytic proliferation and atypia, without reticulin fibrosis >grade 1, accompanied by increased age-adjusted bone marrow cellularity, granulocytic proliferation, and often decreased erythropoiesis
2. Not meeting the WHO criteria for *BCR-ABL1+* CML, PV, ET, myelodysplastic syndromes, or other myeloid neoplasms
3. Presence of *JAK2*, *CALR*, or *MPL* mutation or in the absence of these mutations, presence of another clonal marker, or absence of minor reactive bone marrow reticulin fibrosis

Minor criteria (at least 1 of the following must be present and its presence must be confirmed in 2 consecutive determinations):
1. Anemia not attributed to a comorbid condition
2. Leukocytosis $\geq 11 \times 10^9$/L
3. Palpable splenomegaly
4. LDH increased to above upper normal limit of institutional reference range

Important note:

The WHO revised the criteria of diagnosis and classification of many hematologic malignancies in the year 2016. The criteria for MDS were also revised. I will strongly advice you to go to either their official website or to the website of "Blood" journal and read them up. I will not write them here because they are very nuanced and it will be better to go through the original text. Kindly visit the following:

Arber DA, Orazi A, Hasserjian R, et al. The 2016 revision to the World Health Organization classification of myeloid neoplasms and acute leukemia. Blood 2016; 127:2391.

The previous version of this classification was in 2008, which may be difficult to find. Some questions may still be asked based on that. Notes on the 2008 World Health Organization (WHO) classification system for myelodysplastic syndrome (MDS):

1. Refractory anemia (RA): there are <5 percent bone marrow blasts. It presents with anemia.
2. RA with ring sideroblasts (RARS): there are <5 percent bone marrow blasts. It presents with anemia and ≥15 percent ringed sideroblasts in erythroid precursors
3. MDS with isolated del(5q) (5q- syndrome): there are <5 percent bone marrow blasts. It presents with anemia and normal platelets.
4. Refractory cytopenia with multilineage dysplasia (RCMD): there are <5 percent bone marrow blasts. It presents with bicytopenia or pancytopenia, ring sideroblasts may or may not be there
5. Refractory anemia with excess blasts-1: there are 5 to 9 percent bone marrow blasts. It presents with cytopenias with or without peripheral blood blasts (<5 percent)
6. Refractory anemia with excess blasts-2: there are 10 to 19 percent bone marrow blasts. It presents with cytopenias and peripheral blood blasts

7. Myelodysplastic syndrome, unclassified: there are <5 percent bone marrow blasts. It presents with neutropenia or thrombocytopenia.

Q. Which of the following is not characteristically seen in therapy related AML/MDS:
1. Deletions of chromosome 5
2. -7
3. Del(7q)
4. MLL rearrangement

Answer: MLL rearrangement

Deletions of chromosomes 5 and -7/del(7q) are seen in up to 70 percent cases of therapy-related MDS/AML, particularly those which are induced by alkylating agents and/or radiation therapy.

Q. Which of the following is the most common chromosomal abnormality seen in MDS:
1. Deletion of the long arm of chromosome 5
2. Deletion of the short arm of chromosome 5
3. Deletion of the long arm of chromosome 7
4. Deletion of the short arm of chromosome 7

Answer: Deletion of the long arm of chromosome 5

Note that if you have to answer the question: is deletion of the long arm of chromosome 5 a good prognostic feature? Then the answer will be yes, it is a good prognostic feature.

But if we delve deep into this topic then there are basically two regions where the deletion may take place and these two have different impacts on outcome:
1. Deletion of 5q32-33.1: good prognosis
2. Deletion of 5q31.2: relatively poor prognosis

Q. Which of the following is true about the 5q-syndrome:
1. It is a type of MDS defined by isolated del(5q) or del(5q) plus any one other abnormality
2. The 5q- syndrome has a relatively poor prognosis and has a good chance of responding to treatment with lenalidomide
3. Structural rearrangements of 5q with >1 additional chromosomal change is associated with a worse prognosis
4. All of the above

Answer: Structural rearrangements of 5q with >1 additional chromosomal change is associated with a worse prognosis

Please read the options carefully before answering:
Option 1 is wrong because of the words "any one other chromosomal abnormality". The WHO says that if -7/del(7q) is present with del(5q) then it can not be classified as 5q-syndrome. On the other hand, if any other chromosomal abnormality if present with del5q then it still can be diagnosed as 5q-syndrome.

Q. Which of the following is not a "good" cytogenetic abnormality in an MDS patient according to the International Prognostic Scoring System, Revised (IPSS-R):
1. Normal karyotype
2. del(5q)
3. del(12p)
4. del(11q)

Answer: del(11q)

The del(11q) comes under the "very good" cytogenetic abnormality category.

The "good" cytogenetic abnormalities are: Normal karyotype, del(5q), del(12p), del(20q), double including del(5q).

Notes on the IPSS-R:
This is a very important topic. The IPSS-R score not only predicts the median overall survival but also the evolution of MDS into AML.

Three are five subgroups of cytogenetic abnormalities:
1. Very good: –Y, del(11q). Median survival: 5.4 years
2. Good: Normal, del(5q), del(12p), del(20q), double including del(5q). Median survival: 4.8 years
3. Intermediate: del(7q), +8, +19, i(17q), any other single or double independent clones. Median survival: 2.7 years.
4. Poor: –7, inv(3)/t(3q)/del(3q), double including –7/

del(7q), complex: 3 abnormalities. Median survival: 1.5 years.
5. Very poor: Complex: >3 abnormalities. Median survival: 0.7 years.

The full score of IPSS-R has the following five parameters:
1. Cytogenetics
2. Bone marrow blast percentage
3. Hemoglobin
4. Platelets
5. Absolute neutrophil count

These parameters are given different scores and these scores are added, sum of which gives the final IPSS-R (which divides the patients in very low, low, medium, high and very high risk gorups). It is used for prognostication and treatment decision making.

Its full details can be found in this article: Greenberg PL, Tuechler H, Schanz J, et al. Revised International Prognostic Scoring System (IPSS-R) for myelodysplastic syndromes. Blood 2012.

Q. Most children with JMML have mutations in certain genes which lead to activation of the RAS/MAPK signalling pathway. This activation leads to:
1. Hypersensitivity of myeloid progenitor cells to the GM-CSF
2. Hyposensitivity of myeloid progenitor cells to the GM-CSF
3. Insensitivity of myeloid progenitor cells to the GM-CSF

4. None of the above

Answer: Hypersensitivity of myeloid progenitor cells to the GM-CSF

Q. Which of the following is the treatment of choice for children with JMML:
1. Immediate allogeneic hematopoietic stem cell transplant (HCT)
2. Tyrosine kinase inhibitors (TKIs)
3. Chemotherapy protocols containing multiple drugs and a TKI
4. Immediate autologous HCT followed by TKI maintenance

Answer: Immediate allogeneic hematopoietic stem cell transplant (HCT)

Note that allogeneic HCT is the only potentially curative treatment available for JMML. There are no targeted drugs which have been approved for use in it.

Q. Which of the following statement is not true:
1. For symptomatic patients with MDS, selection of treatment is influenced by the IPSS-R score, level of RBC production based on reticulocyte production index (RPI) but not on serum erythropoietin (EPO) level
2. In a patient with intermediate risk MDS, with im-

paired RBC production (ie, RPI <2) and serum EPO ≤500 mU/mL initial treatment with an ESA is the most appropriate choice
3. In patients with high risk MDS, chronic transfusion therapy, along with definitive treatment is the most appropriate treatment strategy rather than chronic ESA therapy
4. None of the above

Answer: For symptomatic patients with MDS, selection of treatment is influenced by the IPSS-R score, level of RBC production based on reticulocyte production index (RPI) but not on serum erythropoietin (EPO) level

In fact, the treatment of symptomatic patients with MDS the treatment depends on EPO levels too, along with the other two factors.

Notes on treatment of anemia in patients with MDS:

First and foremost consideration is whether or not a patient is symptomatic. If the patients is **asymptomatic,** there is no particular threshold of hemoglobin levels, below which the treatment is indicated. In such patients, clinical judgement dictates the further treatment course.

On the other hand, if the patient is symptomatic then it becomes imperative to do something about the anemia. Then the treatment depends on the above mentioned three parameters (IPSS-R score, level of RBC production based on reticulocyte production index (RPI) and serum erythropoietin (EPO) level), in the following way:

1. **Low/very low/intermediate risk MDS** (ie, IPSS-R ≤4.5 points):

Treatment selection is informed by RPI and EPO levels:

a. RPI <2 **and** serum EPO ≤500 mU/mL: initial treatment with an ESA

b. RPI ≥2 **or** serum EPO >500 mU/mL: RBC transfusions or a trial of an ESA (with or without a myeloid growth factor)

2. **High/very high risk MDS** (ie, IPSS-R >4.5 points): initial treatment is chronic transfusion therapy, along with definitive treatment of the disease

Q. Treatment should be initiated in asymptomatic patients of MDS, because it leads to improvement in survival:
   1. True
   2. False

Answer: false

It is important to remember here that **treatment in not indicated in every patient of MDS.** Treatment has not shown to increase survival outcomes in asymptomatic MDS patients.

Asymptomatic patients are serially followed to monitor the course of the disease. Some clinicians choose to treat asymptomatic patients having severe anemia and/or severe thrombocytopenia.

Q. Which of the following is an indication for treatment in

MDS patients:
1. Symptomatic anemia
2. Symptomatic thrombocytopenia
3. Recurrent infections in the setting of severe neutropenia
4. All of the above

Answer: all of the above

These three are the most common indications of treatment in MDS.

Q. According to the IPSS-R, if a patient of MDS has the score of 6, then he will be diagnosed in which "risk group":
1. Intermediate
2. High
3. Very high
4. Abysmal

Answer: High

Note that there is no such group as "abysmal".

Remember these cutoffs of IPSS-R scores:
1. High risk (>4.5 to 6 points)
2. Very high risk (>6 points)

Q. If a patient of MDS belongs to the high risk subgroup and TP53 gene mutation is present, then which of the following will be the most appropriate treatment option:

1. Azacitidine
2. Decitabine
3. Lenalidomide
4. Cytarabine

Answer: decitabine

Note that in high and very high risk MDS patients who are medically fit, either azacitidine or decitabine is the treatment of choice. But in cases of TP53 mutation, decitabine becomes the drug of choice.

Q. In a patient with high risk MDS, who has IDH2 mutation, which of the following is the drug of choice:

1. Ivosidenib
2. Enasidenib
3. Azacitidine
4. Decitabine

Answer: enasidenib

Enasidenib targets IDH2 and ivosidenib targets IDH1. If in a case of high risk MDS, either of these mutations is present then these are the drugs of choice.

Note here that these drugs are not yet FDA approved for

use in MDS but most experts agree that they should be used whenever possible.

Q. In high risk MDS, not having any additional targetable mutation, which of the following is a treatment option:
1. Allogeneic HCT
2. Intensive chemotherapy
3. Hypomethylating agents
4. All of the above

Answer: all of the above

Note that there is no particular "treatment of choice" in such patients, and the choice depends on clinical factors and patient preference.

Notes on survival outcomes in high- or very high risk MDS patients:
1. Azacitidine: in an international study conducted in "higher risk" MDS, patients were randomised to receive either azacitidine or conventional care (best supportive care, high dose AML like induction chemotherapy or low dose cytarabine). Azacitidine resulted in superior median OS (25 versus 15 months; HR 0.58).
2. Decitabine: in a phase III study, patients with "higher risk" MDS were randomised between decitabine and best supportive care. Decitabine therapy was associated with higher progression-free survival (6.6 versus 3.0 months), but no difference in OS. Note that in a phase II study, decitabine was

found to have a nearly 100% response rate in high risk MDS patients having TP53 mutation.

Q. In patients with high risk MDS having deletion 5q, which of the following is the drug of choice:
1. Lenalidomide
2. Thalidomide
3. Venetoclax
4. Azacitidine

Answer: azacitidine

This is a very important question. Remember that in MDS with del(5q) the treatment depends on the risk category. In very low, low and some intermediate risk patients, lenalidomide is the drug of choice but in high and very high risk categories, lenalidomide is not considered very effective and they are treated similar to those patients of high- or very high risk MDS who don't have the 5q deletion.

Q. In patients with MDS with ringed sideroblasts (MDS-RS) who do not respond adequately to an erythropoiesis stimulating agent, which of the following drug has been recently approved by the FDA:
1. Darbopoietin-twcl
2. Luspatercept
3. Daratumumab
4. Selumetinib

Answer: luspatercept

Notes on treatment of "lower risk MDS":
1. Most experts consider lower-risk MDS to include IPSS-R ≤ 3 points.
2. Asymptomatic patients are just monitored and no active treatment is given.
3. In symptomatic patients, treatment is indicated.
4. Treatment of anemia depends on serum erythropoietin levels. If serum EPO, is ≤500 mU/mL, initial treatment with an erythropoiesis-stimulating agent (ESA) for at least three months is the treatment of choice. If serum EPO is >500 mU/mL, then the patient is treated as a patient of multiple cytopenias (see below).
5. For isolated or predominant, symptomatic thrombocytopenia, a thrombopoietin receptor agonist is initially offered. If there are other features as well then the patient is treated as that of multiple cytopenias.
6. There is no standard treatment for patient of lower risk MDS having multiple cytopenias. Azacitidine, decitabine or lenalidomide have been tried.
7. Patients having 5q deletion are preferably treated with lenalidomide.
8. Patients having IDH1 or IDH2 mutations may be treated with targeted drugs. But they are not FDA approved in this setting.
9. In MDS-RS patients who don't respond to ESAs or who are expected to not respond to ESAs, FDA has approved luspatercept.
10. Monitoring is key in management of lower risk MDS patients.

MYELOPROLIFERATIVE DISORDERS

CML

Q. Which chromosome is known as the Philadelphia chromosome in cases of CML:
1. Chromosome 22
2. Chromosome 9
3. t(9;22)
4. t(22;9)

Answer: chromosome 22

The hallmark of CML is t(9;22); more specifically t(9;22) (q34;q11). This results in the *BCR-ABL1* fusion gene.

But remember that the name "Philadelphia chromosome" was given to the abnormal chromosome 22 by Nowell and Hungerford.

Note that 90 to 95 percent patients demonstrate the t(9;22) (q34;q11.2). The rest of the patients either have some other variant of this translocation or have cryptic translocations.

Q. Which BCR-ABL1 fusion protein is characteristic of CML:
1. p210 BCR-ABL1
2. p190 BCR-ABL1
3. p230 BCR-ABL1
4. p220 BCR-ABL1

Answer: p210 BCR-ABL1

Remember these important points:
1. BCR-ABL1 fusion protein p190 is found in: Philadelphia chromosome positive acute lymphoblastic leukemia
2. BCR-ABL1 fusion protein p210 is found in: CML
3. BCR-ABL1 fusion protein p230 is found in: chronic neutrophilic leukemia

Q. CML is associated with BCR-ABL1 fusion. The BCR gene is found on:
1. Chromosome 9
2. Chromosome 22
3. It results from the fusion of chromosomes 9 and 22
4. It results from the fusion of chromosomes 22 and 9

Answer: chromosome 22

Please remember always:
1. *BCR* gene is found on chromosome 22
2. *ABL1* gene is found on chromosome 9

3. Translocation of chromosome 9 and chromosome 22 results in BCR-ABL1 fusion
4. This fusion gene is then present on chromosome 22

Q. Which of the following is a known risk factor for CML:
1. Ionizing radiation
2. Benzene
3. Polycyclic aromatic hydrocarbons
4. All of the above

Answer: ionizing radiation

Ionizing radiation is the only known risk factor for CML.

Q. Which of the following is the characteristic feature of CML:
1. A greater percent of myelocytes than meta-myelocytes
2. A greater percent of metamyelocytes than myelocytes
3. A greater percent of myelocytes than promy-elocytes
4. A greater percent of promyelocytes than myelocytes

Answer: A greater percent of myelocytes than meta-myelocytes

Q. LAP score in CML is:
1. High
2. Low
3. Indeterminate
4. Variable

Answer: low

Q. Which of the following statement about CML is not correct:
1. Absolute basophilia is present in the blood smears of around 50% patients
2. Absolute eosinophilia is seen in about 90% of cases
3. Absolute monocytosis is common in CML patients
4. All of the above

Answer: Absolute basophilia is present in the blood smears of around 50% patients

In fact, absolute basophilia is present in the blood smears of nearly 100% patients.

Q. Which of the following are characteristically found in bone marrow examination of a patient of CML:
1. Dwarf megakaryocytes
2. Micro megakaryocytes
3. Giant megakaryocytes
4. Normal sized megakaryocytes

Answer: dwarf megakaryocytes

Q. In CML, most commonly the abnormal *BCR-ABL1* fusion transcript is produced is from:
1. A breakpoint in exon 13 or exon 14 in the *BCR* gene, fused to the *ABL1* gene at exon a2
2. A breakpoint in exon 13 or exon 14 in the *BCR* gene, fused to the *ABL1* gene at exon b2
3. A breakpoint in exon 12 or exon 13 in the *BCR* gene, fused to the *ABL1* gene at exon a2
4. A breakpoint in exon 12 or exon 13 in the *BCR* gene, fused to the *ABL1* gene at exon b2

Answer: A breakpoint in exon 13 or exon 14 in the *BCR* gene, fused to the *ABL1* gene at exon a2

Q. Which of the following is not a component of the EURO score used for risk stratification of patients with CML:
1. Age
2. Spleen size below costal margin
3. Blast percentage in the bone marrow
4. Eosinophil count

Answer: Blast percentage in the bone marrow

In fact, blast percentage in the peripheral blood is used (not in the bone marrow).

There are three score of CML risk stratification which have been extensively used:

1. Sokal: age, spleen, platelet count, blasts in peripheral blood
2. Hasford, also known as EURO: age, spleen size [cm below costal margin], percent blasts in peripheral blood, percent eosinophils, basophils, platelet count
3. EUTOS (ELTS): age, spleen size cm below the costal margin, blasts in peripheral blood

Sokal score, for instance, may be low <0.8, intermediate 0.8-1.2 or high >1.2.

The implications of this risk stratification are that they can impact treatment selection. If, for example, the score is low then we may choose imatinib or any other second generation TKIs that have been approved for the treatment of CML in the first line but if the score is high then second generation TKIs become the preferred choice.

Q. Which of the following is not a preferred TKI for treatment of high risk chronic phase CML:

1. Nilotinib
2. Bosutinib
3. Imatinib
4. Dasatinib

Answer: imatinib

Remember:

1. For **low or intermediate risk** CML, imatinib, nilotinib, dasatinib and bosutinib are all equally accept-

able.
2. For **high risk** CML, second generation TKIs (nilotinib, dasatinib and bosutinib) are preferred, but imatinib may also be used.

Remember that no second generation TKI is superior to other second generation TKIs.

However, there are certain risk factors and comorbidities, which if present may make a TKI rather unsuitable, if not entirely contraindicated.

Please read below mentioned adverse effects carefully:
1. Imatinib: fluid retention and edema
2. Nilotinib: coronary, cerebral, and peripheral vascular disease; prolonged QTc interval, hyperglycemia, pancreatitis
3. Dasatinib: pleural effusion, pulmonary hypertension, prolonged QTc interval, platelet dysfunction
4. Bosutinib: pancreatitis

Please note that if a patient is suffering from a coexisting disease which is also a side effect of a TKI, then that TKI is not preferred in that particular patient. For example, if a patient has history of pancreatitis then nilotinib and bosutinib should not be used, because they may cause pancreatitis themselves. Another example is a patient having significant edema; in such a patient imatinib should be avoided because imatinib causes significant fluid retention and edema in many patients.

Q. Imatinib was studied in which of the following trials:
1. IRIS
2. ENESTnd
3. DASISION
4. BELA

Answer: this is a trick question. Imatinib was studied in all of them.

Notes:
1. IRIS trial studied Interferon versus imatinib
2. ENESTnd trial studied nilotinib versus imatinib
3. DASISION trial studied dasatinib versus imatinib
4. BELA trial studied bosutinib versus imatinib

Notes on recommendations for monitoring of CML patients:
1. During treatment:
    1. Quantitative real-time PCR (RQ-PCR) for *BCR-ABL1* transcripts level, every three months until an MMR (BCR-ABL1 ≤ 0.1 percent, or $MR_{3.0}$) has been achieved
    2. Once an MMR has been achieved, RQ-PCR is done every three to six months
    3. If RQ-PCR is not available then CBA of marrow cell metaphases is performed at 3, 6, and 12 months until a CCyR has been achieved
    4. Once CCyR is achieved CBA is done every 12 months.
2. In case of failure or progression:
    1. RQ-PCR
    2. Mutational analysis
    3. CBA of marrow cell metaphases

4. Immunophenotyping in blast crisis

Please always remember these definitions of the response to therapy of CML to TKIs:
1. Optimal responses:
    1. At three months from initiation of TKI: BCR-ABL1 ≤10 percent and/or Ph+ ≤35 percent
    2. At six months from initiation of TKI: BCR-ABL1 <1 percent and/or Ph+ 0
    3. At twelve months from initiation of TKI and beyond: BCR-ABL1 ≤0.1 percent
2. Failure is defined as:
    1. At three months from initiation of TKI: No CHR (complete hematologic response) and/or Ph+ >95 percent
    2. At six months from initiation of TKI: BCR-ABL1 >10 percent and/or Ph+ >35 percent
    3. At twelve months from initiation of TKI: BCR-ABL1 >1 percent and/or Ph+ >0
    4. After 12 months and **at any time** during treatment:
        1. Loss of CHR (complete hematologic response)
        2. Loss of CCyR (complete cytogenetic response)
        3. Confirmed loss of MMR (major molecular response)
        4. Mutations
        5. Clonal chromosome abnormalities in Ph+ cells

All the other parameters, between an optimal response and failure are classified as "warning"

Q. Imatinib inhibits all of the following except:
1. BCR-ABL1 tyrosine kinase
2. PDGFR
3. SRC family kinases
4. KIT

Answer: SRC family kinases

Q. Which of the following TKI is active against the *BCR-ABL1* T315I mutation:
1. Ponatinib
2. Dasatinib
3. Nilotinib
4. All of the above

Answer: ponatinib

Ponatinib is the only TKI which is active against BCR-ABL1 T315I mutation.

Q. The TKIs used in CML are primarily metabolised by:
1. CYP3A4
2. CYP2D6
3. CYP2A2
4. CYP2B5

Answer: CYP3A4

Q. The initial starting dose of imatinib in a patient of chronic phase CML is:
1. 300 mg/day
2. 400 mg/day
3. 600 mg/day
4. 800 mg/day

Answer: 400 mg/day

Preferably imatinib should be taken with food.

Note that in the accelerated phase and in blast crisis, the starting dose of imatinib is 600 mg/day.

Q. In which of the following situation is imatinib dose reduction required:
1. Moderate or severe renal dysfunction
2. Moderate to severe hepatic dysfunction
3. Both of the above
4. None of the above

Answer: both of the above

Q. What is the starting dose of dasatinib is patients of chronic phase CML:

1. 100 mg/day
2. 70 mg/day
3. 140 mg/day
4. 70 mg twice daily

Answer: 100 mg/day

Q. What is the starting dose of dasatinib is patients of accelerated phase or blast crisis CML:
1. 100 mg/day
2. 70 mg/day
3. 140 mg/day
4. 70 mg twice daily

Answer: 70 mg twice daily

This is slightly controversial. But most experts and guidelines agree that a 70 mg twice daily dose is better than 140 mg once daily (although the total dose remains the same).

Always remember that concurrent use of dasatinib and proton pump inhibitors or H2 blockers is **not** recommended.

Q. What is the starting dose of nilotinib for chronic phase CML:
1. 300 mg/day
2. 300 mg twice daily
3. 400 mg/day

4. 400 mg twice daily

Answer: 300 mg twice daily

In cases of imatinib failure, the dose of nilotinib is 400 mg twice daily.

It is very important to remember that nilotinib should be taken **without** food.

Proton pump inhibitors and H2 blockers should not be given with nilotinib because altered gastric acidity may hamper the absorption of nilotinib.

Q. What is the recommended dose of bosutinib in CML:
1. 200 mg/day
2. 300 mg/day
3. 400 mg/day
4. 500 mg/day

Answer: 500 mg/day

Note that bosutinib should be taken **with** food.

Q. What is the approved starting dose of ponatinib in CML:
1. 15 mg/day
2. 30 mg/day
3. 45 mg/day

4. 60 mg/day

Answer: 45 mg/day

Q. Muscle cramps are common with:
1. Imatinib
2. Nilotinib
3. Dasatinib
4. All of the above

Answer: imatinib

Muscle cramps are uncommon with TKIs other than imatinib.

Q. When should imatinib be temporarily withheld in a patient of chronic phase CML:
1. If absolute neutrophil count falls to <1000/microL and/or the platelet count to <50,000/microL during the first months of therapy
2. If absolute neutrophil count falls to <1500/microL and/or the platelet count to <50,000/microL during the first months of therapy
3. If absolute neutrophil count falls to <1000/microL and/or the platelet count to <100,000/microL during the first months of therapy
4. It should never be stopped, regardless of the ANC and platelet counts

Answer: If absolute neutrophil count falls to <1000/microL and/or the platelet count to <50,000/microL during the first months of therapy

Notes:
1. If absolute neutrophil count falls to <1000/microL and/or the platelet count falls to <50,000/microL during the first months of therapy, imatinib should be stopped.
2. We should then wait for ANC to be >1500/microL and the platelet count to be >75 to 100,000/microL. This recovery of blood counts should take four weeks or less. If this happens then imatinib should again be started at full dose.
3. If the above mentioned recovery takes more than 4 weeks then imatinib should be started at 300 mg per day and escalated to the full dose of 400 mg per day after a period of 4 weeks on the lower dose, provided that the recovery is maintained over those 4 weeks.

Q. Which of the following statements is not true:
1. Arterial occlusion is seen in more than one-third of patients of CML on ponatinib
2. Dasatinib is associated with exudative pleural effusion
3. With dasatinib, effusions are seen more commonly in patients with accelerated or blast phase of CML
4. Most effusions with dasatinib occur after the first four to six months of treatment

Answer: Most effusions with dasatinib occur after the first four to six months of treatment

In fact, most effusions with dasatinib occur **within** the first four to six months of treatment.

Q. Which of the following adverse event mandates permanent discontinuation of dasatinib:
  1. Pericardial effusion
  2. Deep venous thrombosis
  3. Sinusoidal obstruction syndrome
  4. Pulmonary arterial hypertension

Answer: pulmonary arterial hypertension

Q. Which TKI used in treatment of CML is associated with increased risk of second malignancies:
  1. Imatinib
  2. Dasatinib
  3. Ponatinib
  4. None of the above

Answer: none of the above

Q. Which of the following is not a WHO criterion for defining accelerated phase CML:
  1. 10 to 19 percent blasts in the peripheral blood
  2. Bone marrow basophils ≥20 percent
  3. Platelets <100,000/microL, unrelated to therapy

4. Progressive splenomegaly, unresponsive to therapy

Answer: Bone marrow basophils ≥20 percent

The criterion of basophils 20% or more is applicable to peripheral blood according to the WHO criteria (not bone marrow).

According to the WHO, if any of these following findings are present in a case of CML, the patents is diagnosed as accelerated phase CML:
1. 10 to 19 percent blasts in the peripheral blood or bone marrow
2. Peripheral blood basophils ≥20 percent
3. Platelets <100,000/microL, unrelated to therapy
4. Platelets >1,000,000/microL, unresponsive to therapy
5. Progressive splenomegaly and increasing white cell count, unresponsive to therapy
6. Cytogenetic evolution: the development of chromosomal abnormalities in addition to the Philadelphia chromosome

Q. Which of the following BCR-ABL1 mutation show only intermediate sensitivity to dasatinib:
1. Y253H
2. E255K
3. F359I
4. V299L

Answer: V299L

The mutational landscape of CML has been studied in detail and specific mutations have been identified in the BCR-ABL1, according to which therapy can be tailored to an individual:

1. The BCR-ABL1 Y253H, E255K/V and F359V/C/I mutations are resistant to imatinib and nilotinib but sensitive to dasatinib.

2. The BCR-ABL1 F317L/V/I/C, V299L, and T315A mutations are sensitive to nilotinib and relatively resistant to imatinib and dasatinib

Q. Which of the following medicine is active against *BCR-ABL1* T315I mutation:
   1. Ponatinib
   2. Omacetaxine
   3. Radotinib
   4. All of the above

Answer: ponatinib and omacetaxine are correct answers

Still, ponatinib is the best choice if you have to choose only one as an answer.

Note that omacetaxine is a protein synthesis inhibitor. It is approved by the FDA for the treatment of accelerated phase CML in adults with resistance or intolerance to two or more

TKIs. It is administered subcutaneously.

Q. According to the WHO, which of the following is the defining feature of CML blast crisis:
1. ≥20 percent blasts in peripheral blood
2. ≥20 percent blasts in bone marrow
3. Extramedullary proliferation of blasts
4. All of the above

Answer: all of the above

These are in fact, the defining criteria according to the WHO. Note that extramedullary proliferation of blasts is also known as a myeloid sarcoma.

Q. Which of the following is a treatment option for a newly diagnosed patient of CML who's in a blast crisis:
1. TKIs
2. Allogeneic HCT
3. Both of the above
4. None of the above

Answer: both of the above

The sequence of initial therapies to be used is somewhat controversial but most experts agree that even if the patient is diagnosed as having CML blast crisis upon first presentation; even then TKIs should be started (preferably second generation TKIs) rather than going directly for allogeneic HCT.

Please remember these criteria of "response" in CML:
1. Complete hematologic response (**all** of the following must be met):
   1. WBC <10 x 10⁹/L
   2. Basophils <5 percent
   3. No myelocytes, promyelocytes, myeloblasts in the differential
   4. Platelet count <450 x 10⁹/L
   5. Spleen nonpalpable
2. Cytogenetic response:
   1. Major: major has two categories:
      1. Complete: No Ph+ metaphases or <1 percent BCR-ABL1-positive nuclei of at least 200 nuclei on FISH
      2. Partial: 1 to 35 percent Ph+ metaphases
   2. Minor: 36 to 65 percent Ph+ metaphases
   3. Minimal: 66 to 95 percent Ph+ metaphases
   4. None: >95 percent Ph+ metaphases
3. Molecular response:
   1. MR4.5: Detectable disease with ratio of BCR-ABL1 to ABL1 (or other housekeeping genes) ≤0.0032 percent (≥4.4 log reduction) on the international scale (IS). MR4.5 may also be defined as undetectable disease in cDNA with ≥32,000 ABL1 transcripts
   2. MR4: Detectable disease with ratio of BCR-ABL1 to ABL1 ≤0.01 percent (≥4 log reduction) on the IS **OR** undetectable disease in cDNA with ≥10,000 ABL1 transcripts
   3. MR3: Detectable disease with ratio of BCR-ABL1 to ABL1 (or other housekeeping genes) ≤0.1 percent (≥3 log reduction) on the IS

Q. The preferred myeloablative regimen for allogeneic HCT in CML is busulfan plus cyclophosphamide:
1. True
2. False

Answer: true

Q. In patients who undergo allogeneic HCT for chronic phase CML, if a molecular remission has been achieved; what should be the next most appropriate strategy:
1. Frequent monitoring for *BCR-ABL1* measurable residual disease
2. Continuing a TKI for 1 more year
3. Continuing a TKI for 2 more years
4. Continuing a TKI indefinitely till progression or unacceptable adverse effects

Answer: Frequent monitoring for *BCR-ABL1* measurable residual disease

Note that this question is about **chronic phase** CML. On the other hand, if a patient is transplanted for **CML blast crisis**, a TKI should be continued for two years after allogeneic HCT.

Q. Which of the following is not a factor in the European Group for Blood and Marrow Transplantation risk assessment score for allogeneic transplantation in chronic myeloid leukemia:

1. Donor type
2. Stage
3. Age
4. BCR-ABL1 load

Answer: BCR-ABL1 load

There are five factor in this system:

1. Donor type
2. Stage
3. Age
4. Sex matching
5. Time to HCT from diagnosis

Polycythemia vera, essential thrombocythemia, primary myelofibrosis

Q. JAK2 mutations are positive in what percent of PV patients:

1. 20-30
2. 30-60
3. 60-90
4. >90

Answer: >90%

Most of the patients have JAK2 V617F mutation.

But note that JAK2 mutations are **not** pathognomonic for PV, because they are found in other myeloproliferative disorders as well, e.g., essential thrombocythemia.

Q. Bone marrow biopsy, in a patient of PV, classically shows:
1. Hypercellularity, trilineage growth with erythroid, granulocytic, and megakaryocytic proliferation
2. Hypocellularity, trilineage growth with erythroid, granulocytic, and megakaryocytic proliferation
3. Hypercellularity, unilineage growth of erythroid lineage and suppressed granulocytic, and megakaryocytic proliferation
4. Hypocellularity, unilineage growth of erythroid lineage and suppressed granulocytic, and megakaryocytic proliferation

Answer: Hypercellularity, trilineage growth with erythroid, granulocytic, and megakaryocytic proliferation

Q. In PV:
1. Stainable iron is absent and reticulin is increased
2. Stainable iron is absent and reticulin is decreased
3. Stainable iron is increased and reticulin is absent
4. Stainable iron decreased and reticulin is absent

Answer: Stainable iron absent and reticulin is increased

Q. In PV, JAK2 mutations occur most commonly in:
1. Either exon 11 or 12
2. Either exon 13 or 12
3. Either exon 14 or 12
4. Either exon 13 or 11

Answer: Either exon 14 or 12

JAK2 V617F mutation is characteristic for PV.

Q. Which of the following is not a 2016 WHO criterion for the diagnosis of PV:
1. Hemoglobin > 16 g/dL in women
2. Hematocrit > 55% in men
3. Serum erythropoietin level below normal
4. Panmyelosis

Answer: Hematocrit > 55% in men

In fact, according to the 2016 WHO criteria, hematocrit should be > 49%.

Notes on WHO criteria for diagnosis of PV:
According to these criteria the diagnosis of PV requires, either the presence of all three major criteria **or** presence of the "first two" major criteria along with the minor criterion.

Major criteria:

1. Increased hemoglobin level (>16.5 g/dL in men or >16.0 g/dL in women), hematocrit (>49 percent in men or >48 percent in women), or other evidence of increased red cell volume
2. Bone marrow biopsy showing hypercellularity for age with trilineage growth (panmyelosis) including prominent erythroid, granulocytic, and megakaryocytic proliferation with pleomorphic, mature megakaryocytes
3. *JAK2 V617F* or *JAK2* exon 12 mutation

Minor criterion:
1. Serum erythropoietin level below the reference range for normal

Q. Which of the following statement about polycythemia vera is not true:
1. For all patients with PV, maintenance of hematocrit <45 percent in men and <42 percent in women is recommended
2. Low-dose aspirin is recommended in all patients with PV, except in those having contraindications for its use
3. In patients of PV with history of thrombosis, treatment with phlebotomy plus cytoreductive agents is recommended
4. In patients of PV without any high risk features, treatment with cytoreductive agents alone is preferred rather than phlebotomy

Answer: In patients of PV without any high risk features, treatment with cytoreductive agents alone is preferred rather than phlebotomy

In fact, just the opposite is true. In patients of PV without any high risk features, treatment with phlebotomy is preferred rather than cytoreductive agents.

Remember these two high risk features of PV:
1. Age >60 years
2. History of thrombosis

Q. Which of the following is the initial pharmacotherapy of choice for majority of patients with PV:
1. Hydroxyurea
2. Pegylated interferon alfa
3. Busulfan
4. Ruxolitinib

Answer: hydroxyurea

Ruxolitinib is JAK2 inhibitor used for treatment of a variety of conditions, including PV. It is generally not used in the first line for treatment of PV. It is used in patients with severe pruritus, symptomatic splenomegaly, or symptoms of post-PV myelofibrosis that failed to respond adequately to first-line therapies.

Q. Which of the following is the most common mutation in essential thrombocythemia:
1. JAK2

2. *CALR*
3. *MPL*
4. FLT3

Answer: JAK2

Around 90% of patients with ET have one of these three mutations: JAK2, CALR or MPL. Note that these mutations are mutually exclusive.

Notes on WHO diagnostic criteria for essential thrombocythemia:
Diagnosis of ET requires meeting all 4 major criteria or the first 3 major criteria and the minor criterion:

Major criteria:
1. Platelet count $\geq 450 \times 10^9/L$
2. Bone marrow biopsy showing proliferation mainly of the megakaryocyte lineage with increased numbers of enlarged, mature megakaryocytes with hyperlobulated nuclei. No significant increase or left shift in neutrophil granulopoiesis or erythropoiesis and very rarely minor (grade 1) increase in reticulin fibers.
3. Not meeting WHO criteria for *BCR-ABL1*+ CML, PV, PMF, myelodysplastic syndromes, or other myeloid neoplasms
4. Presence of *JAK2*, *CALR*, or *MPL* mutation

Minor criterion:
1. Presence of a clonal marker or absence of evidence for reactive thrombocytosis

Q. Which of the following is the most common mutation found in primary myelofibrosis:
1. *JAK2* mutation
2. *CALR* mutation
3. *MPL* mutation
4. None of the above

Answer: JAK2 mutation

Note that in 8 to 10% patients, there is no *JAK2*, *CALR*, or *MPL* mutation. They are known as "triple negative".

Q. Which of the following is not a major diagnostic criterion according to the WHO diagnostic criteria for overt primary myelofibrosis:
1. Presence of megakaryocytic proliferation and atypia, accompanied by either reticulin and/or collagen fibrosis grades 2 or 3
2. Presence of *JAK2*, *CALR*, or *MPL* mutation or, in the absence of these mutations, presence of another clonal marker, or absence of reactive myelofibrosis
3. Palpable splenomegaly
4. Anemia not attributed to a comorbid condition

Answer: options 3 and 4 are correct (they are **not** the major criteria)

Notes on WHO diagnostic criteria for overt primary myelofibrosis (Diagnosis of overt PMF requires meeting all 3 major criteria, and at least 1 minor criterion):

Major criteria (all three must be present):
1. Presence of megakaryocytic proliferation and atypia, accompanied by either reticulin and/or collagen fibrosis grades 2 or 3
2. Not meeting WHO criteria for ET, PV, *BCR-ABL1*+ CML, myelodysplastic syndromes, or other myeloid neoplasms
3. Presence of *JAK2*, *CALR*, or *MPL* mutation or, in the absence of these mutations, presence of another clonal marker, or absence of reactive myelofibrosis

Minor criteria (at least 1 of the following must be present, confirmed in 2 consecutive determinations):
1. Anemia not attributed to a comorbid condition
2. Leukocytosis $\geq 11 \times 10^9$/L
3. Palpable splenomegaly
4. LDH increased to above upper normal limit of institutional reference range
5. Leukoerythroblastosis

Notes on WHO diagnostic criteria for pre-primary myelofibrosis:

Major criteria (all three must be present):
1. Megakaryocytic proliferation and atypia, without reticulin fibrosis >grade 1, accompanied by increased age-adjusted bone marrow cellularity, granulocytic proliferation, and often decreased

erythropoiesis
2. Not meeting the WHO criteria for *BCR-ABL1+* CML, PV, ET, myelodysplastic syndromes, or other myeloid neoplasms
3. Presence of *JAK2*, *CALR*, or *MPL* mutation or in the absence of these mutations, presence of another clonal marker, or absence of minor reactive bone marrow reticulin fibrosis

Minor criteria (at least 1 of the following must be present and its presence must be confirmed in 2 consecutive determinations):
1. Anemia not attributed to a comorbid condition
2. Leukocytosis $\geq 11 \times 10^9$/L
3. Palpable splenomegaly
4. LDH increased to above upper normal limit of institutional reference range

Q. If bone marrow shows loose network of reticulin with many intersections, especially in perivascular areas; what will be WHO grade of such a patient of myelofibrosis;
1. MF-0
2. MF-1
3. MF-2
4. MF-3

Answer: MF-1

Note on WHO grading of myelofibrosis:
1. MF-0: Scattered linear reticulin with no intersections (crossovers) corresponding to normal bone marrow

2. MF-1: Loose network of reticulin with many inter-sections, especially in perivascular areas
3. MF-2: Diffuse and dense increase in reticulin with extensive intersections, occasionally with focal bundles of thick fibers mostly consistent with colla-gen, and/or focal osteosclerosis
4. MF-3: Diffuse and dense increase in reticulin with extensive intersections and coarse bundles of thick fibers consistent with collagen, usually associated with osteosclerosis

Note that in MF-2 and MF-3, additional staining with tri-chrome is recommended.

Q. Which of the following drug is used for symptom control in primary myelofibrosis:
1. Ruxolitinib
2. Fedratinib
3. Hydroxyurea
4. All of the above

Answer: all of the above

Remember that none of the above mentioned drugs can im-prove overall survival in primary myelofibrosis. The only therapy that improves OS in PMF is allogeneic HCT.

Q. In which of the following patient population of PMF pa-tients, treatment is indicated:

1. High risk
2. Low risk, asymptomatic
3. Low risk, symptomatic
4. All of the above

Answer: High risk and low risk, symptomatic

Observation rather than treatment is indicated in low risk, asymptotic patients of PMF.

In high risk patients, allogeneic HCT is the treatment of choice.

In low risk, symptomatic patients, ruxolitinib, fedratinib or hydroxyurea are preferred.

HEMATOPOIETIC CELL TRANSPLANT

Q. Each full sibling potential donor has what chance of being fully HLA-matched with a sibling who requires an HCT:
1. 25%
2. 10%
3. 50%
4. 75%

Answer: 25%

Because of this reason, sibling donors are not the ideal donors in many instances and a search for a fully HLA-matched donor needs to be done.

Q. Which of the following is not true about an unrelated umbilical cord blood (UCB) transplant (compared to other sources of stem cells for allogeneic HCT):
1. A complete human leukocyte antigen (HLA) match is not needed when UCB is used
2. The graft-versus-host disease is more severe for the degree of HLA disparity compared to other stem cell

sources
3. There is an increased risk of graft failure
4. Immune reconstitution is often delayed

Answer: The graft-versus-host disease is more severe for the degree of HLA disparity compared to other stem cell sources

In fact, GVHD is less severe considering the degree of HLA disparity.

Q. Allogeneic HCT may be used in the first remission in all of the following diseases except:
1. AML
2. ALL
3. MDS
4. DLBCL

Answer: DLBCL

In DLBCL, allogeneic HCT is used after failure of autologous HCT.

Q. Allogeneic HCT can be considered for patients with hematologic malignancies > 70 years of age:

1. True
2. False

Answer: true

Previously it was believed that allo-HCT should not be done in patients aged 55 years or older. But with the invention of reduced intensity conditioning, now this age restraint is no longer valid, however with increasing age, chances of having a comorbidity also increase and that does influence the choice of therapy.

Q. Which of the following is not correct:

1. If a patient has DLCO <60 percent then allogeneic HCT is absolutely contraindicated
2. BCNU-based regimens and busulfan are contraindicated in patients having reduced DLCO
3. Patients with a left ventricular ejection fraction (LVEF) <40 percent are not considered candidates for allogeneic HCT
4. Seropositivity for human immunodeficiency virus (HIV) does not exclude patients from undergoing allogeneic HCT

Answer: If a patient has DLCO <60 percent then allogeneic HCT is absolutely contraindicated

While it is true that patients having DLCO <60% are not the ideal candidates for HCT but in many such patients HCT has been successfully done; in other words, it's not an absolute contraindication.

Generally, a corrected DLCO of >35% makes a patient fit enough to go through HCT.

Notes:
There are basically four types of "donors" of stem cells for HCT:

1. An identical twin (syngeneic): in these cases the HLA is identical
2. A sibling, relative, or unrelated donor: they can be HLA identical, haploidentical, or mismatched
3. Umbilical cord blood: it can also be HLA identical, haploidentical, or mismatched
4. The patient him/herself (autologous): in this case HLA is identical

Q. Which of the following is not an HLA class I antigen:

1. HLA-A

2. HLA-C

3. HLA-DRB1

4. HLA-DQB2

Answer: options 3 and 4 are correct

There are basically five HLA antigen types that are most important for "matching" between the donor and the recipient: A, B, C, DRB1 and DQB1. Out of these, A, B and C antigens belong to class I and HLA-DRB1 and -DQB1 belong to class II.

Very important points to remember:

1. There are various methods for HLA matching.

2. Serologic typing is used for antigen matching. This method is not preferred by most centres nowadays and molecular typing is considered a better option.

3. Molecular typing, used for allele matching. It can be of low or high resolution types.

4. Remember the following definitions:

A. 12/12 HLA match: donor-recipient pairs matched for HLA-A, HLA-B, HLA-C, HLA-DRB1, HLA-DQB1, and HLA-DP1 at the allele level

B. 10/10 HLA match: donor-recipient pairs matched for HLA-A, HLA-B, HLA-C, HLA-DRB1, and HLA-DQB1 at the allele level

C. 9/10 HLA match: pairs with a single allele or anti-gen mismatch at either HLA-A, HLA-B, HLA-C, HLA-DRB1, or HLA-DQB1

D. 8/8 HLA match: donor-recipient pairs matched for HLA-A, HLA-B, HLA-C, and HLA-DRB1 at the allele level

E. 7/8 HLA match: pairs with a single allele or antigen mismatch at either HLA-A, HLA-B, HLA-C, or HLA-DRB1

F. 6/6 HLA match: donor-recipient pairs matched for HLA-A, HLA-B, and HLA-DRB1 at the allele level.

Antigen mismatches can be further characterized as being in the "graft-versus-host" direction or the "host-versus-graft" direction:

Q. If the recipient of allogeneic HCT possesses one or more alleles not present in the donor, it is known as:

1. A graft-versus-host direction mismatch

2. A host-versus-graft direction mismatch

3. A graft-versus-host flow mismatch

4. A host-versus-graft flow mismatch

Answer: A graft-versus-host direction mismatch

On the other hand a "host-versus-graft direction mismatch" means that the donor possesses one or more alleles not present in the patient.

Q. Which of the following is true about the minimum matching criteria for allogeneic HCT:

1. Unrelated adult donor transplant requires an at least 7 of 8 HLA match

2. UCB transplant allows for a 4 of 6 matched UCB unit

3. Haploidentical donors are matched at least at 1 of 6 loci

4. All of the above

Answer: options 1 and 2 are true and option 3 is false

Haploidentical donors are matched at 3 of 6 foci

Q. For patients undergoing peripheral blood progenitor cell

transplant, which of the following antigen mismatch coneys the worst prognosis:

1. HLA-A

2. HLA-B

3. HLA-C

4. HLA-DR

Answer: HLA-C

On the other hand, for patients undergoing bone marrow transplant, allele or antigen mismatch at HLA-B or HLA-C may be better tolerated than HLA-A or HLA-DR.

Q. While performing the HLA match, the patient's full biological siblings may avoid typing for which of the following HLA antigen:

1. A

2. B

3. C

4. None of the above

Answer: C

This is because B and C are tightly linked together on their location on chromosome 6. That being said, ideally a full high resolution matching exercise is the best way to proceed.

Q. Which of the following is not true:

1. Patients who receive HCT from an identical sibling donor are at higher risk of relapse of any underlying malignant disease than similar patients transplanted with HLA-matched but nonidentical sibling donors
2. Patients who receive HCT from an identical sibling donor, do not develop GVHD and thus don't require pre-transplant immunosuppression
3. The survival is almost similar with either syngeneic or allogeneic transplant
4. HLA-DQ mismatch is associated with worse outcomes compared with HLA-DR mismatch

Answer: HLA-DQ mismatch is associated with worse outcomes compared with HLA-DR mismatch

Another interesting antigen is HLA-DPB1. In the previous era, this antigen was not routinely studied but now it is believed that it may help in further narrowing the search. Although the long term impact on survival outcomes of this antigen is not clear.

Q. MHC-I MICA is tightly linked to:
1. HLA-B locus
2. HLA-A locus
3. HLA-DPB1 locus
4. None of the above

Answer: HLA-B locus

MICA matched transplant may be helpful in reduction of GVHD and it is especially beneficial when reduction in GVHD is desperately needed.

Q. The KIR gene complex encodes for natural killer cell receptors that recognise epitopes of HLA antigens. Which of the following KIR haplotype is inhibitory;
1. A
2. B
3. C
4. None of the above

Answer: A

There are two main haplotypes of KIR. KIR-haplotype A encodes inhibitory receptors while KIR-haplotype B encodes activating receptors. But remember that these terms (activating and inhibitory) are not absolute as both A and B haplotypes code for both types of epitopes, it's just that they encode "predominantly" one type of epitope.

KIR matching is helpful when many HLA matched donors are available. Remember that KIR is a "non-HLA" matching parameter.

Notes on haploidentical transplants:
1. The most important advantage of this type of transplant is that the donors are readily available
2. Other advantages are availability of donors for repeated transplants, adequate doses of stem cells and graft-versus-tumor effect
3. The disadvantages are increased risk of graft failure, increased incidence of all grades of acute GVHD and chronic GVHD
4. Many methods are used to circumvent some of the above mentioned issues:
a. T cell depletion (TCD) with "mega-dose" CD34+ cells
b. The "GIAC" strategy (**G**CSF-stimulation of the donor; **I**ntensified immunosuppression post-transplantation; **A**nti-thymocyte globulin added to conditioning to help prevent GVHD and aid engraftment; and **C**ombination of peripheral blood stem cell and bone marrow allografts)

 c. High dose, post-transplantation cyclophosp-
hamide(PTCy)

 d. Immune reconstitution is superior with GIAC strategy and PTCy method compared with the TCD
method

Note that immune reconstitution is slightly slower after
HLA-haploidentical HCT but non-relapse mortality is not
significantly increased compared with matched sibling
HCT.

Q. In a patient of a hematologic malignancy, who received a
haploidentical HCT and has relapsed, there is no loss of expression of the mismatched HLA haplotype. Which of the
following is an accepted treatment option for such a patient:

 1. Donor lymphocyte infusion

 2. Another haploidentical HCT

 3. Both of the above

 4. None of the above

Answer: donor lymphocyte infusion

Note that the most important words in this question are "no
loss of expression." If a patient has "loss of expression of the
mismatched HLA haplotype", he is a candidate for another

haploidentical HCT from a relative who is mismatched for certain antigens from the initial donor. But if loss of expression of mismatched HLA haplotype is not there then DLI is the most acceptable option and such a patient will not be a candidate for another haploidentical HCT.

Q. When selecting a donor for HLA-haploidentical HCT, which of the following will not constitute a major ABO incompatibility:
  1. Recipient blood type O: Donor type A, B, or AB
  2. Recipient blood type A: Donor blood type B or AB
  3. Recipient blood type B: Donor blood type A or AB
  4. Recipient blood type AB: Donor blood type A or B

Answer: Recipient blood type AB: Donor blood type A or B

It is important to note that with recipient blood type AB, there are no major ABO incompatibilities, whatever the blood group of the donor may be.

So basically, there are three types of major ABO incompatibilities, they are option 1, 2 and 3.

The most optimal combination is when the recipient and donor are of the same blood group. If the donor and the recipient are not of the same blood group and there are no major incompatibilities either then all of the other possible combination are known as "minor" ABO incompatibilities.

Q. Which of the following is the correct phenotype of human hematopoietic stem cells:
1. CD34+, Lin-, Thy-1+, Dr-, CD38-
2. CD34-, Lin-, Thy-1+, Dr-, CD38-
3. CD34+, Lin+, Thy-1-, Dr+, CD38-
4. CD34+, Lin-, Thy-1-, Dr-, CD38+

Answer: CD34+, Lin-, Thy-1+, Dr-, CD38-

The most relevant and important markers for a clinician are CD34+ and Thy-1+

Notes on stem cell collection from bone marrow harvest technique:
1. Bone marrow is generally aspirated from the posterior iliac crests. General anaesthesia is preferred by some but local anaesthesia is also frequently used.
2. The goal of bone marrow harvest is collecting up to 10 to 15 mL of marrow per kilogram of recipient body weight
3. Heparin or acid-citrate-dextran-A can be used to anti-coagulate bone marrow products

4. Before cryopreservation, red blood cells must be washed off

5. In some patients who are heavily pretreated, the yield of peripheral blood stem cells may be suboptimal and the yield of bone marrow harvest may also not be sufficient. In such cases, GCSF may be used for 3 to 4 days prior to bone marrow harvest (not PBSC). According to some reports this practice may be associated with reduced incidence of GVHD.

6. A nucleated cell dose of 2×10^8/kg is generally considered to be adequate for an HCT.

Notes on stem cell collection from peripheral blood:

1. Normally the numbers of hematopoietic stem cells (HSCs) are very very low in the peripheral blood

2. To raise the numbers of HSCs is the peripheral blood, there are four commonly used strategies: G-CSF, GM-CSF, plerixafor and chemotherapy.

3. Sometimes the yield of PBSCs is low despite adequate attempts at mobilization. There are some factors that are associated with a low yield, like low circulating CD34+ cells, older donor age, and decreased total blood volume.

4. G-CSF mobilisation is the most commonly used method. The usual doe of G-CSF is 10 to 16 mcg/kg per day, with HSC mobilization usually occurring between days four and six.

5. When chemotherapy is used for the purpose of stem cell mobilisation, cyclophosphamide is the most commonly used drug at a dose of 3 to 4 g/m2 along with G-CSF 10 mcg/kg.

6. G-CSF is superior to GM-CSF and the combined, sequential use of G-CSF and GM-CSF is also superior to GM-CSF alone. In summary, G-CSF is the drug of choice.

7. At least 2 x 106 CD34+ cells/kg of recipient body weight must be collected.

Q. What is the mechanism of action of plerixafor:
1. It inhibits the interaction between stromal-cell-derived factor 1 (SDF-1) and its receptor CXCR4
2. It facilitates the interaction between stromal-cell-derived factor 1 (SDF-1) and its receptor CXCR4
3. It inhibits the interaction between stromal-cell-derived factor 2 (SDF-2) and its receptor CXCR4
4. It facilitates the interaction between stromal-cell-derived factor 2 (SDF-2) and its receptor CXCR4

Answer: It inhibits the interaction between stromal-cell-derived factor 1 (SDF-1) and its receptor CXCR4

It is used when mobilisation with G-CSF or G-CSF plus chemotherapy fails. The primary reason for its infrequent use is its prohibitively high cost.

Plerixafor is begun after the patient has received G-CSF for a minimum of four days. Subcutaneous plerixafor (240 mcg/kg based on actual body weight) and G-CSF (10 mcg/kg) are administered in the evening, followed by collection the next day. Plerixafor may be administered daily till the desired results are achieved but for a maximum of 4 days.

Q. Which of the following statement is wrong:
1. Hematopoietic colony assays are the fastest method for the determination of CD34+ cell content in an apheresis sample
2. Following infusion of the mobilized PBPCs, neutrophil recovery takes 8 to 10 days
3. Following infusion of mobilized PBPCs, platelet recovery takes 10 to 12 days for platelet recovery
4. A dose of 2 x 10^6 CD34+ cells/kg appears to be adequate for autologous HCT

Answer: Hematopoietic colony assays are the fastest method for the determination of CD34+ cell content in an apheresis sample

The hematopoietic colony assays are the best way to determine the CD34+ cell content but they are cumbersome and take a lot of time, that's why in most of the centres world-wide the CD34+ cell content is assayed by fluorescence acti-vated cell sorting (FACS). This is a rapid and reliable method.

The last option needs to be clarified. We must read the question very carefully. If the examiner asks, what is the ad-equate dose of CD34+ cells for an autologous HCT then 2 x 10_6 CD34+ cells/kg is the correct answer. But if the examiner asks about an matched sibling allo-HCT or haploidentical HCT then the dose is different; 2-5 x 10_6 CD34+ cells/kg and 10-20 x 10_6 CD34+ cells/kg, respectively. If these options are not provided then we may still choose 2 x 10_6 CD34+ cells/kg as our answer.

Notes on peripheral blood progenitor cells (PBPCs) versus bone marrow as source of stem cells:

1. For autologous HCT, generally PBPCs are preferred
2. For allogeneic HCT, the choice is more complicated
3. Engraftment is more rapid with PBPCs
4. When deciding which to use for an allogeneic HCT, PBSCs may be preferred for those at high risk of graft failure or infections in the early post-transplanta-tion period. The reason is that because as engraft-ment is more rapid with PBPCs, hematopoietic re-covery will be faster.
5. PBPCs are associated with higher rates of GVHD
6. The choice of stem cell source (PBPC or BM) does not appear to impact overall survival, disease-free sur-vival, or non-relapse or transplant-related mortal-

ity.

7. Some studies suggest that graft-versus-tumor effect is more pronounced with PBPCs and this may translate into better long-term outcomes.

Notes on conditioning regimens:

There are basically these following kinds of preparatory (also known as "conditioning") regimens:

1. Myeloablative conditioning (MAC) regimen: they result in profound pancytopenia which is long-lasting and usually irreversible. After MAC infusion of hematopoietic stem cells is a must

2. Nonmyeloablative (NMA) regimen: they result in minimal cytopenia and may not require stem cell support

3. Reduced intensity conditioning (RIC) regimen: they are an intermediate category of regimens that do not fit the definition of myeloablative or nonmyeloablative but they generally require stem cell support

Q. Which of the following is not an example of myeloablative conditioning:

1. Cy/TBI
2. Bu4/Cy
3. Flu/Bu2

4. BEAM

Answer: Flu/Bu2

Note that Flu/Bu4 is MAC but Flu/Bu2 is RIC.

The exact doses and schedules are out of the scope of this book and the reader is advised to go through a standard textbook to learn these protocols.

Other examples of MAC are melphalan (200 mg/m2), CVP regimen (carmustine, etoposide, cyclophosphamide) etc.

Q. Total body irradiation (TBI) is commonly used in the preparatory regimens of HCT. What is the maximally tolerated dose of TBI:
1. 10 Gy
2. 15 Gy
3. 20 Gy
4. 25 Gy

Answer: 15 Gy

Notes on NMA and RIC regimens:

1. In a nutshell, these approaches are different from the MAC regimens in their mechanism of action. The NMA and RIC regimens rely more on donor cellular immune effects (the graft versus tumor effect or GVT effect) and less on the cytotoxic effects of the preparative regimen to control the underlying disease.

2. They are associated with reduced transplant related mortality. And because they are better tolerated, they can be used in those patients, who can not tolerate MAC regimens.

3. The choice of these therapies should be carefully contemplated in context of the underlying disease and its biology. Not all cancer types are equally susceptible to the GVT effect. For example, Hodgkin's lymphoma and ALL are not as sensitive to the GVT effect.

4. Examples of NMA regimens include: Flu/TBI, TLI/ATG

5. Commonly used RIC regimens include: Flu/Mel, Flu/Bu2, Flu/Cy, Flu/Bu/TT and melphalan 140 mg/m2 or less.

6. As far as the comparison between NMA/RIC and MAC is concerned, there are no clear cut guidelines and the therapy depends more on the clinical factors and on a case by case basis. Generally, MAC regimens achieve superior relapse-free survival (RFS), but are associated with increased treatment-related mortality (TRM); as a result, overall survival (OS) is comparable with the two approaches.

Q. Which of the following is true about GVHD:
1. Classic acute GVHD cases present within 100 days of HCT and display features of acute GVHD. The diagnostic and distinctive features of chronic GVHD should be absent
2. Late onset acute GVHD cases present greater than 100 days post-HCT with features of acute GVHD. The diagnostic and distinctive features of chronic GVHD should be absent
3. Classic chronic GVHD cases may present at any time post-HCT but there should be no features of acute GVHD
4. All of the above

Answer: all of the above

Sometimes, acute and chronic GVHD are present simultaneously, these cases are known as the overlap syndrome or simply, "acute and chronic GVHD."

Some clinicians use the term hyper acute GVHD for patients developing acute GVHD within first 14 days of HCT.

Q. Which is the characteristic skin lesion found in acute GVHD:
1. Morbilliform rash
2. Purpuric patches
3. Maculopapular rash
4. Generalised eczema

Answer: maculopapular rash

Notes on staging of skin manifestations of acute GVHD:

1. Stage 1 – Maculopapular rash over <25 percent of body area
2. Stage 2 – Maculopapular rash over 25 to 50 percent of body area
3. Stage 3 – Generalized erythroderma
4. Stage 4 – Generalized erythroderma with bullous formation, often with desquamation

Q. The diagnosis of gastrointestinal involvement by acute GVHD requires pathologic evaluation of the tissue:
1. True
2. False

Answer: true

Although a negative biopsy doesn't rule out acute GVHD.

Notes on staging of acute GVHD involving GI tract:
1. Stage 1 – Diarrhea 500 to 1000 mL/day
2. Stage 2 – Diarrhea 1000 to 1500 mL/day
3. Stage 3 – Diarrhea 1500 to 2000 mL/day
4. Stage 4 – Diarrhea >2000 mL/day or pain or ileus

Notes:
Acute GVHD primarily involves skin, GI tract and liver. The involvement of liver alone is usually not seen and some degree of skin and/or GI tract involvement is there. To diagnose liver involvement by acute GVHD, biopsy is the procedure of choice but it may sometimes be tricky due to the risk of bleeding.

Staging of acute GVHD involving liver:
1. Stage 1 – Bilirubin 2 to 3 mg/dL

2. Stage 2 – Bilirubin 3 to 6 mg/dL
3. Stage 3 – Bilirubin 6 to 15 mg/dL
4. Stage 4 – Bilirubin >15 mg/dL

Q. Which of the following is not true about the IBMTR grading system for acute GVHD:
1. Grade A is stage 1 skin involvement alone with no liver or gastrointestinal involvement
2. Grade B is stage 2 skin involvement without gut or liver involvement
3. Grade C is stage 3 involvement of any organ system
4. Grade D is stage 4 involvement of any organ system

Answer: Grade B is stage 2 skin involvement wihout gut or liver involvement

In fact, grade B is stage 2 skin involvement **with or without stage 1 or 2** gut or liver involvement

There are many methods used for grading of acute GVHD. The most widely used ones are the Glucksberg grade (I-IV) and the International Bone Marrow Transplant Registry (IBMTR) grading system (A-D).

In both of the systems skin, gut and liver involvement is accounted for and in the Glucksberg system patient's performance status is also added.

Q. Which of the following cells are primarily responsible for development of acute GVHD:
1. T cells

2. B cells
3. Dendritic cells
4. Mast cells

Answer: T cells

Q. Clinically significant acute GVHD occurs in approximately what percent of patients who receive an allogeneic HCT, despite receiving intensive prophylaxis:
1. 10-20
2. 20-50
3. 60-80
4. >80%

Answer: 20-50%

Q. GVHD is a feared and common complication of allogeneic HCT. Which of the following is not true about acute GVHD:
1. Prophylaxis is a must to prevent GVHD but prophylaxis only decreases the risk, it doesn't eliminate the risk
2. The prophylaxis used for prevention of GVHD may lead to reduction of graft versus tumour (GVT) as well
3. The severity of acute GVHD is proportional to re-

duced survival outcomes
4. Increasing degrees of acute GVHD increase the risk of relapse

Answer: Increasing degrees of acute GVHD increase the risk of relapse

In fact, increasing degrees of acute GVHD **reduce** the risk of relapse.

An important point here is that GVHD and GVT share some common mechanisms and at present it is not entirely possible to separate these two. Allogeneic HCT has many advantages over autologous HCT, and one of the most important mechanism of action of allo-HCT is the GVT effect. So in future if such strategies may be devised that enable us to suppress only acute GVHD but spare GVT effect, then it would be the optimal situation.

Q. Which of the following is not true about acute GVHD:
1. The incidence of acute GVHD is more in those who receive HLA mismatched transplant
2. The incidence of acute GVHD is higher with male donor
3. Its incidence is lower with reduced intensity conditioning regimens

4. Its incidence is lower with umbilical cord blood compared with peripheral blood allogeneic HCT

Answer: The incidence of acute GVHD is higher with male donor

In fact the incidence in generally higher with female donor.

Notes on risk factors of acute GVHD:
1. Increasing degree of HLA mismatch
2. Female donor: if choice is available then male donor should be used. If female donor must be used then nulliparous females are preferred over parous female donors to reduce the risk of an anamnestic response to antigen exposure during pregnancy
3. Myeloablative conditioning regimens. However if the disease requires myeloablative conditioning then it has to be done and certain things can be done to reduce the intensity and severity of acute GVHD. A bone marrow or umbilical cord graft may be preferred in the setting of myeloablative conditioning, while peripheral blood progenitor cells may be preferred in the setting of reduced intensity conditioning.
4. Higher with peripheral blood or bone marrow than umbilical cord blood.

Notes on prophylaxis of acute GVHD:

I must say that this topic is very complex and an entire book may be written about just this topic. I will try to highlight the most important points here, and I would like to encourage you to go through a standard textbook for a better understanding of the subject.

1. There are two basic methods of prophylaxis of acute GVHD: T cell depletion and immunosuppressive therapy.

2. The most commonly used schedules are:

a. A short course of intravenous methotrexate (eg, given on days +1, +3, +6, and +11 after HCT) is combined with a six-month tapered course of cyclosporine

b. Methotrexate plus tacrolimus. This combination is considered at least as effective as methotrexate plus cyclosporine

c. Mycophenolate mofetil plus cyclosporine or tacrolimus. This combination is associated with reduced oral mucositis

3. Another strategy is T cell depletion. Note that T cell depletion is associated with significant lower grade III and IV acute GVHD compared with pharmacotherapy listed above. But these two modalities are associated with similar rates of chronic GVHD, transplant related mortality and relapse rates.

4. A combination of pharmacotherapy and T cell depletion is often used. Sometimes ATG may also be combined with these two, especially in cases at an excessively high risk of developing acute GVHD.

5. The most widely used regimen is methotrexate plus

cyclosporine. Cyclosporine is given IV for initial few days because the absorption of oral cyclosporine is erratic due to the presence of oral or gastrointestinal mucositis. The target concentration of cyclosporine is 200 to 300 mcg/L during the first three to four weeks then it may be reduced to 100 to 200 mcg/L if there is no GVHD. This concentration is maintained for three months and then it is tapered further.

6. Methotrexate in this regimen is administered on days +1, +3, +6, and +11. Leucovorin is used variably; some institutes use leucovorin routinely after 24 hours of each methotrexate dose while some measure levels of methotrexate and use if the measurements are higher than expected.

7. There are many side effects of both methotrexate and cyclosporine. Extreme precaution must be taken.

Notes on methods of T cell depletion:

1. Physical separation techniques
2. Density gradients
3. Selective depletion with lectins
4. Cytotoxic drugs
5. Anti T cell serum or monoclonal antibodies like anti-CD52, anti-CD2, anti-CD3, and anti-CD5 antibodies or antibodies with more restricted reactivity like anti-CD8 and anti-CD25.
6. In-vivo T cell depletion may be achieved with antithymocyte globulin or alemtuzumab

Q. HCT is associated with which of the following:

1. Expansion of Enterobacteriaceae population in the gut
2. Increased numbers of Clostridia in the gut
3. Reduction in bacterial diversity
4. All of the above

Answer: options 1 and 3 are correct

In fact, HCT is associated with **reduced** numbers of anti-inflammatory bacteria like Clostridia.

Many studies have been done on the subject of use of antibiotics to alter the gut bacteria population and its association with acute GVHD. Most experts use a quinolone, most often ciprofloxacin, starting a day before conditioning therapy and continuing till the engraftment has taken place.

Some studies showed superiority of a combination antibiotic regimen but this approach is not commonly used.

Q. Which is the most effective drug for the treatment of acute GVHD:

1. Methotrexate plus cyclosporine
2. Azathioprine plus infliximab
3. Prednisone
4. Methotrexate plus prednisone

Answer: prednisone

Read the question very carefully, it is asking what is the most effective drug for the **treatment**, not prophylaxis.

Note that while prednisone is the most effective drug for the treatment of acute GVHD, its role in prophylaxis of acute GVHD is not established.

Q. An experimental approach for reducing acute GVHD while maintaining graft versus tumour effect is TLI/ATG. It acts on which basic principle:
1. The regulatory T cells are relatively insensitive to radiation
2. Host natural killer cells are decreased by giving total lymphoid irradiation
3. Both of the above
4. None of the above

Answer: the regulatory T cells are relatively insensitive to radiation

The number of host natural killer cells are actually **increased** by giving total lymphoid irradiation (TLI). TLI in this setting is often combined with ATG.

Q. Which organ is least commonly affected in acute GVHD:
1. Skin
2. Gastrointestinal tract
3. Liver
4. Lung

Answer: lung

Three most commonly involved organs in acute GVHD are: skin, GI tract and liver. By definition acute GVHD presents within first 100 days of HCT, though most often it manifests within the first three weeks.

Q. Which of the following is not true:
1. Grade I acute GVHD by definition involves patients with a maculopapular rash over ≤10 percent of their body surface area
2. Evidence of liver or gastrointestinal tract involve-

ment must not be present in a patient with grade I acute GVHD

3. The most appropriate treatment of acute GVHD of grade I is control of local symptoms and optimisation of prophylaxis
4. None of the above

Answer: Grade I acute GVHD by definition involves patients with a maculopapular rash over ≤10 percent of their body surface area

In fact, grade I acute GVHD by definition involves patients with a maculopapular rash over ≤50 percent of their body surface area

Notes:
1. As we have noted above, grade I acute GVHD by definition involves patients with a maculopapular rash over ≤50 percent of their body surface area **and** there should be no involvement of liver or GI tract. All other manifestations are categorised as grade II or higher.
2. Grade I acute GVHD generally don't require a specific treatment. The management of grade I GVHD is directed towards treatment of symptoms and optimisation of prophylaxis regimen
3. Grade II or higher acute GVHD require treatment.

They are treated with glucocorticoids. Many drugs have been studied for treatment of acute grade II or higher GVHD, in combination with glucocorticoids but the results are not promising. Thus glucocorticoids alone remain the mainstay of treatment.

4. Methylprednisolone is the most commonly used steroid for treatment and the usual dose is 2 mg/kg per day in divided doses. It is important to gradually taper steroids when symptoms improve.

5. When acute GVHD is treated with steroids, the complete response rates range from 25 to 40 percent.

6. In patients having acute grade II or higher GVHD, involving the intestinal tract, a combination of systemic and oral **non-absorbable** steroids like budesonide and beclomethasone is used. Use of oral steroids in this setting is more effective than systemic steroids alone and allows for reduced doses of systemic steroids, thus reducing the associated toxicity.

Q. Which of the following patients with acute GVHD will be considered glucocorticoid resistant:

1. A patient having no response by day 5 of steroid course

2. A patient having worsening of GVHD by day 3 of steroid course

3. A patient having no response by day 7 of steroid course

4. A patient having worsening of GVHD by 2 weeks of

steroid course

Answer: a patient having no response by day 7 of steroid course

Although the assessment of response is a continuous process when treating a patient of acute GVHD with steroids but day 5 and day 7 are most important. If a patient has GVHD worsening on day 5 of steroid course **or** has no response on day 7 of steroid course, then he is considered steroid resistant.

The most commonly used drug in steroid resistant patients is MMF.

Options for treatment of steroid resistant acute GVHD:
1. Mycophenolate mofetil
2. Etanercept
3. Pentostatin
4. Sirolimus
5. Ruxolitinib
6. Alpha-1-antitrypsin
7. ATG
8. IL-2 receptor antibodies (daclizumab and basiliximab)
9. Brentuximab
10. Alemtuzumab

11. Tocilizumab
12. Mesenchymal stromal cells
13. Extracorporeal plasmapheresis

Notes on chronic graft-verus-host disease (GVHD):
Essential clinical features of chronic GVHD:

1. Skin involvement (the skin lesions in chronic GVHD resemble lichen planus or scleroderma)
2. Dry oral mucosa which is often associated with ulcerations and sclerosis
3. Gastrointestinal tract effects
4. Increasing levels of serum bilirubin

Q. Which of the following is not true:

1. Chronic GVHD can occur even while acute GVHD is going on
2. Higher degree of HLA mismatching is associated with increased incidence of chronic GVHD
3. Chronic GVHD is more common when the donor is male and recipient is female
4. When PBPCs are used as source of stem cells the incidence of chronic GVHD is higher compared with bone marrow or umbilical cord blood

Answer: Chronic GVHD is more common when the donor is male and recipient is female

In fact, just the opposite is true, i.e., chronic GVHD is more common when the donor is female and recipient is male

Notes on risk factors predisposing to chronic GVHD:
1. Higher degree of HLA mismatching
2. Older age of donor and/or recipient
3. Donor and recipient gender disparity (female donor to male recipient)
4. Alloimmunization of the donor (history of pregnancy, transfusions)
5. Source of stem cells (peripheral blood precursor cells [PBPC] rather than bone marrow or umbilical cord blood)
6. Prior acute GVHD
7. Administration of unirradiated donor buffy coat transfusions (eg, donor lymphocyte infusions)
8. Previous splenectomy
9. Cytomegalovirus seropositivity (donor and/or recipient)
10. Donor Epstein-Barr virus seropositivity

There are many other risk factors but the above mentioned ones are the most established.

Q. Which of the following organ is commonly involved in chronic GVHD but not in acute GVHD;

1. Skin

2. Liver

3. Lung

4. None of the above

Answer: lung

Skin, liver and gastrointestinal tract are commonly involved in both acute and chronic GVHD; although the manifestations are different. Lungs, on the other hand are one of the principal target organs involved in patients with chronic GVHD but they are only rarely affected in acute GVHD.

Q. Which of the following is not true about the skin manifestation of chronic GVHD:

1. Skin involvement is the most common clinical feature of chronic GVHD

2. Poikiloderma is not a diagnostic feature of chronic GVHD in itself

3. Depigmentation is not considered an unequivocal feature of chronic GVHD

4. A maculopapular rash may be seen in both acute and chronic GVHD

Answer: Poikiloderma is not a diagnostic feature of chronic GVHD in itself

Poikiloderma is in fact a diagnostic feature. When we say that a clinical feature is "diagnostic" for chronic GVHD, it means that we don't need to do any further tests before labelling the lesion as a manifestation of chronic GVHD. Other clinical features that are considered diagnostic of chronic GVHD involving skin are:

1. Lichen planus-like features

2. Sclerotic features

3. Morphea-like features

4. Lichen sclerosis-like features

Note that many patients who undergo HCT have changes in hairs and nails due to chronic GVHD but none of them are "diagnostic."

Q. Which of the following is not a "diagnostic" gynecologic manifestation of chronic GVHD:

1. Lichen planus-like features

2. Vaginal scarring

3. Vaginal stenosis

4. Vaginal ulcers

Answer: vaginal ulcers

Q. The presence of an esophageal web and strictures or stenosis in the upper to mid third of the esophagus is diagnostic of chronic GVHD:
1. True
2. False

Answer: true

Q. Which of the following is not a diagnostic criteria of bronchiolitis obliterans in an HCT recipient:
1. Forced expiratory volume in 1 second (FEV1)/forced vital capacity (FVC) ratio <0.7 **or** FEV1 <75 percent of predicted
2. Evidence of air trapping or small airway thickening or bronchiectasis on high resolution chest computed tomography, residual volume >120 percent, or pathologic confirmation of constrictive bronchiolitis
3. Absence of infection in the respiratory tract, documented with investigations directed by clinical

symptoms

4. Histologically, the bronchioles are destroyed with fibrous obliteration of the lumen; granulation tissue frequently extends into the alveolar ducts

Answer: Forced expiratory volume in 1 second (FEV1)/ forced vital capacity (FVC) ratio <0.7 **or** FEV1 <75 percent of predicted

I must admit that this question is a very difficult one. The option labelled wrong here is not entirely wrong, the only word wrong in the sentence is the word "**or**". One of the diagnostic criteria of BO is forced expiratory volume in 1 second (FEV1)/forced vital capacity (FVC) ratio <0.7 **and** FEV1 <75 percent of predicted.

Note here that a diagnosis of bronchiolitis obliterans requires **all** of the four above mentioned criteria.

Notes on the NIH consensus criteria for diagnosis of chronic GVHD:

1. Chronic GVHD can occur at any time point following allogeneic HCT
2. Chronic GVHD is a diagnosis of exclusion
3. There are "diagnostic features", which if present, establish the diagnosis of chronic GVHD without need of further investigation

4. On the other hand, there are "distinctive features". They are present in chronic GVHD but not in acute GVHD. But their presence is not sufficient for diagnosis of chronic GVHD and further testing has to be done to confirm the diagnosis.

5. To make a diagnosis of chronic GVHD, at least one diagnostic clinical sign of chronic GVHD must be present **or** at least one distinctive manifestation must be confirmed by pertinent biopsy or other relevant tests (eg, Schirmer test) in the same or another organ

Notes on grading system for chronic GVHD:

There are many grading systems available for chronic GVHD but only the NIH system has been prospectively validated, the details of which are as follows:

1. Mild: Involves two or fewer organs/sites with no clinically significant functional impairment

2. Moderate: Involves three or more organs/sites with no clinically significant functional impairment or at least one organ/site with clinically significant functional impairment, but no major disability

3. Severe: Major disability caused by chronic GVHD

Notes on prophylaxis of GVHD in patients receiving **myeloablative conditioning**:

1. The standard prophylaxis when using myeloabla-

tive conditioning is cyclosporine plus short course of methotrexate.

2. The initial dose of cyclosporine is 3 mg/kg/day and it is started on day -1. Initially it is given IV and when oral intake becomes possible, it is given orally. The first oral dose is **twice** the IV dose. Each daily dose is divided in two equal quantities and given at an interval of 12 hours.

3. The dose of cyclosporine in this setting needs to be modified depending on the serum levels of cyclosporine or toxicity. The serum levels should be monitored 12 hours after the dose, before giving a new dose. So, when we talk about the cyclosporine levels, we are referring the "trough" or lowest level before the next dose.

4. The target serum concentration of cyclosporine is 200 to 300 microgram/L for the initial four weeks of initiation and then 100 to 200 microgram/L for upto 3 months post HCT. After 3 months, if there is no GVHD then the dose is slowly tapered. The total duration of cyclosporine therapy is 6 months if there is no GVHD. Note that the tapering of the dose can not be done if GVHD is still present at 3 months.

5. The first dose of methotrexate is 15 mg/m2 by IV route, and it is given on day +1. Three additional doses of 10 mg/m2 are given by IV route are given on days +3, +6 and +11.

6. The dose of methotrexate is not modified but in some patients the day +11 dose may be omitted in case there is grade II or higher toxicity.

7. Most experts recommend that leucovorin should be

given when using methotrexate prophylaxis. Leu-covorin administration is started 24 hours after each methotrexate dose. The dosage is 15 mg x 3 given every six hours after methotrexate adminis-tration on day +1, the same dose x 4 given every six hours after methotrexate doses on days +3, +6 and +11.

8. ATG may be given in selected patients, especially those receiving transplant from an unrelated donor. ATG reduces the incidence of chronic GVHD and also improves quality of life. It is administered on days -3, -2 and -1. There are two formulations available, the dose of thymoglobulin is 2.5 mg/kg for three days (total 7.5 mg/kg).

Notes on prophylaxis of GVHD in patients receiving **reduced intensity conditioning**:

1. The most commonly used regimen is cyclosporine plus MMF.
2. The principles of administering cyclosporine are exactly the same as in patients receiving myeloa-blative conditioning when the IV followed by oral route is chosen (see above).
3. In many patients receiving reduced intensity condi-tioning, it is possible to directly use the oral route. When such is the case the dose is 12 mg/kg/day. This dose should be divided into two equal parts and ad-ministered 12 hours apart.
4. The dose of MMF is 30 mg/kg/day and it is started on

day +1. The dose should be divided into two equal parts and given 12 hours apart.

5. The dose of MMF needs to be adjusted according to toxicity.

6. The duration of mycophenolate mofetil prophylaxis is one month in sibling transplantations, and three months in transplantations from unrelated or mis-matched donor.

7. The dose of ATG, when used in patients receiving reduced intensity conditioning is the same as those who receive myeloablative conditioning (see above).

Notes on prophylaxis of GVHD in patients receiving umbilical cord blood transplant:

1. The prophylaxis in these patients is exactly the same as those receiving reduced intensity conditioning (see above).

Notes on **treatment** of acute GVHD:

1. Treatment is indicated in acute GVHD grade II or higher.

2. Methylprednisolone is the drug of choice.

3. The dose of methylprednisolone is 2 mg/kg per day, divided in two doses. The initial treatment is continued for 7 days and during this time dose modification is not done.

4. Methylprednisolone should be continued till all signs of acute GVHD have resolved and the dose

should be slowly tapered.

5. Failure of methylprednisolone is defined as no response after 7 days of therapy or clear progression after 5 days of therapy.

6. When acute GVHD involves skin, topical steroids may be used and when acute GVHD involves GIT, non-absorbable oral steroids, like budesonide 9 mg/kg/day as a single dose, are given.

7. In cases of failure of methylprednisolone, many second line drugs are available. But there is **no standard second line therapy** (discussed elsewhere).

Notes on **treatment** of chronic GVHD:

1. There are only two recommended treatment options for chronic GVHD: corticosteroids and cyclosporine

2. If the patient is not on any immunosuppressive drugs then corticosteroids are the drug of choice

3. If the patient is already on cyclosporine and develops chronic GVHD, corticosteroids are the drug of choice

4. If the patient is already on corticosteroids then cyclosporine is added and the dose of corticosteroids is increased

5. If the patient is already on both corticosteroids and cyclosporine, there is no standard treatment option

6. It is important to note that at least one month is required for a therapy to work, once chronic GVHD settles in. So changing therapy due to lack of re-

sponse, or sometimes even progression, during the first month, is not advisable

7. There are many second line options available and are routinely used, but none of them is a standard option

Q. Which of the following is not true about donor lymphocyte infusion (DLI):

1. The main mechanism of action of DLI is induction of a graft-versus-tumor (GVT) effect
2. DLI is thought to mediate GVT primarily via reversal of T cell exhaustion in resident CD4+ T cells
3. Patients who respond to DLI usually demonstrate a clinical response within two to three months, but a full response may take one year or longer
4. Cell doses <0.01 x 108 T cells/kg appear to be suboptimal and doses above 4.5 x 108 T cells/kg do not appear to improve response

Answer: DLI is thought to mediate GVT primarily via reversal of T cell exhaustion in resident CD4+ T cells

In fact, DLI is thought to mediate GVT primarily via reversal of T cell exhaustion in resident **CD8+ T cells.**

Q. When using PBPCs for allogenic HCT, when will the engraftment take place sufficiently to support hematopoiesis:
1. 14 to 21 days
2. 10 to 14 days
3. 28 to 36 days
4. 7 to 10 days

Answer: 10 to 14 days

If bone marrow is used then generally 14 to 21 days are needed.

Q. In allogeneic HCT recipients, if blood product transfusion is indicated then why it is recommend that blood products should be irradiated:
1. To reduce transmission of infections
2. To prevent graft versus host disease
3. To reduce chances of TRALI
4. To enhance graft versus tumor effect

Answer: to prevent graft versus host disease

It should be clearly understood that irradiation of blood products in this setting has many benefits but the primary reason for irradiating is to deplete the leukocytes of the donor from the blood product. If these leukocytes are not depleted then they will enter the immunocompromised recipient and will produce a **transfusion associated graft versus host disease (ta-GVHD).**

Q. Which of the following is true:
1. All cytomegalovirus (CMV)-negative patients who receive bone marrow cells from a CMV-negative donor should receive seronegative blood products
2. Platelet transfusion is indicated for platelet counts less than 50,000/microL or for higher values if clinical bleeding is present
3. G-CSF or GM-CSF may be used in the setting of allogeneic HCT in patients who are experiencing delayed neutrophil recovery
4. Erythropoietin (EPO) does not appear to be of benefit immediately following allogeneic or autologous transplant

Answer: Platelet transfusion is indicated for platelet counts less than 50,000/microL or for higher values if clinical bleeding is present

There are no concrete guidelines for platelet transfusions in the setting of HCT, but many experts and the centres worldwide believe that platelet transfusions are indicated for platelet counts less than **10,000/microL** or for higher values if clinical bleeding is present.

Q. Which of the following is a relative contraindication of allogeneic HCT in follicular lymphoma (FL):
1. Relapsed or refractory FL
2. FL with histologic transformation
3. Chemotherapy-resistant disease
4. Relapse after chemoimmunotherapy

Answer: Chemotherapy-resistant disease

Note that the patient has to have **chemotherapy sensitive disease,** if optimal outcomes are to be expected after allogeneic HCT. That being said, allogeneic HCT has been done in chemotherapy resistant disease also but the results have been suboptimal. Hence chemotherapy resistant disease is a relative contraindication to allogeneic HCT in follicular lymphoma.

Generally, **autologous** HCT is performed in follicular lymphoma. Autologous HCT is chosen for patients with relapsed disease, especially in those who have had short remissions (eg, significantly less than the mean PFS for an individual treatment regimen, often <2 years). The disease should be chemotherapy sensitive, if autologous HCT is to be performed.

Q. In relapsed follicular lymphoma, autologous HCT has

been associated with a treatment-related mortality rate and a potential cure rate of:
1. <10% and 25 to 40%, respectively
2. <5% and 50 to 60%, respectively
3. 10 to 15% and 10 to 30%, respectively
4. >20% and <30%, respectively

Answer: <10% and 25 to 40%, respectively

Q. A patient of relapsed follicular lymphoma undergoes an autologous HCT, which results in complete remission. What will be the most appropriate strategy following transplantation:
1. Observation
2. 6 cycles of chemoimmunotherapy
3. Rituximab maintenance
4. Ibrutinib maintenance

Answer: rituximab maintenance

Notes on HCT in specific situations:
1. Allogeneic (HCT) is commonly used as part of the post-remission therapy of patients with acute lymphoblastic leukemia (ALL). The indictions for this depend on the guidelines that an institute follows; it is usually done in those who demonstrate high-risk features, such as the presence of the Philadelphia chromosome. It can be performed in the first or second complete remission. Total body irradiation (TBI) plus cyclophosphamide is the most com-

monly used regimen but many others, including RIC regimens, are also being used. An interesting point is that the GVL (graft versus leukaemia) effect is not very pronounced in ALL.

2. Allogeneic HCT may be used for young patients with clinically aggressive relapsed or refractory CLL or those with high-risk genetic factors including 17p13 abnormalities and TP53 mutation. Another important indication is the Richter's transformation. But note that neither auto- nor allo-HCT are routinely used in CLL and because many newer molecules are available now, the indications for performing an HCT are gradually shrinking. If HCT must be done, then most of the times an RIC regimen is used because most of the patients who reach that stage are elderly, have comorbidities and are often heavily pretreated.

3. The topic of allogeneic HCT in CML is a difficult one, because such good TKIs are now available that most of the centres don't use HCT till all options have been exhausted. When it is to be done, then BuCy is the conditioning regimen of choice. Cure rates depend on the stage of disease, with long term survival being upto 80%, 50% and 30% in CML-CP, CMP-AP and CML-BC, respectively.

4. Autologous HCT has an impressive cure rate of about 50% in patients with classical Hodgkin's lymphoma that relapse after initial complete response (CR) or failed to achieve initial CR (primary refractory cHL). For conditioning of the patient for auto-HCT, BEAM is the preferred regimen and PBPCs are the preferred source of stem cells. In some patients of classical HL, allogeneic HCT may be used.

5. If a patient of classical Hodgkin's lymphoma undergoes auto-HCT and is at high risk of relapse or progression (ie, primary refractory disease, relapse

<12 months after initial therapy, or relapse with ex-tranodal disease), maintenance therapy with bren-tuximab vedotin till progression is preferred ra-ther than observation. Brentuximab can't be used in those who already have received brentuxiamb and progressed on it, before undergoing an auto-HCT.

6. Most experts recommend proceeding directly to al-logeneic HCT in patient with severe or very severe aplastic anemia who are under age 50 years (rather than using immunosuppressive therapy). In patients with AA who are candidates for HCT, bone marrow is the preferred source of stem cells (rather than per-ipheral blood).

7. In children with Fanconi anemia, who cannot toler-ate the supportive measures, androgens and growth factors; or who have developed severe bone mar-row failure, myelodysplasia, or acute myeloid leuke-mia, allogeneic HCT is the only treatment option. Fludarabine is an important conditioning agent for this indication.

8. Allogeneic HCT is the only curative therapy for thalassemia. It is usually used in patients who have undergone therapy with transfusion support and iron chelation. PBPCs are **not** the preferred source of stem cells in this setting and stem cells either from bone marrow or umbilical cord blood are preferred. Many centres use the Pesaro system for risk stratifi-cation of thalassemia patients, this system is based on iron overload. There is more than 90 percent like-lihood of cure, especially in children less than 14 years of age. Standard myeloablative conditioning regimens include busulfan and cyclophosphamide. It is important to note that stabilisation of hemato-poiesis after HCT may take upto 2 years.

9. Allogeneic HCT offers a potentially curative option in patients with sickle cell disease. It is indicated

in patients who have vaso-occlusive complications that are not well controlled with medical therapy. A 96% cure rate can be achieved in carefully selected patients. It is important to note here that PBPCs are **not** the preferred source of stem cells.

10. Allogeneic HCT is effective in the treatment of Diamond Blackfan anemia unresponsive to glucocorticoid therapy. Long-term survival is achieved in approximately 75% of patients.

11. Multiple myeloma:

a. High-dose therapy followed by autologous HCT is considered the standard of care. It may be done early (which is done after a fixed number of cycles of chemotherapy) or it may be done in "delayed" fashion (in which chemo is continued till relapse and once the patient relapses then auto-HCT is done).

b. Note that auto-HCT is **not curative** for multiple myeloma. It improves the survival outcomes compared with standard myeloma directed therapy alone.

c. On the other hand, allogeneic HCT in myeloma may prove to be curative but is associated with substantial transplant related mortality.

d. Induction chemotherapy is administered for approximately four months prior to stem cell collection. Regimens used are many, but the most common ones are VRd and VCd. It is important to note that melphalan containing regimens should not be used, because melphalan causes stem cell damage. Another important point to remember is that more than four months of initial therapy should also not be given, because prolonged initial therapy may also harm stem cells.

e. Both PBPCs and bone marrow may be used for auto-HCT but PBPCs are preferred. Either G-CSF or G-CSF plus cyclophosphamide may be used for mobilising stem cells for collection from peripheral blood. Plerixafor is a reserved agent.

f. Apheresis is begun when the peripheral CD34+ counts reach 10 CD34 cells/microL. The goal of aphaeresis is collecting at least 3 x 106 CD34+ cells/kg if only one transplant is being considered, or at least 6 x 106 CD34+ cells/kg if two transplants are being considered. (2 x 106 CD34+ cells/kg is considered essential for one transplant).

g. PBPCs are cryopreserved in 5 percent dimethylsulfoxide. They should be thawed at the bedside at the time of infusion.

h. These collected cells are contaminated with tumor cells. Some experts suggest purging of tumor cells from the collected PBPCs. There are two methods for this: 1. cells can be identified and isolated by CD34+ or CD34+/Thy1+ selection. 2. Tumour cells can be purged by using a combination of monoclonal antibodies. But remember that there is no evidence of a clinical benefit with these methods and thus, most centres don't attempt to purge myeloma cells from PBPC collections.

i. Basically there are two options, once patient has received around 4 months of initial therapy. They can proceed directly with HCT (early transplant) or they can continue induction therapy with transplant being done at the time of early relapse (delayed transplant).

j. In many trials, early transplantation resulted in deeper responses and improved progression-free survival (PFS), but no clear overall survival (OS) benefit. This benefit is most apparent in patient with **high-risk** multiple myeloma.

k. Some times a second (tandem) preplanned transplant may be done. When it is contemplated, it should be done within 6 to 12 months of the first transplant. Tandem transplantation has not improved outcomes in standard-risk myeloma. In high-risk myeloma some studies have suggested better outcomes compared with single transplant, but the evidence is very flimsy and that's why most centres **do not** perform tandem HCT.

l.   The standard conditioning regimen used for HCT in MM isf melphalan at a dose of 200 mg/m2. Dose may be reduced depending on the age and comorbidities.

m.   Trials have compared 200 mg/m2 melphalan with variants like a) melphalan 140 mg/m2 plus 8 Gy TBI and b) melphalan 100 mg/m2. In both of these trials melphalan 200 mg/m2 resulted in better outcomes.

n.   Most experts recommend that the dose of melphalan should be reduced to 140 mg/m2 if creatinine is >2 mg/dL. Melphalan is generally used at dose of 140 mg/m2 in patients more than 70 years of age.

o.   After approximately 24 hours after completion of the preparative chemotherapy, peripheral blood progenitor cells (PBPCs) are reinfused in the patient.

p.   Neutrophil engraftment usually occurs by day 12 and platelet counts are expected to recover to greater than 20,000/microL by day 16.

q.   About 40 percent of patients with multiple myeloma undergoing autologous HCT will experience febrile neutropenia. Prophylactic antibacterial, antifungal and antiviral therapies are indicated in these patients.

r.   It is important to understand, once again, that autologous HCT is **not curative** for multiple myeloma. Thus even after a patient undergoes auto-HCT, some form of therapy should be given as maintenance therapy. Maintenance therapy has consistently shown improved outcomes in studies.

s.   Most experts recommend **a minimum of 2 years**

of maintenance therapy. For standard-risk patients, lenalidomide is used, whereas for high risk patients, bortezomib is indicated. Ixazomib may be used in patients who are not able to tolerate bortezomib.

t. Monitoring of the disease after transplant must be done. International myeloma working group criteria are used worldwide for this purpose.

u. If a patient of multiple myeloma relapses after autologous HCT, the treatment options are not well defined. Options include a second autologous HCT (experts recommend not performing another auto-HCT in a patient who relapses within 12 to 18 months of first auto-HCT), nonmyeloablative allogeneic HCT, or treatment with salvage chemotherapy.

Q. Which of the following statement is not true about CMV infection and allogeneic HCT:

1. Patients should undergo testing with CMV quantitative polymerase chain reaction (PCR) two weeks prior to commencing the conditioning regimen and should receive anti-CMV therapy if found to have CMV viremia

2. The development of CMV infection prior to allogeneic transplantation is associated with a high risk of death after HCT

3. Ganciclovir, valganciclovir or foscarnet may be used to prevent CMV disease

4. The conditioning regimen may be started during antiviral therapy with ganciclovir or valganciclovir but not with foscarnet, because foscarnet has add-

itional myelosuppressive effects

Answer: The conditioning regimen may be started during antiviral therapy with ganciclovir or valganciclovir but not with foscarnet, because foscarnet has additional myelosuppressive effects

This important concept needs to be understood. It is very important that CMV infection should be cleared or controlled before starting the conditioning regimen but in some cases we may proceed with conditioning regimen while the anti-CMV therapy is ongoing.

If we choose to give conditioning regimen while anti-CMV therapy is being given then we must switch the patient to foscarnet, before we start conditioning regimen. This is so because ganciclovir and valganciclovir have myelosuppressive effects and giving these drugs with the conditioning regimen will lead to excessive toxicity.

Notes on infections present in the **donor,** which make the hematopoietic cell donation contraindicated:
1. HIV infection
2. Acute cytomegalovirus (CMV) or Epstein-Barr virus (EBV) infection
3. Acute hepatitis A infection (as determined by a positive hepatitis A IgM)

4. Zika virus
5. Acute toxoplasmosis
6. Active tuberculosis (until it is well controlled)
7. An acute tickborne infection, such as Rocky Mountain spotted fever, babesiosis, anaplasmosis, ehrlichiosis, Q fever, or Colorado tick fever
8. Active or past history of Chagas disease
9. Acute or recent West Nile Virus infection

There are many other infections, which may be present in a donor and will make the donor not a suitable candidate if another donor is available. But apart from the above mentioned infections, no other infection present in the donor is an absolute contraindication.

Q. HCT candidates should receive live virus vaccines:
1. ≥4 weeks prior to the initiation of the conditioning regimen
2. ≥6 weeks prior to the initiation of the conditioning regimen
3. ≥8 weeks prior to the initiation of the conditioning regimen
4. They should not receive live virus vaccines before successful engraftment

Answer: ≥4 weeks prior to the initiation of the conditioning regimen

If the patient is to receive **inactivated** virus vaccines then the he should receive them ≥2 weeks prior to the initiation of the conditioning regimen

Q. Which of the following statement is not true:
1. Inactivated vaccines are less immunogenic in HCT recipients compared with immunocompetent individuals
2. Live virus vaccines should not be administered during the first 24 months following HCT
3. MMR vaccine should be given beginning 24 months following transplantation, especially in those patients who are receiving immunosuppression for acute GVHD
4. Recombinant zoster vaccine is indicated in autologous HCT recipients ≥18 years of age, with the first dose given 50 to 70 days following transplant and a second dose given one to two months later

Answer: MMR vaccine should be given beginning 24 months following transplantation, especially in those patients who are receiving immunosuppression for acute GVHD

MMR vaccine should indeed be given beginning 24 months following transplantation but **there must be no ongoing**

GVHD and the patient must not be receiving any immuno-suppression.

Q. Which of the following is not associated with an increased risk of HCT related infections:
1. HCT in a patient with CLL who has been treated with a purine analog previously
2. Iron deficiency
3. Myeloablative conditioning regimens
4. T cell depletion

Answer: iron deficiency

In fact, iron **overload** is associated with an increased risk of infections.

Q. Which of the following is not true:
1. In the pre-engraftment period, diarrhea is commonly caused by *Clostridioides difficile*
2. Diffuse pulmonary infiltrates during the preengraftment period are mostly due to noninfectious causes
3. In the early postengraftment period, hemorrhagic cystitis is most commonly due to adenovirus
4. During the late postengraftment period, sinopulmonary infections, are frequently caused by encap-

sulated bacteria

Answer: In the early postengraftment period, hemorrhagic cystitis is most commonly due to adenovirus

In fact, it is due to BK polyoma virus.

Notes:
There are three periods:
1. Preengraftment – From transplantation to approximately day 30
2. Early postengraftment – From engraftment to day 100
3. Late postengraftment – After day 100

Q. Which of the following is not true:
1. Fluoroquinolone prophylaxis is recommended for allogeneic HCT recipients who have received myeloablative conditioning regimen
2. Levofloxacin is favoured in patients with increased risk for oral mucositis-related *Streptococcus viridans* infection
3. Reduced intensity conditioning regimens do not require antibiotic prophylaxis generally
4. Antibiotic prophylaxis with a fluoroquinolone should not be given in autologous HCT patients

Answer: Antibiotic prophylaxis with a fluoroquinolone

should not be given in autologous HCT patients

While it's true that autologous HCT patients do not routinely require antibiotic prophylaxis, but the statement that **fluoroquinolone should not be given,** is wrong. Fluoroquinolone prophylaxis is given in autologous HCT patients, especially those having hematologic malignancies and in whom the chemotherapy regimen used is expected to produce significant mucosal injury or if comorbidities are such that will lead to increased toxicity from the procedure.

Q. Cytokine release syndrome is associated with:
1. Chimeric antigen receptor (CAR)-T cell therapy
2. Monoclonal antibodies
3. Haploidentical allogeneic transplantation
4. All of the above

Answer: all of the above

Q. Cytokine release syndrome is commonly associated with CAR-T cell therapy. Its incidence is highest in which of the following malignancies:
1. ALL
2. CLL
3. NHL
4. Multiple myeloma

Answer: ALL

Q. Which of the following cells are primarily responsible for cytokine release syndrome:
1. T cells
2. B cells
3. Dendritic cells
4. Bone marrow stromal cells

Answer: T cells

Q. Cytokine release syndrome usually begins when after haploidentical hematopoietic cell transplantation:
1. Within 1 to 3 days
2. After 3 days but before 7 days
3. After 7 to 14 days
4. After engraftment

Answer: within 1 to 3 days

Although the clinical course is variable, CRS in this setting usually resolves after a few days, as opposed to many weeks in certain other scenarios.

Q. In cytokine release syndrome manifestations, the term ICANS is used for involvement of which organ:
1. Bone marrow
2. CNS
3. Muscles
4. Kidneys

Answer: CNS

The term ICANS stands for immune effector cell-associated neurotoxicity syndrome (ICANS).

It is also known as cytokine release encephalopathy syndrome (CRES).

Q. Which of the following is an essential criterion for diagnosis of cytokine release syndrome:
1. Fever ($\geq 38.0°C$)
2. Hypotension
3. End-organ dysfunction
4. All of the above are essential criteria

Answer: Fever ($\geq 38.0°C$)

Note that only fever is a manifestation that **must** be present. All other manifestations may or may not be there, depending on the severity of CRS.

Q. If a patient who has undergone haploidentical HCT, presents with CRS having hypotension that can be managed with one pressor, it will be classified as which grade according to NCI-CTCAE:
1. Grade 1
2. Grade 2
3. Grade 3
4. Grade 4

Answer: grade 3

Notes on NCI-CTCAE grading of CRS associated with HCT (note that there are different criteria for CAR-T cell associated CRS):
1. Grade 1: Fever, with or without constitutional symptoms
2. Grade 2: Hypotension responding to fluids. Hypoxia responding to <40 percent FiO2
3. Grade 3: Hypotension managed with one pressor. Hypoxia requiring ≥40 percent FiO2
4. Grade 4: Life-threatening consequences; urgent intervention needed

Q. For treatment of haploidentical HCT related severe cytokine release syndrome, which of the following is the drug of choice:

1. Corticosteroids
2. Tocilizumab
3. Corticosteroids plus tocilizumab
4. Infliximab with or without corticosteroids

Answer: corticosteroids

In case of severe CRS associated with CAR-T cell therapy, the combination of corticosteroid plus tocilizumab is the preferred option. In all other indications, corticosteroids alone are the drug of choice.

Q. Hepatic sinusoidal obstruction syndrome (SOS) most often occurs in:

1. Patients undergoing HCT
2. Use of high dose melphalan
3. Ingestion of alkaloid toxins
4. High dose radiation therapy

Answer: patients undergoing HCT

Hepatic sinusoidal obstruction syndrome (SOS) is also seen in other conditions mentioned above. Another important cause of hepatic sinusoidal obstruction syndrome (SOS) is liver transplantation.

Gemtuzumab and inotuzumab may lead to hepatic sinusoidal obstruction syndrome (SOS).

Q. In hepatic sinusoidal obstruction syndrome (SOS), the hepatic venous outflow obstruction is due to occlusion of:
1. Terminal hepatic venules
2. Hepatic sinusoids
3. Hepatic veins
4. Inferior vena cava

Answer: 1 and 2 both are correct

But the single most correct answer will be terminal hepatic venules.

The most basic mechanism of development of hepatic sinusoidal obstruction syndrome (SOS) is injury to hepatic venous endothelium.

Q. Which of the following statement is wrong about hepatic sinusoidal obstruction syndrome (SOS) associated with HCT:

1. It is more common in patients with pre-existing liver disease
2. It's incidence is higher with high dose cyclphosphamide
3. It is more common in patients with poor baseline performance status
4. The rates are higher in adolescents and adults compared to children

Answer: The rates are higher in adolescents and adults compared to children

In fact the rates are higher in children, especially those < 7 years of age.

There are many risk factors for hepatic sinusoidal obstruction syndrome (SOS), some important ones are:

1. Preexisting liver diseases like hepatitis, cirrhosis, hepatitis B or C infections
2. High dose chemotherapy, especially high dose cyclophosphamide. But other regimens used in conditioning like busulfan may lead to hepatic sinusoidal obstruction syndrome (SOS). Another important risk factor for the development of Hepatic

sinusoidal obstruction syndrome (SOS) is sirolimus, especially when used in combination with busulfan.
3. Drugs like gemtuzumab and inotuzumab
4. Reduced lung diffusion capacity
5. Female sex

Q. The most common time of onset of hepatic sinusoidal obstruction syndrome (SOS) after HCT is:
1. Within 3 weeks of HCT
2. After 3 weeks but within 3 months
3. After 3 months but within one year
4. It is more of a delayed complication, seen after prolonged periods of time

Answer: within 3 weeks of HCT

In one study the peak incidence was noted at 12 days after HCT.

Q. Which of the following is not true:
1. Weight loss is one of the earliest signs of hepatic sinusoidal obstruction syndrome (SOS)
2. A transjugular liver biopsy should be used instead of a percutaneous biopsy when liver biopsy is used to confirm the diagnosis of Hepatic sinusoidal obstruction syndrome (SOS)

3. A hepatic venous pressure gradient greater than 10 mmHg is highly correlated with the presence of Hepatic sinusoidal obstruction syndrome (SOS)
4. Abnormalities of hemostasis are commonly seen in Hepatic sinusoidal obstruction syndrome (SOS)

Answer: weight loss is one of the earliest signs of hepatic sinusoidal obstruction syndrome (SOS)

In fact, **weight gain** is one of the earliest signs of hepatic sinusoidal obstruction syndrome (SOS).

Q. The modified Seattle criteria used to define hepatic sinusoidal obstruction syndrome (SOS) include all of the following except:
1. Serum conjugated bilirubin > 3 mg/dL
2. Hepatomegaly
3. Right upper quadrant pain
4. > 2% increase in the baseline body weight

Answer: serum conjugated bilirubin > 3 mg/dL

The Seattle criteria are used to define hepatic sinusoidal obstruction syndrome (SOS). The diagnosis is considered when two or more of the following three features are present within the first 20 days of HCT. If should be noted that all other aetiologies must be ruled out.

1. Serum **total** bilirubin concentration greater than 2 mg/dL
2. Hepatomegaly or right upper quadrant pain
3. Sudden weight gain due to fluid accumulation (>2 percent of baseline body weight)

Q. Which of the following is not a feature of the Baltimore criteria used to define hepatic sinusoidal obstruction syndrome (SOS):

1. Bilirubin >2 mg/dL within 21 days of HCT

2. Hepatomegaly

3. Ascites

4. Weight gain >2 percent from pre-HCT weight

Answer: weight gain >2 percent from the pre-HCT weight

The Baltimore criteria for defining hepatic sinusoidal obstruction syndrome (SOS) are: the presence of bilirubin >2 mg/dL within 21 days of HCT with two or more of the following:

1. Hepatomegaly
2. Ascites
3. Weight gain >**5%** from pre-HCT weight

We must note here that hepatic sinusoidal obstruction syndrome (SOS) is a clinical diagnosis. Imaging studies and liver biopsy or other invasive procedures are usually not needed for diagnosis of Hepatic sinusoidal obstruction syndrome (SOS).

Q. Which of the following is not true about prophylaxis of hepatic sinusoidal obstruction syndrome (SOS) in patients undergoing allogeneic HCT:

1. Ursodeoxycholic acid 12 mg/kg daily is used by many experts, starting from the day preceding the preparative regimen and continued for the first month of transplantation

2. For most patients undergoing autologous HCT, low dose heparin is an effective prophylactic agent

3. Defibrotide has demonstrated efficacy in the prevention of Hepatic sinusoidal obstruction syndrome (SOS) in children at high risk of developing Hepatic sinusoidal obstruction syndrome (SOS) but not in adults

4. Low dose heparin prophylaxis, when used, should be continued till engraftment

Answer: Ursodeoxycholic acid 12 mg/kg daily is used by many experts, starting from the day preceding the preparative regimen and continued for the first month of transplantation

The dose here is correct but the timing is not. In fact, UDCA is continued for the **first three months** of transplantation.

Give special attention to the third option. While its true that studies have not found as robust efficacy of defibrotide in adults as in children but it is still used in adults, especially in severe cases.

Q. Which of the following is not correct:
1. In patients undergoing myeloablative conditioning therapy, oral cryotherapy helps in prevention of oral mucositis
2. Photobiomodulation using laser is recommended by NCCN guidelines for prevention of HCT associated oral mucositis
3. Palifermin, a recombinant keratinocyte growth factor, is useful in prevention of not only in HCT induced oral mucositis but also in control of mucosal toxicity in other parts of GI tract
4. Clinical practice guidelines recommend the use of palifermin for prophylaxis of oral mucositis in patients undergoing autologous HCT

Answer: Palifermin, a recombinant keratinocyte growth

factor, is useful in prevention of not only in HCT induced oral mucositis but also in control of mucosal toxicity in other parts of GI tract

Palifermin is approved for use in prevention of **oral mucositis only.** It does not have any significant action on other parts of GI tract. Most experts don't use it because of its prohibitively high cost and its lack of activity on other parts of GI tract.

Note here that G-CSF/GM-CSF, parenteral glutamine and pentoxyfylline have **no role** in prevention of oral mucositis induced by HCT.

Q. Which of the following is the most common cause of persistent acute diarrhoea following allogeneic HCT:
1. CMV infection
2. Clostridium infection
3. Acute GVHD
4. Mucositis induced by conditioning regimen

Answer: acute GVHD

So, we must be alert of this possibility and immunosuppressive medications have to be started if the clinical suspicion is sufficiently high. Infections are less common causes of post-HCT diarrhoea but it is very important to exclude them before starting immunosuppressive medicines for acute GVHD.

Q. Which of the following is not a feature of the cord colitis syndrome:
1. It is seen in recipients of umbilical cord blood grafts
2. Viral and bacterial cultures are negative
3. Colon biopsy shows chronic active colitis
4. Granulomas are characteristically absent in biopsy specimens from colon

Answer: Granulomas are characteristically absent in biopsy specimens from colon

Colon biopsy shows chronic active colitis and **granulomas are sometimes present.**

Q. Which of the following is not correct:
1. Acute kidney injury following HCT most often develops 10 to 21 days after HCT
2. Myeloablative regimens are associated with a higher incidence of AKI compared with nonmyeloablative regimens

3. The majority of patients who have AKI as a consequence of HCT do not require dialysis
4. The long-term renal prognosis of AKI following total body irradiation (TBI) is very very poor

Answer: The long-term renal prognosis of AKI following total body irradiation (TBI) is very poor

In fact, the long-term renal prognosis of AKI following total body irradiation (TBI) is good.

Q. In cases of thrombotic microangiopathy after HCT, plasma exchange is a helpful treatment strategy:
1. True
2. False

Answer: false

The fact is that the results of plasma exchange in this setting are disappointing, despite it being an effective modality for the treatment of thrombotic microangiopathy induced by other etiologies like TTP.

Q. All of the following second malignancies usually occur more than 3 years after HCT except:
1. Solid tumors
2. Acute leukaemia
3. Myelodysplastic syndromes
4. Post-transplant lymphoproliferative disease

Answer: PTLD

PTLD usually occurs within one year of HCT.

Q. Which of the following is not correct:
1. When lenalidomide is used as maintenance in multiple myeloma patients post-HCT, it increases the chances of developing a second malignancy
2. Generally patients undergoing HCT have a two-fold increased risk of developing a second malignancy compared with general population
3. Patients who have undergone HCT, are at a higher risk of developing melanoma of skin and to a lesser extent basal cell carcinoma of skin
4. Most of the leukemias that develop in survivors of HCT, as a consequence of HCT, are of myeloid lineage

Answer: Patients who have undergone HCT, are at a higher risk of developing melanoma of skin and to a lesser extent basal cell carcinoma of skin

In fact, the chances of developing non-melanoma skin cancer (NMSC) are higher than melanoma in patients who have undergone HCT.

Q. Which of the following is not true about post-transplant lymphoproliferative disease developing after HCT:
1. It is associated with Epstein-Barr virus (EBV)
2. About 50% of cases occur within the first year of HCT
3. PTLD is associated with T cell depletion during HCT
4. The highest incidence in seen in the first five months post-HCT

Answer: about 50% of cases occur within the first year of HCT.

This important concept should be understood clearly that PTLD mostly occurs within the first year post HCT and after the first year the incidence of PTLD exponentially declines. The majority of cases occur within the first five months.

Q. Which of the following is not true:
1. The risk of secondary malignancy is not higher in

    patients who have undergone transplantation for severe aplastic anemia compared to general population

2. Female HCT survivors should undergo screening for breast cancer beginning no later than age 40 years
3. Woman who received radiation to the chest between the age of 10 and 35 years should undergo screening with both annual breast magnetic resonance imaging (MRI) and mammography
4. The cumulative incidence rates of developing second solid cancers in allogeneic HCT survivors is 1 to 2 percent at 10 years

Answer: The risk of secondary malignancy is not higher in patients who have undergone transplantation for severe aplastic anemia compared to general population

In fact, the risk is especially high in aplastic anemia patients who have undergone HCT.

Q. The halo sign on chest imaging is seen in which of the following pulmonary infection post-HCT:
1. Nocardia
2. Aspergillus
3. CMV
4. All of the above

Answer: aspergillus

The halo sign is produced by *Aspergillus,* which is a surrounding ground glass opacity. This ground glass opacity results from angioinvasion and hemorrhage into the surrounding tissue. But note that this sign may be seen with other fungi as well.

Q. Patients with severe hepatic veno-occlusive disease can present with:
1. Cardiogenic pulmonary edema
2. Noncardiogenic pulmonary edema
3. Pleural effusion
4. All of the above

Answer: all of the above

Q. Which of the following is not true about engraftment syndrome:
1. It is more common with autologous HCT and only rarely seen after allogeneic HCT
2. It develops around 7 to 11 days following HCT during the time of neutrophil recovery
3. The dermal biopsy of skin lesions due to engraft-

    ment syndrome characteristically shows presence of lymphocytic infiltration
4. None of the above

Answer: The dermal biopsy of skin lesions due to engraftment syndrome characteristically shows presence of lymphocytic infiltration

Note that engraftment syndrome is more common in autologous HCT (around 10% incidence) but only rarely it is seen after allogeneic HCT.

Q. Which of the following is true:
1. Hyperacute GVHD occurs in the first 14 days post-transplant
2. Hyper acute GVHD is associated with noncardiogenic pulmonary edema but skin involvement is not there
3. Acute GVHD develops in the first 100 days following autologous HCT
4. Pulmonary involvement is commonly seen in acute GVHD

Answer: hyperacute GVHD occurs in the first 14 days post-transplant

Read each option carefully. The other three options are wrong.

Q. Which of the following is not true about idiopathic pneumonia syndrome:

1. It generally occurs after four months of HCT
2. The alveolar-arterial oxygen gradient is increased
3. Lower respiratory tract infections are absent
4. It is more common with myeloablative regimens compared with reduced intensity conditioning regimens

Answer: It generally occurs after four months of HCT

In fact, it generally occurs **within** four months after HCT.

Q. Diffuse alveolar haemorrhage occurs more commonly with:

1. Autologous HCT
2. Allogeneic HCT with myeloablative conditioning
3. Allogeneic HCT with reduced intensity conditioning
4. UCB transplant

Answer: autologous HCT

DAH is a rare complication of HCT and is more commonly seen with **autologous** HCT than with allogeneic HCT.

Q. Which of the following is not true about pulmonary veno-occlusive disease:
1. It generally occurs early in the course, usually within the first 100 days
2. Kerley B lines are often present on a chest radiograph
3. CT pulmonary angiography shows no evidence of pulmonary emboli
4. Right-sided heart catheterisation is necessary for documentation of the combination of pulmonary hypertension and a normal pulmonary artery occlusion pressure

Answer: it generally occurs early in the course, usually within the first 100 days

In fact, it generally occurs **late** in the course, usually **after** the first 100 days.

Q. In what percent of patients receiving autologous HCT is

peri-engraftment respiratory distress syndrome (PERDS) reported:

1. 1-2
2. 3-5
3. 5-7
4. 7-12

Answer: 3-5%

TRANSFUSION MEDICINE

Q. Which of the following is true about cryoprecipitate:
1. It is insoluble
2. It is produced by thawing the frozen plasma
3. It is rich in fibrinogen
4. All of the above

Answer: all of the above

Notes on preparation of one unit of cryoprecipitate:
1. Take 250 mL of Fresh Frozen Plasma (FFP) from one unit of whole blood
2. Thaw it at 4°C (range 1 and 6°C) for 24 hours
3. Separate the insoluble precipitate from the liquids by centrifugation
4. Refreeze the separated insoluble precipitate at -18°C in a concentrated volume of approximately 10 to 20 mL
5. This yields one unit of cryoprecipitate

Q. All of the following are constituents of one unit of cry-

oprecipitate (5 to 20 mL), except:
1. Fibrinogen: 150 to 250 mg
2. Factor VIII: 80 to 150 units
3. Factor XIII: 150 to 300 units
4. von Willebrand factor: 100 to 150 units

Answer: Factor XIII: 150 to 300 units

In fact, the concentration of factor XIII is around 50 units.

Apart from these four constituents, fibronectin is another one. But there is no specified concentration required to be present in one unit of cryoprecipitate.

Q. Each unit of cryoprecipitate raises the plasma fibrinogen concentration by:
1. 5 to 10 mg/dL
2. 1 to 2 mg/dL
3. 10 to 20 mg/dL
4. 20 to 50 mg/dL

Answer: 5 to 10 mg/dL

A typical dose of cryoprecipitate in many situations is one unit (bag) per 10 kg of body weight.

Q. Cryoprecipitate must be thawed before infusion. Once thawed, it must be transfused within what time frame:
  1. Within 6 hours
  2. Within 24 hours
  3. Within 48 hours
  4. Within one hour

Answer: within 6 hours

Q. Before administering cryoprecipitate, which of the following compatibilities need to be checked:
  1. ABO
  2. Rh
  3. Both of the above
  4. None of the above

Answer: ABO

Rh compatibility testing is not required before cryoprecipitate infusion.

Q. In which of the following situation cryoprecipitate will be effective:

1. Factor VIII deficiency
2. Factor IX deficiency
3. Von Willebrand factor deficiency
4. In reversing warfarin induced anticoagulation

Answer: options 1 and 3 are correct

Remember that cryoprecipitate is not helpful in **all kinds** of factor deficiencies. It has four main factor concentrates: factor VIII, XIII, fibrinogen and von Willebrand factor.

Some examples where cryoprecipitate will **not** be helpful:

1. Deficiency of any factor other than those mentioned above.
2. Bleeding due to thrombocytopenia
3. Warfarin induced bleeding

Remember these facts:

1. One unit of whole blood = 500 mL
2. One unit of packed RBCs = 350 mL
3. One unit of FFP = 200 to 300 mL
4. One unit of cryoprecipitate = 10 to 20 mL
5. 1 unit of apheresis platelets = 200 to 300 mL

Remember these facts:

1. One unit of packed RBCs increases Hb by 1 g/dL and hematocrit by 3%
2. One unit of cryoprecipitate **per 10 kg body weight** (5 units in an adult weighing 50 kg) will increase plasma fibrinogen by approximately 50 mg/dL
3. One unit of aphaeresis platelets (or 5 to 6 units of whole blood-derived platelets) will increase the platelet count by 30,000/microL.

Q. All of the following may be used for vitamin K dependent coagulation factor replacement except:

1. FFP
2. PF24
3. Thawed Plasma
4. Cryoprecipitate

Answer: cryoprecipitate

As we have already discussed above, cryoprecipitate has only a few coagulation factors and it can't be used for vitamin K dependent coagulation factor replacement, for example in control of bleeding caused by warfarin..

Q. Which of the following factor has the shortest plasma half

life:
1. Factor VII
2. Factor VIII
3. Factor IX
4. Factor X

Answer: factor VII

Factor VII has a plasma half life of about 4 to 6 hours.

Q. Which of the following criteria should be met, if granulocyte transfusion is to be given:
1. Absolute neutrophil count (ANC) < 500 cells/microL
2. Evidence of bacterial or fungal infection
3. Unresponsiveness to antimicrobial treatment for at least 48 hours
4. Any of the above
5. All of the criteria 1, 2 and 3 should be met

Answer: all of the criteria 1, 2 and 3 should be met

Q. For emergency surgery requiring massive transfusion, red blood cell (RBC) units, fresh frozen plasma (FFP), and platelets are transfused in what ratio, respectively:
1. 1:1:1

    2. 2:1:1

    3. 1:2:1

    4. 2:1:2

Answer: 1:1:1

They are transfused in almost equal ratios.

Q. Each unit of cryoprecipitate has how much fibrinogen:

    1. 150 to 250 mg

    2. 700 to 800 mg

    3. 15 to 25 mg

    4. 70 to 80 mg

Answer: 150 to 250 mg

Each unit of FFP has 700 to 800 mg fibrinogen.

Q. Which of the following is used for pathogen inactivation of blood products:

    1. Amotosalen plus ultraviolet light

    2. Riboflavin plus UV light

    3. Methylene blue plus visible light

    4. UV light alone

Answer: all of the above

All of them are used for pathogen inactivation. Note that three of them use UV light but the methylene blue method uses visible light (not UV light).

Q. Which of the following pathogen inactivation methods is used for whole blood:
1. Solvent/detergent method
2. Amotosalen plus UV light
3. Riboflavin plus UV light
4. Methylene blue plus visible light

Answer: riboflavin plus UV light

Notes on methods of pathogen inactivation and their uses:
1. Solvent/detergent method: used for plasma
2. Amotosalen plus UV light: used for plasma and platelets
3. Riboflavin plus UV light: used for plasma, platelets and whole blood
4. Methylene blue plus visible light: used or plasma
5. UV light alone: used for platelets

Q. Which of the following is a "three factor" prothrombin complex concentrate:
1. Kcentra
2. Profilnine SD
3. FEIBA NF
4. All of the above

Answer: Profilnine SD

The other two are "4 factor" complex concentrates.

Out of these three, only the FEIBA NF is an activated prothrombin complex concentrate. The other two are un-activated.

Q. All of the following make a donor unfit for blood donation, except:
1. Hemoglobin less than 12.5 g/dL for women
2. Blood pressure above 180 mmHg systolic
3. Pulse rate more than 100 beats/minute
4. None of the above

Answer: options 1, 2 and 3 are correct

These all are criteria, which make the donor unfit. For men the lower limit of hemoglobin is 13 g/dL.

Q. To prevent post blood donation vasovagal reactions, the donation should be restricted to what percent of donor's estimated blood volume:
    1. 15%
    2. 20%
    3. 25%
    4. 5%

Answer: 15%

A donor must have an estimated blood volume of > 3500 mL to be eligible for donating blood.

Q. Which of the following is not a clinically significant alloantibody against RBCs:
    1. Rh
    2. Kidd
    3. Lewis
    4. Lutheran

Answer: Lewis

The following are clinically significant alloantibodies against RBCs: ABO, Rh, Duffy, Kidd, Kell, SsU and Lutheran.

Q. Which of the following red blood cell antigen has the lowest reactive immunogenicity:

1. A
2. B
3. Fy
4. Jk

Answer: Jk

A and B antigens have 100% reactive immunogenicity, whereas Rh(D) has 80% immunogenicity. Jk has 0.1% reactive immunogenicity.

Q. Fibrin sealants are composed of all of the following except:

1. Factor XIII
2. Factor VII
3. Fibrinogen
4. Calcium

Answer: factor VII

Fibrin sealants have two components:
1. Concentrated fibrinogen and factor XIII
2. Thrombin and calcium

The component 1 is mixed with component two, which results in formation of coagulum.

Q. Blood products and collection methods often utilise citrate. Which of the following is a clinically significant complication of citrate:
1. Hypocalcemia
2. Hypercalcemia
3. Hypokalaemia
4. Hyperkalemia

Answer: hypocalcemia

Citrate binds to ionised calcium, resulting in hypocalcemia.

Q. Which of the following is the definition of refractoriness to platelet transfusion:

1. Platelet count response significantly less than expected following two or more platelet transfusions
2. Platelet count response significantly less than expected following three or more platelet transfusions
3. Platelet count response significantly less than expected following four or more platelet transfusions
4. Platelet count response significantly less than expected following five or more platelet transfusions

Answer: Platelet count response significantly less than expected following two or more platelet transfusions

The "expected" response is defined as a rise in platelet count of approximately 30,000/microL in 10 to 60 minutes, with a return to baseline at two to three days. Some centres also use the criteria of immediate response, according to which if the platelet count increases by >10,000/microL within an hour of transfusion, it is considered an accepted response.

Q. Which of the following has the highest threshold hemoglobin value mandating RBC transfusion:

1. Myocardial ischemia
2. GI bleeding
3. Cardiac surgery

4. Oncology patients undergoing treatment

Answer: Myocardial ischemia

The hemoglobin threshold for transfusion in symptomatic myocardial ischemia patients is 10 g/dL. For all the other situations, usually the threshold is 7 to 8 g/dL.

Q. Each unit of whole blood has how many leukocytes:
1. 2 to 5×10^9
2. 5 to 10×10^9
3. 10 to 20×10^9
4. 5 to 10×10^8

Answer: 2 to 5×10^9

In certain indications, like febrile non hemolytic transfusion reactions and HLA alloimmunization, leukoreduction is indicated. The goal of modern day leukoreduction techniques is to reduce the leukocytes below 1×10^6.

Q. Which of the following oxygen carrier is approved by the

FDA for clinical use:
1. Hemoglobin-based carriers (HBOCs)
2. Perfluorocarbons (PFCs)
3. Both of the above
4. None of the above

Answer: none of the above

There are two types of oxygen carriers under active research, HBOCs and PFCs. But neither of these has been approved by the FDA.

Q. All of the following are features of TRALI and not of TACO, except:
1. Raised body temperature
2. Normal ejection fraction
3. Transient leukopenia
4. Hypertension

Answer: hypertension

In TRALI, generally hypotension is present.

TRALI is transfusion-related acute lung injury and TACO is transfusion-associated circulatory overload.

Some contrasting features of TRALI and TACO are:

Feature	TRALI	TACO
Body temperature	Fever may be there	Normal
BP	Hypotension	Hypertension
Signs and symptoms of heart failure	Usually absent	Usually present
EF	Normal	Decreased
Pulmonary fluid	Exudate	Transudate
WBC	Transient leukopenia	Normal
BNP	Low	Very high

Q. Which of the following statement is wrong:

1. Acute hemolytic transfusion reactions occur during the transfusion or within the first 24 hours after transfusion
2. Febrile nonhemolytic transfusion reactions (FNHTR) are more common than febrile hemolytic transfusion reactions
3. FNHTR is caused by white blood cells or cytokines in the transfused product
4. Premedication is often used to prevent FNHTR

Answer: Premedication is often used to prevent FNHTR

In fact, the use of premedication may itself lead to certain reactions. Most centres do not use premedication for prevention of FNHTR.

Q. Delayed hemolytic transfusion reactions occur due to:
  1. ABO incompatibility
  2. Rh incompatibility
  3. Anamnestic response
  4. Kell antigen mismatch

Answer: Anamnestic response

Q. Which of the following is not a diagnostic criterion for TRALI:
  1. ARDS risk factor present at time of transfusion
  2. Onset within 6 hours of transfusion
  3. Bilateral infiltrates on a chest radiograph
  4. No evidence of left atrial hypertension

Answer: ARDS risk factor present at time of transfusion

Remember that any risk factors for ARDS or ALI must be **ab-**

sent, if a diagnosis of TRALI is to be made. If a patient fulfils all the diagnostic criteria for TRALI but has any risk factor for ARDS or ALI at the time of transfusion then the diagnosis will be **possible** TRALI.

The diagnostic criteria for TRALI are:
1. Acute onset (during or within six hours of transfusion)
2. Hypoxemia
3. Bilateral infiltrates on frontal chest radiograph
4. No evidence of circulatory overload/left atrial hypertension
5. No pre-existing ALI/ARDS before transfusion

Note that TRALI and possible TRALI are older terms, which are still frequently used. A new classification of TRALI has now come into effect:

TRALI type I:
No risk factors for ARDS and **all** the following criteria are met:
1. Acute onset; Hypoxemia ($PaO_2/FiO_2 \leq 300$ mmHg or $SpO_2 < 90\%$ on room air); Clear evidence of bilateral pulmonary edema on imaging; No evidence of left atrial hypertension or, if left atrial hypertension is present, it is judged to not be the main contributor to the hypoxemia
2. Onset during or within 6 hours of transfusion

3. No temporal relationship to an alternative risk factor for ARDS

TRALI type II:

Risk factors for ARDS are present (but ARDS has not been diagnosed) or mild ARDS at baseline but with respiratory status deterioration that is judged to be due to transfusion based on both of the following:

1. Findings as described in categories a and b of TRALI type I
2. Stable respiratory status in the 12 hours before transfusion

RED BLOOD CELL DISORDERS

Thalassemias

Q. Thalassemia is the most common hemoglobinopathy:
1. True
2. False

Answer: true

Around 5 percent of the world's population has at least one thalassemia variant allele.

Q. Thalassemias are characterized by:
1. Reduced production of the alpha or beta globin chains
2. Increased production of the alpha or beta globin chains
3. Increased production of defective alpha or beta globin chains
4. Increased production of unstable alpha or beta globin chains

Answer: Reduced production of the alpha or beta globin chains

Remember that thalassemias are "quantitative" disorders of globin chain production, which means that either alpha or beta globin chains is produced in reduced quantities or not produced at all. But the chains which are produced, have normal structure.

Q. There are how many alpha globin genes:
  1. 1
  2. 2
  3. 3
  4. 4

Answer: 4

Alpha thalassemia occurs due to **deletion** of any number of these four genes (not due to mutations).

Q. Hydrops fetalis occurs due to:
  1. Loss of all four alpha globin genes
  2. Gain of all four alpha globin genes
  3. Loss of all four beta globin genes
  4. Gain of all four beta globin genes

Answer: loss of all four alpha globin genes

Q. In hydrops fetalis, a disease caused by loss of all four alpha globin genes, a special kind of hemoglobin is produced known as "hemoglobin Barts". This hemoglobin is composed of:

1. Tetramers of gamma globin
2. Tetramers of beta globin
3. Tetramers of delta globin
4. Defective dimers of alpha globin

Answer: Tetramers of gamma globin

Hydrops fetalis is incompatible with live birth.

Q. Hemoglobin H disease results from:

1. Loss of three alpha-chain genes
2. Loss of four alpha-chain genes
3. Loss of three beta-chain genes
4. Loss of four beta-chain genes

Answer: loss of three alpha-chain genes

Patients with HbH disease have loss of three alpha-chain genes. It is important to note that these patients usually are "transfusion independent" but some may deteriorate and become transfusion dependent.

Q. Alpha thalassemia minima results from:

1. Loss of three alpha-chain genes
2. Loss of two alpha-chain genes
3. Loss of one alpha-chain genes
4. Loss of four alpha-chain genes

Answer: loss of one alpha-chain genes

Alpha thalassemia minima patients are known as the silent carriers.

On the other hand, alpha thalassemia "minor" results from loss of two alpha chain genes.

Q. How many beta globin genes are there:
    1. 1
    2. 2
    3. 3
    4. 4

Answer: 2

Q. The genes coding for alpha globin chains are located on which chromosome:
    1. 11
    2. 12
    3. 14
    4. 16

Answer: 16

Q. The genes coding for beta globin chains are located on which chromosome:
1. 11
2. 12
3. 14
4. 16

Answer: 11

Q. What is the usual age of manifestation of beta thalassemia:
1. At birth
2. Before birth
3. Four to six months
4. Two to five years

Answer: four to six months

Remember that newborns are asymptomatic in this disease. This happens because HbF is the major hemoglobin present in newborns (which does not contain beta chains).

Q. In which of the following, beta globin chain production is minimal or absent:

1. Beta thalassemia major
2. Cooley's anemia
3. Mediterranean anemia
4. Transfusion-dependent thalassemia

Answer: all of the above

In fact, all of these four are synonyms.

These patients require treatment and expert care, because if they are left untreated, more than 85% of them die by the age of 5 years.

Q. The usual age of presentation of beta thalassemia intermedia is:
1. At birth
2. 4 to 6 months
3. 6 to 12 months
4. 24 to 48 months

Answer: 24 to 48 months

Beta thalassemia intermedia is also known as non-transfusion-dependent thalassemia. It may be caused by homozygosity or compound heterozygosity for a beta+ thalassemia mutation or by heterozygosity for a beta0 thalassemia mutation.

The clinical course is variable in these patients. Usually they become transfusion dependent in the third or fourth decade of life. But in some patients this dependence may come early.

Q. Which of the following is false about beta thalassemia minor:
1. It is also called beta thalassemia trait
2. It is an asymptomatic carrier state
3. A minority of patients exhibit microcytosis
4. None of the above

Answer: A minority of patients exhibit microcytosis

In fact, **most of the patients** exhibit microcytosis.

Q. Hereditary persistence of fetal hemoglobin (HPFH) results in:
1. Lessened severity of beta thalassemia
2. Heightened severity of beta thalassemia
3. Has no effect on severity of beta thalassemia
4. It is particularly lethal in beta thalassemia

Answer: lessened severity of beta thalassemia

The fetal hemoglobin (HbF) doesn't have beta globin chains, hence it acts independently of beta thalassemia disease biology. In this way, when it occurs with beta thalassemia, it results in reduced severity of beta thalassemia.

Q. Which of the following is not seen in beta thalassemia patients:
1. Frontal bossing
2. Delayed pneumatization of the sinuses
3. Marked undergrowth of the maxillae
4. Increased prominence of the malar eminences

Answer: marked undergrowth of the maxillae

In fact, there is **marked overgrowth** of maxillae

The characteristic facial appearance in beta thalassemia is called "chipmunk face" appearance.

Q. The "hair-on-end" radiographic appearance of skull in thalassemia results due to:
1. Widening of the diploic spaces in the skull
2. Narrowing of the diploic spaces in the skull
3. Scalloping of the diploic spaces in the skull
4. Destruction of the diploic spaces in the skull

Answer: Widening of the diploic spaces in the skull

Q. Hypogonadism in thalassemia results from:
1. Pituitary iron deposition
2. Pituitary ischemia
3. Hypothalamic iron deposition

4. Mini strokes of mid brain

Answer: pituitary iron deposition

Notes on high performance liquid chromatography (HPLC) findings in thalassemia:
1. Alpha thalassemia
    1. In newborns suffering from alpha thalassemia major, which may occur in one of two forms: hydrops fetalis or alpha thalassemia intermedia (HbH disease); HPLC shows Hb Barts.
    2. In older children with HbH disease, HbF and HbH are increased.
    3. In alpha thalassemia minor, only a small amount of Hb Barts is present on HPLC or it may be normal.
2. Beta thalassemia:
    1. In beta thalassemia major and intermedia, HPLC shows increased HbF and HbA2. In beta thalassemia major HbA2 is 5% or more; HbF is up to 95% and there is no HbA. Whereas in beta thalassemia intermedia, HbA2 is 4% or more and HbF is up to 50%.
    2. In beta thalassemia trait (also known as carrier) HbA2 level is increased and in some patients HbF is also increased. In this disease HbA2 is 4% or more and HbF is up to 5%.
    3. In some patients of beta thalassemia, there may be concomitant mutation of other globin chain genes as well which may lead to a normal level of HbA2.

Q. Which of the following is a hallmark of thalassemia:
1. Hypochromic microcytic anemia
2. Normochromic microcytic anemia
3. Normochromic normocytic anemia
4. Hyperchromic microcytic anemia

Answer: hypochromic microcytic anemia

Q. In thalassemia the red cell distribution width (RDW) is typically:
1. Low
2. Large
3. Normal
4. Variable

Answer: low

Q. Which of the following supplementation should be done in cases of thalassemia:
1. Folic acid
2. Iron
3. Vitamin B12
4. Copper and zinc

Answer: folic acid

Folic acid supplementation is even more necessary if on-going hemolysis is there.

Q. In patients with beta thalassemia requiring chronic transfusion, which of the following is the most commonly used pretransfusion nadir hemoglobin level range:
1. 9.5 to 10.5 g/dL
2. 8.5 to 9.5 g/dL
3. 7.5 to 8.5 g/dL
4. 6.5 to 7.5 g/dL

Answer: 9.5 to 10.5 g/dL

So, a patient of thalassemia should be transfused when the hemoglobin nadir reaches 9.5 to 10.5 g/dL. Using a lower or higher nadir hemoglobin level for guiding transfusion results in suboptimal outcomes. This is based on trial data and clinical experience.

Q. Which of the following is not true about allogeneic HCT in thalassemia:
1. After HCT for thalassemia, it may take upto two years for hematopoiesis to stabilize
2. Mixed chimerism after HCT is a risk factor for graft rejection
3. There is not a need to promote graft-versus-tumor effect in thalassemia
4. Iron stores must be assessed following engraftment, and if excess of iron is present then chelation should be started

Answer: Iron stores must be assessed following engraftment, and if excess of iron is present then chelation should be started

Note that it is important to assess iron stores and to give appropriate treatment for the excess iron but this assessment and treatment should be done after around 18 months of transplant or after 6 months of stopping all transplant related medications. It is **not** done immediately after transplant.

Q. Which of the following statement is not true about allogeneic hematopoietic cell transplantation in thalassemia:
1. Allogeneic HCT is the only curative therapy for thalassemia
2. HCT outcomes are best for individuals who have not undergone blood transfusions leading to iron overload
3. Peripheral blood is not the preferred source of stem cells in thalassemia
4. For risk stratification, the Pesaro system is used in this setting

Answer: HCT outcomes are best for individuals who have not undergone blood transfusions leading to iron overload

In fact, HCT outcomes are best for individuals who **have undergone** blood transfusions and iron chelation therapy for iron overload treatment.

Q. Luspatercept is helpful in children with thalassemia to reduce blood transfusion dependence but it is not helpful in adults:
1. True
2. False

Answer: false

Luspatercept is a red blood cell maturation agent.

In fact, luspatercept is an option for older adolescents and adults.

Q. Which of the following is the most preferred source of stem cells for HCT in patients with thalassemia:
1. Bone marrow
2. Peripheral blood
3. Umbilical cord blood
4. Any of the above

Answer: bone marrow

Umbilical cord blood is the second best option. Peripheral blood is not chosen because it is associated with high incidence and severity of graft versus host disease compared with the other two sources.

Q. What is the standard myeloablative conditioning regimens for thalassemia patients:
1. Busulfan and cyclophosphamide
2. Busulfan and fludarabine
3. Fludarabine and cyclophosphamide
4. Busulfan with TBI

Answer: busulfan and cyclophosphamide

Q. Which of the following is not a factor in the Pesaro risk stratification system used in thalassemia:
1. Hepatomegaly
2. Splenomegaly
3. Liver fibrosis
4. Iron chelation therapy

Answer: splenomegaly

Notes on the Pesaro system:
1. This system is most useful in paediatric thalassemia patients.
2. It is used for risk stratification and prognostication of patients of thalassemia undergoing allogeneic HCT.
3. There are three risk factors:
a. Hepatomegaly (>2 cm from costal arch is considered an adverse feature and if it is 2 cm or less then it is considered a favorable feature)
b. Liver fibrosis (if present, it is considered an adverse feature)
c. Iron chelation therapy (if it has been given on an ir-

regular basis, it is an adverse prognostic feature and if it has been given on a regular basis, it is a favourable prognostic feature)

4. There are three risk classes based on these three risk factors:
a. Class I: all three risk factors are favourable
b. Class II: there are one or two adverse risk factors
c. Class III: all three risk factors are adverse

Sickle cell disorders

Q. Which of the following is not true about sickle cell anemia:

1. Hemoglobin S (HbS) results from a point mutation in the beta globin gene
2. The substitution of a valine for glutamic acid as the sixth amino acid of the beta globin chain results in HbS
3. The hemoglobin tetramer (alpha2/beta S2) in sickle cell anemia becomes poorly soluble when oxygenated
4. The pathological polymerization of HbS is essential to vaso-occlusive phenomena

Answer: The hemoglobin tetramer (alpha2/beta S2) in sickle cell anemia becomes poorly soluble when oxygenated

In fact, the hemoglobin tetramer (alpha2/beta S2) in sickle cell anemia becomes poorly soluble when **de**oxygenated (not oxygenated).

Q. Which of the following is not true about sickle cell disorders (SCD):
1. Clinical manifestations of SCD are not present at birth
2. SCD can be diagnosed in the prenatal time using fetal DNA samples obtained by chorionic villus sampling
3. New born screening is usually performed after 72 hours of life by "heel stick" filter paper screen method
4. In very premature babies the incorrect diagnosis of hemoglobin S/beta+ thalassemia is an often encountered lab error

Answer: New born screening is usually performed after 72 hours of life by "heel stick" filter paper screen method

In fact, new born screening is usually performed **within** 72 hours of life by "heel stick" filter paper screen method (not **after** 72 hours).

Q. Which is not a pattern of hemoglobin in sickle cell disorders:
1. FS pattern
2. FAS pattern
3. FSA pattern
4. FSS pattern

Answer: FSS pattern

There are basically three patterns of hemoglobin in sickle cell disorders:
1. FS
2. FAS
3. FSA

Notes on these patterns:
1. FS pattern: seen in newborns with homozygous sickle cell anemia (HbSS). They have predominantly HbF with a small amount of HbS. There is no HbA.
2. FAS pattern: seen in newborns with sickle cell trait. They have HbF, HbA, and HbS. The quantity of HbA is greater than that of HbS.
3. FSA pattern: if this pattern is found then the presumptive diagnosis is sickle cell-beta+ thalassemia. Here HbF, HbA and HbS are found but the quantity of HbS is greater than that of HbA.

Q. Which of the following is the preferred method for the diagnosis of sickle cell disorders:
1. High performance liquid chromatography
2. Thin-layer isoelectric focusing
3. Cellulose acetate electrophoresis
4. Sickledex solubility test

Answer: high performance liquid chromatography

Methods using sodium metabisulfite are now obsolete and

of historic interest only.

Q. Which of the following is not true:
1. In sickle cell trait, the usual pattern is: >50 percent HbA, 35 to 45 percent HbS, and <2 percent HbF
2. In sickle cell anemia, the usual pattern is: 0 percent HbA, <2 percent HbF, normal amounts of HbA2, and the remainder HbS
3. In sickle cell-beta+ thalassemia, there is 5 to 30 percent HbA, increased HbA2, with the remainder HbS.
4. In sickle cell-betao thalassemia, there is 10 to 20 percent HbA, along with variable amounts of HbF, increased amounts of HbA2, with the remainder HbS

Answer: In sickle cell-betao thalassemia, there is 10 to 20 percent HbA, along with variable amounts of HbF, increased amounts of HbA2, with the remainder HbS

This question seems difficult but is very easy. In sickle cell-betao thalassemia, there is **0** percent HbA, along with variable amounts of HbF, increased amounts of HbA2, with the remainder HbS. The name "betao thalassemia" implies that there is no HbA in such a patient.

Q. Which of the following statement is wrong about treatment of sickle cell disorders:
1. Hydroxyurea has been demonstrated to improve survival
2. L-glutamine is effective in patients of SCD in whom the pain of veno-occlusive disease is not controlled

by hydroxyurea
3. Opioids are needed many times in patients having chronic veno-occlusive disease induced pain
4. None of the above

Answer: none of the above

All of the above mentioned statements are correct.

There are some other medical treatment options besides hydroxyurea and L-glutamine, like voxelotor and crizanlizumab.

Q. Which of the following is the preferred source of stem cells for allogeneic HCT in sickle cell disorder patients:
1. Bone marrow
2. Umbilical cord blood
3. Peripheral blood
4. Chimeric lab grown cells

Answer: bone marrow

Umbilical cord blood is the second best option. Peripheral blood is not preferred as a stem cell source because it is associated with high incidence of graft versus host disease.

Q. Hydroxyurea, when used in sickle cell disease, is associ-

ated with which of the following:
1. Reduction in pain
2. Decreased hospitalisation rates
3. Improved overall survival
4. All of the above

Answer: all of the above

Remember that in sickle cell disease, hydroxyurea not only relieves symptoms but also improves survival.

Also remember that hydroxyurea is **not** curative. The only curative option available at present is hematopoietic cell transplantation.

Q. Which of the following is true about antibiotic prophylaxis in sickle cell disease patients:
1. All individuals with SCD should begin antibiotic prophylaxis within the first three months of life and continue for at least five years
2. All individuals with SCD should begin antibiotic prophylaxis after the first three months of life and continue for at least five years
3. All individuals with SCD should begin antibiotic prophylaxis after the first twelve months of life and continue for at least five years
4. All individuals with SCD should begin antibiotic prophylaxis with in the first twelve months of life and continue for at least ten years

Answer: All individuals with SCD should begin antibiotic prophylaxis within the first three months of life and continue for at least five years

The drug of choice for prophylaxis is penicillin. If the patient is allergic to penicillin then erythromycin should be used.

Q. Supplementation of which of the following is usually not recommended in sickle cell disease:
   1. Folic acid
   2. Vitamin D
   3. Calcium
   4. Iron

Answer: iron

Q. For patient with sickle cell disease presenting with acute pain due to vaso-occlusive disease; which of the following is not a first line therapy:
   1. Oral hydration
   2. Intravenous hydration
   3. Oral or intravenous opiate
   4. Non steroidal anti-inflammatory drugs

Answer: Non steroidal anti-inflammatory drugs

Remember that in this clinical scenario the WHO pain ladder is not usually followed. We should directly start an opioid drug in them.

Porphyria

Q. Which of the following is known as the Swedish porphyria:
1. Acute intermittent porphyria (AIP)
2. Hereditary coproporphyria (HCP)
3. Variegate porphyria (VP)
4. 5-aminolevulinic acid dehydratase (ALAD) porphyria

Answer: acute intermittent porphyria (AIP)

Q. Which of the following is found in HCP but not in AIP:
1. Elevated urinary PBG
2. Blistering photosensitivity
3. Increased fecal porphyrins
4. All of the above

Answer: blistering photosensitivity

This is a confusing question and some may differ from my opinion and may choose "all of the above". Here is my logic behind choosing blistering photosensitivity:

1. Both HCP and AIP are characterized by elevated urinary PBG, but PBG elevation in HCP may be less marked and more transient in HCP than in AIP.
2. HCP may have blistering photosensitivity, which is absent in AIP.
3. Fecal porphyrins are elevated in both AIP and HCP but this elevation is much more in HCP. In HCP, especially the levels of coproporphyrin III are very high.

So, as we can see here that while degrees of elevation differ, urinary PBG and fecal porphyrins are elevated in both AIP and HCP. The options nowhere describe the degree of elevation that's why I have chosen blistering photosensitivity. If degree of elevation were provided then the answer would have been different.

Q. Which of the following porphyria is associated with increased plasma porphyrins with a characteristic peak fluorescence at 626 nm:
1. Acute intermittent porphyria (AIP)
2. Hereditary coproporphyria (HCP)
3. Variegate porphyria (VP)
4. 5-aminolevulinic acid dehydratase (ALAD) porphyria

Answer: Variegate porphyria (VP)

Q. Which of the following porphyria is not associated with elevated urinary PBG:
1. Acute intermittent porphyria (AIP)

2. Hereditary coproporphyria (HCP)
3. Variegate porphyria (VP)
4. 5-aminolevulinic acid dehydratase (ALAD) porphyria

Answer: 5-aminolevulinic acid dehydratase (ALAD) porphyria

In ALAD porphyria, urinary ALA is elevated and urinary PBG is not elevated.

Q. Which of the following porphyria is the most common one:
1. Acute intermittent porphyria (AIP)
2. Hereditary coproporphyria (HCP)
3. Variegate porphyria (VP)
4. 5-aminolevulinic acid dehydratase (ALAD) porphyria

Answer: Acute intermittent porphyria (AIP)

These four are the most common acute (neurovisceral) porphyrias and AIP is the most common out of these four.

Q. Which of the following porphyria is caused by an inherited deficiency of porphobilinogen deaminase:
1. Acute intermittent porphyria (AIP)
2. Hereditary coproporphyria (HCP)
3. Variegate porphyria (VP)

4. 5-aminolevulinic acid dehydratase (ALAD) porphyria

Answer: Acute intermittent porphyria (AIP)

AIP has autosomal dominant inheritance with variable penetration.

The enzyme porphobilinogen deaminase is also called hydroxymethylbilane synthase.

The PBGD activity is tested in the erythrocytes.

Q. What is the treatment of choice for a patient of acute intermittent porphyria having an acute episode:
1. Intravenous hemin
2. Oral hemin
3. Carbohydrate loading
4. Pyrophosphate

Answer: intravenous hemin

Panhematin is given in doses of 3 to 4 mg/kg in 25 percent human albumin IV as a single dose for 4 days.

Q. How many enzymes are there in the heme synthetic pathway? Please enumerate these enzymes in a sequential manner (from first step to last step).

Answer: there are eight enzymes in the heme synthetic pathway. Their names (sequentially) are as follows:
1. ALA synthase (ALAS)
2. ALA dehydratase (ALAD)
3. PBG deaminase (PBGD)
4. Uroporphyrinogen synthase (UROS)
5. Uroporphyrinogen decarboxylase (UROD)
6. Coproporphyrinogen oxidase (CPOX)
7. Protoporphyrinogen oxidase (PPOX)
8. Ferrochelatase (FECH)

Q. Which of the following enzyme of heme biosynthetic pathway is mitochondrial:
1. ALAS
2. ALAD
3. PBGD
4. UROS

Answer: ALAS

There are total eight enzymes in the heme synthetic pathway. Four of them are mitochondrial and four are cytoplasmic.
1. Mitochondrial enzymes: ALAS, CPOX, PPOX, FECH
2. Cytoplasmic enzymes: ALAD, PBGD, UROS, UROD

Q. Which of the following porphyria is not a hepatic por-

phyria:
1. ADP
2. AIP
3. PCT
4. XLP

Answer: XLP

Porphyrias are classified in many ways, like hepatic or erythropoietic; acute or cutaneous etc.

The following three are erythropoietic porphyrias:
1. CEP: congenital erythropoietic porphyria
2. EPP: erythropoietic protoporphyria
3. XLP: X-linked protoporphyria

The following six are hepatic porphyrias:
1. ADP: delta-aminolevulinic acid (ALA) dehydratase porphyria
2. AIP: acute intermittent porphyria
3. HCP: hereditary coproporphyria
4. VP: variegate porphyria
5. PCT: porphyria cutanea tarda
6. HEP: hepatoerythropoietic porphyria

Notes on inheritance patterns of porphyrias:
1. Autosomal dominant: AIP, HCP, VP, PCT
2. Autosomal recessive: ADP, HEP, CEP, EPP
3. X-linked: XLP

Notes on porphyrias and the enzyme deficiencies that cause them:

1. ADP (delta-aminolevulinic acid [ALA] dehydratase) porphyria is caused by ALAD (ALA dehydratase) deficiency.
2. AIP (acute intermittent porphyria) is caused by P-BGD (porphobilinogen [PBG] deaminase) deficiency.
3. HCP (hereditary coproporphyria) is caused by CPOX (coproporphyrinogen oxidase) deficiency.
4. VP (variegate porphyria) is caused by PPOX (proto-porphyrinogen oxidase) deficiency.
5. PCT (porphyria cutanea tarda) is caused by UROD (uroporphyrinogen decarboxylase) deficiency.
6. HEP (hepatoerythropoietic porphyria) and CEP (congenital erythropoietic porphyria) are caused by UROS (uroporphyrinogen III synthase) deficiency.
7. EPP (erythropoietic protoporphyria) is caused by FECH (ferrochelatase) deficiency.
8. XLP (X-linked protoporphyria) is caused by ALAS2 (ALA synthase 2) deficiency.

Q. Hydroxychloroquine is most useful in the treatment of which of the following porphyria:

1. PCT
2. AIP
3. EPP
4. All of the above

Answer: PCT

Hemin and carbohydrate loading are mainstays of treatment of AIP. EPP, on the other hand, is treated with β-carotene and afamelanotide.

Q. The most common symptom of acute intermittent porphyria is:
   1. Abdominal pain
   2. Vomiting
   3. Tachycardia
   4. Muscle weakness

Answer: abdominal pain

Abdominal pain is present in around 90% patients.

Q. Which of the following is the standard of care for the
treatment of PCT:
   1. Phlebotomy
   2. Low-dose hydroxychloroquine
   3. High-dose hydroxychloroquine
   4. Hemin

Answer: there are two correct answers, phlebotomy and
low-dose hydroxychloroquine.

These two options are highly effective in treatment of PCT
and they are unique, because they are not useful in any other
type of porphyria.

Q. In a patient of PCT with substantial iron overload, which of the following is the preferred treatment option:
1. Phlebotomy
2. Low dose hydroxychloroquine
3. Hemin
4. Splenectomy

Answer: phlebotomy

As we have noted in the previous question, both phlebotomy and low dose hydroxychloroquine are standard of care in PCT. But if the patient has substantial iron overload, phlebotomy is the preferred option. On the other hand, if the patient doesn't have iron overload either phlebotomy or low dose hydroxychloroquine may be used.

Phlebotomy is preferred in cases with homozygosity or compound heterozygosity for *HFE* mutations.

Q. For management of HEP, which of the following is the most important treatment strategy:
1. Folate supplementation
2. Avoidance of sunlight
3. Periodic phlebotomhy
4. Pulse administration of hemin and glucose

Answer: avoidance of sunlight

Reducing the hepatic iron stores does not benefit the patients of HEP.

APLASTIC ANEMIA

Q. In approximately what percent of children with aplastic anemia, the cause remains unknown:
1. 90
2. 70
3. 30
4. <10

Answer: 70%

In the remaining 30% of patients, etiology may be known. The most common etiologies in children are post viral hepatitis, certain infections, drugs and toxins and ionising radiation.

Q. Which age group is least affected by aplastic anemia:
1. 2 to 5 years
2. 5 to 15 years
3. 20 to 25 years
4. 55 to 60 years

Answer: 5 to 15 years

Aplastic anemia has a triphasic age distribution. The three peaks are seen at: 2 to 5 years, 20 to 25 years and 55 to 60 years or more.

Q. Which of the following chemical is associated with development of aplastic anemia:
1. Benzene
2. Lindane
3. Both of the above
4. None of the above

Answer: both of the above

Q. Which of the following is not true about hepatitis and aplastic anemia:
1. After an episode of acute hepatitis, aplasia develops within seven months
2. Approximately 15% of patients with seronegative acute liver failure develop aplastic anemia
3. Hepatitis A, B and C are major etiologic agents in development of aplastic anemia due to viral hepatitis
4. T cell activation plays a major role in aplastic anemia genesis due to viral hepatitis

Answer: Hepatitis A, B and C are major etiologic agents in development of aplastic anemia due to viral hepatitis

Note that the virus responsible for aplastic anemia development, post viral hepatitis is not precisely known. Most experts agree that hepatitis A, B, C and G **do not** play a role.

Q. The aplastic anemia associated with pregnancy is usually self limiting and resolves after pregnancy:
  1. True
  2. Fasle

Answer: true

Q. For patients with severe aplastic anemia, which of the following is the treatment of choice:
  1. Matched sibling allogeneic HCT
  2. Autologous HCT
  3. Immunosuppressive therapy
  4. Matched unrelated HCT

Answer: matched sibling allogeneic HCT

If a matched sibling donor is not available then the next best approach is using immunosuppressive therapy rather than alternative donor transplant.

Q. Which of the following is not a component of the initial immunosuppressive therapy used in the treatment of severe aplastic anemia:
  1. Antithymocyte globulin
  2. Cyclosporine

3. Prednisone
4. Methotrexate

Answer: methotrexate

The combination of options 1, 2 and 3 is the most commonly used immunosuppressive therapy in aplastic anemia. This cocktail is sometimes called "triple immunosuppression".

In this protocol G-CSF is also added for a short time but it doesn't act as an immunosuppressive agent.

Q. Which of the following is not a diagnostic criterion of severe aplastic anemia:
1. Bone marrow cellularity <25 percent
2. Peripheral blood absolute neutrophil count <1000/ microL
3. Peripheral blood platelet count <20,000/microL
4. Peripheral blood reticulocyte count <20,000/ microL

Answer: Peripheral blood absolute neutrophil count <1000/ microL

In fact, peripheral blood absolute neutrophil count **<500/ microL** is a diagnostic criterion.

Notes on diagnostic criteria of aplastic anemia:

The definition of aplastic anemia is pancytopenia with a hypocellular bone marrow in the absence of an abnormal infiltrate or marrow fibrosis. The most important part of this definition is "the absence of an abnormal infiltrate or marrow fibrosis", because there are many conditions that have pancytopenia with a hypocellular bone marrow. In other words, aplastic anemia is a diagnosis of exclusion.

Diagnostic criteria of severe aplastic anemia (both of the following criteria must be met):

1. Bone marrow cellularity <25 percent (or 25 to 50 percent if <30 percent of residual cells are hematopoietic)
2. At least two of the following:
a. Peripheral blood absolute neutrophil count <500/microL
b. Peripheral blood platelet count <20,000/microL
c. Peripheral blood reticulocyte count <20,000/microL

Diagnosis criteria of very severe severe aplastic anemia (both of the following criteria must be met):

1. Bone marrow cellularity <25 percent (or 25 to 50 percent if <30 percent of residual cells are hematopoietic)
2. At least two of the following:
a. Peripheral blood absolute neutrophil count <200/microL
b. Peripheral blood platelet count <20,000/microL
c. Peripheral blood reticulocyte count <20,000/microL

The only difference between severe and very severe aplastic anemia is the ANC count.

Non severe aplastic anemia:
In this category, the patient has pancytopenia with a hypocellular bone marrow in the absence of an abnormal infiltrate or marrow fibrosis; but the criteria for severe and very severe aplastic anemia are not met.

Q. For patients with aplastic anemia, which of the following is the preferred source of hematopoietic stem cells:
1. Bone marrow
2. Peripheral blood
3. Umbilical cord blood
4. Any of the above

Answer: bone marrow

Peripheral blood is the least preferred source due to the highest incidence and severity of graft versus host disease in its recipients. Remember that in **benign** hematological conditions, if hematopoietic cell transplantation is indicated then we should not choose peripheral blood as a source of stem cells. The reason behind this recommendation has two main aspects:
1. We don't need graft versus tumor (GVT) effect in these patients (because these are benign conditions).
2. We need the least amount of graft versus host disease (GVHD) to reduce transplant related mortality

and morbidity.

In malignant hematologic conditions, we need GVT effect (also known as graft versus leukemia effect) that's why we have to accept some level of GVHD too. Thus in malignant cases, peripheral blood is the most commonly used stem cell source.

MISCELLANEOUS TOPICS

Q. X-linked sideroblastic anemia (XLSA) is the most common congenital sideroblastic anemia:
1. True
2. False

Answer: true

Congenital sideroblastic anemias have many modes of inheritance and varied presentations.

Q. Which of the following type of RBCs are least commonly seen in acquired sideroblastic anemias:
1. Normocytic
2. Macrocytic
3. Microcytic
4. All are seen with equal frequency

Answer: microcytic

Most commonly RBCs are either macrocytic or normocytic.

Q. The hemolytic disease of the fetus and newborn (HDFN) may occur due to the maternal exposure to an allogeneic red blood cell antigen by:
1. Prior transfusion
2. Previous pregnancy
3. Sharing of needles
4. Fetomaternal hemorrhage

Answer: all of the above

These all are mechanisms, which may lead to development of HDFN.

Actually, the mechanism of development of HDFN from a previous pregnancy is fetomaternal haemorrhage.

Q. Which of the following is not true about HDFN:
1. Fetal RBC antigens arise from expression of a maternally inherited gene
2. IgG antibodies are responsible for fetal hemolysis
3. Fetal anemia occurs primarily via phagocytosis of antibody-coated RBCs
4. Major sites on destruction of RBCs in HDFN are liver and spleen

Answer: Fetal RBC antigens arise from expression of a maternally inherited gene

In fact, fetal RBC antigens arise from expression of a **paternally** inherited gene

Q. Which of the following is true:
1. HDFN may result from alloantibodies to antigens other than RhD
2. Maternal alloantibodies to non-RhD antigens are seen in approximately 1.5 to 2.5 percent of pregnancies
3. Antibodies against the K antigen of the Kell system, causes a more severe HDFN compared with other types
4. All of the above

Answer: all of the above

Q. Which for the following is not true:
1. Routine screening for antibodies to RBC antigens in pregnancy should be typically done at the first prenatal visit
2. The antibody level to an RBC antigen is predictive of the likelihood or severity of HDFN
3. Doppler scanning of the fetal middle cerebral artery peak systolic velocity (MCA-PSV) is the best tool for noninvasive assessment for fetal anemia
4. None of the above

Answer: The antibody level to an RBC antigen is predictive of the likelihood or severity of HDFN

While it is important to know, whether or not the antibody is present above a certain threshold but the level of antibody is not predictive of the likelihood of development of HDFN or the severity of HDFN, if it develops.

Q. If a woman's first pregnancy is affected by RhD alloimmunization, what are the chances of development of severe fetal anemia:
1. 2%
2. 5%
3. 15%
4. 25%

Answer: 15%

The key word here is: **first pregnancy**.

If severe anemia develops, it usually occurs in the third or late second trimester.

Q. Which of the following is incorrect about HDFN:
1. An RhD-negative fetus is not at risk for hemolytic disease

2. If the father of the fetus is RhD-negative, the fetal RHD type is determined by cfDNA testing
3. If the father is an *RHD*-positive homozygote, further testing for fetal RhD type is unnecessary
4. If the father is an RHD-positive heterozygote, there is a 50% chances of an offspring being RHD-positive

Answer: If the father of the fetus is RhD-negative, the fetal RHD type is determined by cfDNA testing

Remember that the inheritance of RhD blood group is paternal and the Rh blood group of mother plays no role. If the father is RhD-negative then the fetus **can't be** RhD-positive, so further testing of RHD of fetus is unnecessary.

Some notes on the first pregnancy affected by RhD allo-immunization:
1. If the father is RhD-negative then the fetus **can't be** RhD-positive, so further testing of RHD of fetus is unnecessary.
2. If the father is an *RHD*-positive homozygote, further testing for fetal RhD type is unnecessary
3. If the father is an RHD-positive heterozygote, there is a 50% chances of an offspring being RHD-positive
4. If the fetus is *RHD*-positive, the indirect Coombs titer (ie, indirect antiglobulin test) is repeated monthly and if this titer begins to rise then it should be tested every 2 weeks.
5. There is no absolute value above which the risk for development of severe anemia and hydrops fetalis becomes universally apparent. In most centres an anti-D titer between 16 and 32 is considered critical.
6. If the critical value is found upon testing then we

must determine the status of anemia in the fetus. For this purpose, Doppler study the fetal middle cerebral artery (MCA) peak systolic velocity (PSV) is the test of choice.

7. The MCA-PSV monitoring is done at one to two weeks interval. The results are recorded in the multiples of the median (MoMs). If the MCA-PSV is ≤1.5 MoMs for gestational age, then we can continue observation and schedule delivery at 37 to 38 weeks of gestation.

8. If MCA-PSV is >1.5 MoMs for gestational age, sampling of fetal blood by cordocentesis is indicated and if the fetal hemoglobin is two standard deviations below the mean value for gestational age, an intrauterine blood transfusion is indicated. If the pregnancy has crossed 35 weeks, then delivery is considered a better option than intrauterine blood transfusion.

Note that in a woman having history of HDFN in the previous pregnancy, the management is similar to the above mentioned recommendations. The difference is in the frequency of monitoring and urgency of interventions, both of which depend on the clinical situation.

Q. If a D-negative pregnant woman tests negative for RhD-antibody screening at first prenatal visit, when should a repeat screening be performed:
1. There is no need to perform a repeat screening
2. 28 weeks
3. 32 weeks
4. After administration of anti-D immune globulin

Answer: 28 weeks

Remember that antibody screening is a must in all D-negative pregnant women. The initial antibody screen is done at the first prenatal visit and if the initial screen is negative, a repeat screen at 28 weeks of gestation should be performed prior to the administration of anti-D immune globulin.

Notes on management of women who are D-negative whose fetus is D-positive (confirmed or presumed):
1. The ideal course is routine administration of anti-D immune globulin 300 micrograms at 28 weeks of gestation. There are many other schedules available. Using this protocol reduces the incidence of antenatal alloimmunization from 1 to 2 percent to 0.1 to 0.3 percent.
2. In cases where the risk of fetomaternal haemorrhage is there, anti-D immune globulin 300 micrograms as soon as possible within 72 hours of the event should be administered.
3. After delivery of an D-positive infant, 300 microgram anti-D immune globulin should be administered within 72 hours of delivery. Sometimes additional doses may be required if excessive fetomaternal bleeding is there.

Q. Which of the following is correct:
1. A serum vitamin B12 level below 148 pmol/L is consistent with deficiency
2. A serum folate level below 4.5 nmol/L is consistent with deficiency

3. If the level of MMA is normal and homocysteine is elevated, it signifies vitamin B12 deficiency
4. All of the above

Answer: only options 1 and 2 are correct. Option 3 is not correct.

Notes:
1. Remember the following values of serum vitamin B12
   d. Above 300 pg/mL (above 221 pmol/L): Normal
   e. 200 to 300 pg/mL (148 to 221 pmol/L): Borderline
   f. Below 200 pg/mL (below 148 pmol/L): Low
2. Remember the following values of serum folate:
   a. Above 4 ng/mL (above 9.1 nmol/L): Normal
   b. From 2 to 4 ng/mL (from 4.5 to 9.1 nmol/L): Borderline
   c. Below 2 ng/mL (below 4.5 nmol/L): Low

In some cases the values of both serum vitamin B12 and folate may be borderline, or there may be other confounding factors which may make the diagnosis difficult. In these situations, MMA and homocysteine levels may help in reaching a final diagnosis:
1. If MMA and homocysteine are normal then it suggests that there in no deficiency of vitamin B12 or folate.
2. If both MMA and homocysteine are elevated, then it most probably suggests a deficiency of vitamin B12. But in some cases this may be associated with folate deficiency.
3. If MMA is normal and homocysteine is elevated then

it suggests a deficiency of folate and **no deficiency** of vitamin B12.

Q. If a patient of vitamin B12 deficiency has neuropsychiatric symptoms, which of the following is the most appropriate treatment regimen:
1. Vitamin B12 1000 mcg by deep subcutaneous or intramuscular injection once weekly for one month followed by 1000 mcg once per month
2. Oral vitamin B12 1000 to 2000 mcg daily
3. Sublingual vitamin B12 1000 to 2000 mcg daily
4. Any of the above

Answer: Vitamin B12 1000 mcg by deep subcutaneous or intramuscular injection once weekly for one month followed by 1000 mcg once per month

Note that the question is about "the most appropriate treatment regimen", not about "treatment options". While it's true that oral and sublingual routes are almost equally effective compared with the SC/IM route; the SC/IM route is the best.

Q. What is the typical dose of folic acid in patients at risk for folate deficiency:
1. 1 mg orally daily
2. 1 mg orally every alternate day
3. 5 mg orally daily
4. 5 mg orally every alternate day

Answer: 1 mg orally daily

Note that this dose is not for pregnant women. This is for at risk populations, like chronic alcoholics and certain types of malabsorption syndromes.

Q. What is the dose of folic acid in patients having folic acid deficiency:
1. 1 to 5 mg orally daily
2. 1 to 5 mg IV daily
3. 1 to 5 mg IM daily
4. 1 to 5 mg SC daily

Answer: 1 to 5 mg orally daily

This dose is continued for one to four months or until there is laboratory evidence of hematologic recovery. In some patients therapy may need to be continued indefinitely.

In the treatment of vitamin B12 or folate deficiency, once the treatment in started, reticulocytosis is seen over one to two weeks and resolution of anemia generally takes four to eight weeks.

Complete resolution of neuropsychiatric and some other manifestations may take much longer and the recovery may be incomplete.

Q. Which of the following finding on cardiac MRI are suggestive of iron overload:
1. Cardiac T2* by MRI < 20 milliseconds
2. Cardiac T2* by MRI > 20 milliseconds
3. Cardiac T1* by MRI < 20 milliseconds
4. Cardiac T1* by MRI > 20 milliseconds

Answer: Cardiac T2* by MRI < 20 milliseconds

Notes on some other findings suggestive of iron overload:
1. Increased serum ferritin without significant inflammation
2. Increased TSAT
3. Liver MRI suggestive of liver iron concentration > 3 to 7 mg per gram of dry liver weight

Q. Which of the following is the most common HH gene mutation responsible to hereditary hemochromatosis:
1. HFE C282Y
2. HFE H63D
3. HFE C28Y
4. HFE H36D

Answer: HFE C282Y

Q. Clinical manifestation of hereditary hemochromatosis generally become apparent:
1. After 40 years of age

2. After 10 years age
3. Within first 5 years of life
4. In the seventh decade

Answer: after 40 years of age

To begin with, the symptoms and signs are nonspecific. If left untreated, patients may develop cirrhosis, hepatocellular cancer (HCC), heart failure, type 2 diabetes, hypogonadism, bronze-colored skin etc.

There are many screening tests available that assess iron overload in suspected patients but to confirm the diagnosis of HH, an individual must have iron overload and biallelic HFE mutations.

Q. Which of the following is not a treatment option for hereditary hemochrombtosis:
1. Phlebotomy
2. Iron chelation
3. Erythrocytapheresis
4. Hemin and carbohydrate loading

Answer: hemin and carbohydrate loading

Q. A serum ferritin level <30 ng/mL is considered confirmatory for iron deficiency:
1. True

2. False

Answer: true

Q. Which of the following is the formula used for calculating hemoglobin iron deficit:
1. Hemoglobin iron deficit (mg) = body weight x (14 - hemoglobin concentration in g/dL) x (2.145) + iron to replenish stores if desired (mg)
2. Hemoglobin iron deficit (mg) = body weight x (15 - hemoglobin concentration in g/dL) x (2.145) + iron to replenish stores if desired (mg)
3. Hemoglobin iron deficit (mg) = body weight x (14 - hemoglobin concentration in g/dL) x (2.415) + iron to replenish stores if desired (mg)
4. Hemoglobin iron deficit (mg) = body weight x (15 - hemoglobin concentration in g/dL) x (2.415) + iron to replenish stores if desired (mg)

Answer: Hemoglobin iron deficit (mg) = body weight x (14 - hemoglobin concentration in g/dL) x (2.145) + iron to replenish stores if desired (mg)

Once the haemoglobin iron deficit is calculated in the above mentioned manner, we have to calculate the volume of product required. There are various formulations available in market which have different concentrations of iron.

The final volume of product is calculated follows: hemoglobin iron deficit (mg)/C.

"C" is the per mL concentration of iron in the parenteral preparation of iron like: iron dextran: 50 mg/mL; iron sucrose: 20 mg/mL; ferric gluconate: 12.5 mg/mL; ferumoxytol: 30 mg/mL; ferric carboxymaltose: 50 mg/mL.

HEMOLYTIC ANEMIA

Q. Which of the following is not a laboratory finding of haemolytic anemia:
1. Reticulocytosis
2. High LDH level
3. High haptoglobin level
4. High bilirubin level

Answer: high haptoglobin level

In fact, haptoglobin levels are low in hemolytic anemia.

Q. Which of the following is not true about warm autoimmune hemolytic anemia:
1. Approximately half of warm AIHA cases are primary and the other half are secondary
2. The autoantibodies are almost always IgM
3. The hemolysis in warm AIHA typically occurs extravascularly
4. The autoantibodies are directed against multiple RBC antigens

Answer: The autoantibodies are almost always IgM

In fact, the autoantibodies are almost always IgG.

Q. What is the treatment of choice for warm AIHA:
1. Observation with periodic transfusion
2. Glucocorticoids alone
3. Glucocorticoids plus rituximab
4. Allogeneic bone marrow transplant

Answer: glucocorticoids plus rituximab

Apart from this combination, there are many second line options available but the standard of care is not known in the second line setting and beyond.

Note that it is important to add folic acid 1 mg daily orally, in patients having continued hemolysis.

Q. Which of the following disease typically presents in childhood:
1. Paroxysmal cold hemoglobinuria
2. Cold agglutinin disease
3. Cryoglobulinemia
4. All of the above

Answer: Paroxysmal cold hemoglobinuria

The other two diseases usually present after 60 years of age.

Q. Which of the following is caused by antibody against the P antigen:
1. Paroxysmal cold hemoglobinuria
2. Cold agglutinin disease
3. Cryoglobulinemia
4. All of the above

Answer: Paroxysmal cold hemoglobinuria

Q. Which of the following is caused primarily by IgM anti-bodies:
1. Paroxysmal cold hemoglobinuria
2. Cold agglutinin disease
3. Cryoglobulinemia
4. All of the above

Answer: Cold agglutinin disease

Notes on paroxysmal cold hemoglobinuria (PCH):
1. Caused by antibodies against "P" antigen, the anti-body is usually polyclonal, of Ig**G** type and it's **cold** reacting.
2. It causes hemolysis upon rewarming
3. Another name for this antibody is Donath-Land-

steiner antibody.

Notes on cold agglutinin disease (CAD):
1. Caused by antibodies against "I" antigen, the antibody may be polyclonal or monoclonal, of IgM type and it's **cold** reacting.
2. The titer of antibody is higher in cold agglutinin disease than in paroxysmal cold hemoglobinuria.

Notes on cryoglobulinemia:
1. A mixture of antibodies is present. IgG, IgM and/or IgA types are there.
2. The antibodies may be polyclonal or monoclonal.
3. The important thing about these antibodies is that they don't bind to RBCs. In contrast, the antibodies present in PCH and CAD bind to RBCs.

Q. Which of the following is associated with intravascular hemolysis:
1. Paroxysmal cold hemoglobinuria
2. Cold agglutinin disease
3. Cryoglobulinemia
4. All of the above

Answer: Paroxysmal cold hemoglobinuria

CAD is associated with extravascular hemolysis and cryoglobulinemia is not associated with hemolysis at all.

Q. Which of the following has the lowest upper limit of normal of MCV of RBCs:
1. Preterm infants
2. Term newborns
3. Infants
4. Adults

Answer: infants

When MCV is more than the upper limit of normal, macrocytosis is present. However, upper limit of normal varies by age. The following are the upper limits of normal MCV by age:
1. Preterm infants born at ≤25 weeks of gestation: 119 ± 7 fL
2. Term newborns (cord blood): 106 ± 4 fL
3. Infants and young children: 90 fL
4. Adults: 96 to 100 fL

Please memorise these facts about normal haematology parameters of adults:
1. Hemoglobin (g/dL): 13.6 to 16.9 in males, 11.9 to 14.8 in females
2. Hematocrit (%): 40 to 50 in males, 35 to 43 in females
3. RBC count ($\times 10_6$/microL): 4.2 to 5.7 in males, 3.8 to 5.0 in females
4. MCV (fL): 82.5 to 98 in both males and females
5. MCHC: 32.5 to 35.2 in both males and females
6. RDW (%): 11.4 to 13.5 in both males and females

7. Reticulocyte count (x 10^6/microL): 16 to 130 in males, 16 to 98 in females
8. Platelet count ($\times$ 10^3/microL): 152 to 324 in males, 153 to 361 in females
9. WBC count ($\times$ 10^3/microL): 3.8 to 10.4 in both males and females

Q. Which of the following is an example of a non-eluting label used for estimation of RBC life span:
1. Biotin
2. Chromium-51
3. Both of the above
4. Carbon-14

Answer: biotin

The mean lifespan of RBCs in an adult is 110 to 120 days. There are many methods for determination of this, the most advanced methods are known as "random RBC labelling techniques". For these labelling techniques, special agent are used, like biotin or chromium-51. Biotin is a non-eluting label, which is also known as "perfect label". On the other hand, ^{51}Cr is an eluting label. These methods calculate the "RBC half time".

Notes on methemoglobinemia:
1. In this condition hemoglobin becomes altered, i.e., the ferrous (Fe^{2+}) iron in heme is oxidized to the ferric (Fe^{3+}) state.
2. Methemoglobin is unable to bind to oxygen and it alters affinity of other molecules to oxygen as well,

thus making oxygen delivery to tissues difficult.

3. RBCs have an enzyme, cytochrome b5 reductase (Cyb5R), which keeps the level of methemoglobin in check.

4. When total methemoglobin exceeds 1.5 g/dL, clinically cyanosis becomes apparent.

5. Congenital methemoglobinemia is caused by biallelic pathogenic variants in the *CYB5R3* gene. It is an autosomal recessive disorder. When there is reduced Cyb5R in RBCs only, it's known as type I congenital methemoglobinemia. Rarely, Cyb5R enzyme activity is reduced in cells other than RBCs as well, which leads to "type II disease"; this is a very serious illness.

6. Oral methylene blue or ascorbic acid are mainstays for the management of congenital methemoglobinemia.

7. Acquired methemoglobinemia has many etiologies. The most important ones are dapsone, aniline dyes and nitrites and nitrates. The diagnosis of acquired methemoglobinemia is confirmed by documenting a methemoglobin level >5 percent.

8. The drug of choice for acquired methemoglobinemia is methylene blue. In some cases, like those with G6PD deficiency or patients on serotonergic medication, methylene blue is contraindicated. In cases where methylene blue can't be used, ascorbic acid is the next best choice.

PLATELET DISORDERS

Q. Which is the gold standard method of platelet counting:
1. Manual count, using phase contrast microscopy
2. Automated cell counters with phase contrast
3. Platelet counting machines using optical interference
4. Flow cytometry methods

Answer: Manual count, using phase contrast microscopy

But it should be kept in mind that manual count is imprecise and thus, it hasn't been feasible to incorporate it in modern automated counters.

Note that the method which is most accurate at low platelet counts (<10,000/microL) is the flow cytometry method.

Optical methods are also very precise at low platelet counts but if the count drops below 1000-2000/microL then they become less sensitive than flow cytometry methods.

Q. The automated cell counters used today, overestimate the platelet count in all of the following conditions except:
1. Thalassemia
2. Leukemias
3. Thrombotic thrombocytopenic purpura

4. Immune thrombocytopenia

Answer: Immune thrombocytopenia

In ITP, the platelet count is underestimated. In all of the other above mentioned conditions, cellular debris are present which the machines mistake for platelets.

Q. The flow cytometry methods for platelet counting use which fluorescent monoclonal antibody directed against an antigen on the surface of the platelets:
1. Anti-CD61
2. Anti-CD41a
3. Both of the above
4. None of the above

Answer: both of the above

Q. Which of the following is a platelet agonist used in platelet function testing:
1. Collagen
2. ADP
3. Epinephrine
4. All of the above

Answer: all of the above

Another platelet agonist is ristocetin.

A panel having many such agents is used in modern aggregometry.

Q. The VerifyNow method is useful in platelet function testing in context of all of the following drugs except:
  1. Aspirin
  2. Clopidogrel
  3. Abciximab
  4. P2Y13

Answer: P2Y13

The cartridge for this assay is available for P2Y**12.**

Q. The Duke and Ivy techniques are for assessment of bleeding time:
  1. In vivo
  2. In vitro
  3. Both of the above
  4. None of the above, as they are methods of calculating the clotting time

Answer: in vivo

Q. The force exerted by activated platelets on the fibrin network is known as:
  1. Platelet contractile force
  2. Elastic modulus
  3. Platelet retraction potential
  4. Brush against impedance

Answer: platelet contractile force

The elastic modulus (clot rigidity) is a measure of the physical structure of the fibrin/cellular network.

Q. Platelet contractile force is decreased in all except:
1. Thrombocytopenia
2. Uremia
3. Glanzmann thrombasthenia
4. Coronary artery disease

Answer: coronary artery disease

Q. The platelet-specific proteins, platelet factor 4 and beta thromboglobulin, are released from which granules upon platelet activation:
1. Alpha granules
2. Beta granules
3. Gamma granules
4. Epsilon granules

Answer: alpha granules

Q. Clotting time is measured:
1. From start of sample to 2 mm clot amplitude
2. From start of sample to 20 mm clot amplitude
3. From 2 mm to 20 mm clot amplitude
4. None of the above

Answer: From start of sample to 2 mm clot amplitude

There are many important definitions:
1. Clotting time: From start of sample to 2 mm clot

amplitude
2. Clot formation time: Time from 2 mm to 20 mm clot amplitude
3. Alpha angle: Angle of tangent line from 2 mm to 20 mm clot formation
4. Maximal clot strength/firmness: Amplitude measured at peak clot strength
5. Clot lysis: Percentage of loss of amplitude at fixed time after maximal amplitude

Q. Which of the following is a test of global hemostasis:
1. Bleeding time
2. Aggregometry by turbidimetric methods
3. Aggregometry and luminescence
4. Thromboelastography

Answer: thromboelastography

Notes on platelet function:
1. Step 1 is platelet adherence. The whole process is initiated by exposure of the vascular subendothelium following injury to the endothelial surface. Many molecules become exposed on the subendothelium due to an injury like collagen, fibronectin, von Willebrand factor (VWF), fibrinogen, and thrombospondin and platelets bind to them with help of glycoprotein receptors on the platelet surface.
2. Step 2 is platelet activation. This activation happens as a result of the above mentioned binding of the factors and it leads to release of many substances from alpha granules and dense granules present in the platelets. The alpha granules contain VWF, platelet factor 4, thrombospondin, fibrinogen, beta-thromboglobulin, and platelet-derived growth factor; whereas the dense granules contain adenosine diphosphate and serotonin.
3. Step 3 is platelet aggregation. This step is made

possible by binding of fibrinogen to the conforma-
tionally altered integrin αIIbβ3 receptor on two or
more adjacent platelets. There are many other factors responsible for this step.
4. Step 4 is the interaction with coagulation factors.

Q. Large platelets are seen in the peripheral smear in all of
the following disorders except:

1. Accelerated platelet turnover
2. Bernard-Soulier disease
3. Giant platelet syndromes
4. Wiskott-Aldrich syndrome

Answer: Wiskott-Aldrich syndrome

Remember that in Wiskott-Aldrich syndrome the platelets
are characteristically small.

Q. Which of the following is not true about "gray" platelets:

1. They appear hypergranulated on the peripheral
blood smear examination
2. They indicate a congenital deficiency in alpha granules
3. They may be seen myelodysplastic syndrome
4. They are characteristically pale

Answer: They appear hypergranulated on the peripheral
blood smear examination

In fact, they are **hypo**granulated.

Q. Which of the following is not true about aspirin:

1. Aspirin acetylates cyclooxygenase irreversibly and thereby inhibits the first step in prostanoid synthesis
2. It blocks thromboxane A2 production due to which platelet aggregation and vasoconstriction are inhibited
3. Much larger doses of aspirin are required for anti-platelet activity than for anti-inflammatory effects
4. Aspirin inhibits COX-1 to a greater degree than COX-2

Answer: Much larger doses of aspirin are required for anti-platelet activity than for anti-inflammatory effects

The fact is that much higher doses of aspirin are required for anti-inflammatory effects (COX-2) as compared with anti-platelet activity (COX-1), due to aspirin's greater inhibition of COX-1 compared with COX-2.

Q. What is the absolute increase in major bleeding events in patients using aspirin in doses upto 100 mg daily:

1. 0.3 to 1.7 per 1000 patient-years
2. 1.7 to 5.7 per 1000 patient-years
3. 0.3 to 1.7 per 100 patient-years
4. 1.7 to 5.7 per 100 patient-years

Answer: 0.3 to 1.7 per 1000 patient-years

This figure is based on data from one of the largest trials ever done on the subject.

Q. Which of the following is not true:

1. Dipyridamole is an effective antithrombotic agent but it has scarce anti-inflammatory effects
2. Clopidogrel and ticlopidine inhibit the P2Y12 receptor
3. Ticagrelor is a direct P2Y12 receptor blocker
4. Blockade of the integrin αIIbβ3 receptor with agents such as abciximab and eptifibatide leads to a thrombasthenic state

Answer: Dipyridamole is an effective antithrombotic agent but it has scarce anti-inflammatory effects

The fact is that dipyridamole is not considered an effective antithrombotic agent. Except for one trial, it has never been demonstrated to have a significant antithrombotic activity in clinical use.

Q. Which of the following is not correct regarding disorders of hemostasis in organ dysfunction:

1. Thrombocytopenia can be quite severe in cases of acute hepatitis
2. Chronic liver disease with cirrhosis often leads to modest thrombocytopenia
3. Severity of renal failure correlates with abnormal platelet aggregation
4. In renal failure, correction of the anemia with erythropoietin may decrease the incidence of bleeding

Answer: Severity of renal failure correlates with abnormal platelet aggregation

In fact, the severity of renal failure does not correlate with abnormal platelet aggregation.

Q. Which of the following is not associated with decreased platelet reactivity:

1. Hepatic failure
2. Uremia
3. Diabetes mellitus
4. Cardiopulmonary bypass

Answer: diabetes mellitus

Q. Acquired Glanzmann thrombasthenia can occur in all except:

1. Pregnancy
2. Systemic lupus erythematosus
3. ITP
4. Use of abciximab

Answer: none of the above

It can occur in all of the above mentioned situations.

Q. Which of the following is not an inherited syndrome with giant platelets:

1. Bernard-Soulier syndrome
2. Gray platelet syndrome
3. Wiskott-Aldrich syndrome

4. Montreal platelet syndrome

Answer: Wiskott-Aldrich syndrome

This question has been asked many times, so there is no excuse for getting this wrong. Note that in most of the inherited syndromes the platelet size is either large or normal and there are just two syndromes: WAS and X-linked thrombocytopenia, in which the platelet size is small. The list of the disorders with normal or large platelet size is very long, so there is no point in going on memorizing all of them.

Montreal platelet syndrome is a variant of VWD.

Another inherited syndrome with giant platelets is the May-Hegglin anomaly.

Q. Which of the following is not true about Glanzmann thrombasthenia:

1. It is an autosomal dominant bleeding disorder
2. The underlying basic defect is in the platelet integrin αIIbβ3
3. There is presence of mucocutaneous bleeding and a normal platelet count
4. Hematopoietic cell transplantation has successfully cured many patients with this disorder

Answer: it is an autosomal dominant disorder

It is an autosomal recessive disorder

Q. A "scramblase" defect in response to platelet activation signals is seen in:
1. Scott syndrome
2. May-Hagglin anomaly
3. Glanzmann thrombasthenia
4. Wiskott-Aldrich syndrome

Answer: Scott syndrome

Q. Which of the following is not correct:
1. Desmopressin is used to correct the hemostatic defect in von Willebrand disease
2. Conjugated estrogens are used for treatment of uremic bleeding
3. Erythropoietin has been used in uremic patients to both reduce and prevent bleeding
4. rFVIIa is approved in Europe for use in patients with Glanzmann thrombasthenia to reduced dependence on platelet transfusions

Answer: rFVIIa is approved in Europe for use in patients with Glanzmann thrombasthenia to reduced dependence on platelet transfusions

Recombinant factor VIIa is approved in Europe for management of Glanzmann thrombasthenia in patients who are **refractory** to platelet transfusions.

Q. In Bernard-Soulier syndrome platelet aggregation is seen in response to all of the following except:
1. Primary ADP

2. Secondary ADP
3. Collagen
4. Ristocetin

Answer: ristocetin

It is an important point to remember because in Glanzmann thrombasthenia the platelet aggregation response is seen **only** with ristocetin and not with primary and secondary ADP and collagen. So it's an important differentiating feature.

In VWD the response is seen with primary ADP, secondary ADP and collagen; the response to ristocetin is variable.

Q. Which of the following enzyme is constitutive:
1. COX-1
2. COX-2
3. Both of the above
4. None of the above

Answer: COX-1

Note that COX-1 is also known as PGHS-1 and COX-2 as PGHS-2.

Q. In uremic patients all of the following findings are present except:

1. Decreased platelet aggregation
2. Impaired platelet adhesiveness
3. Intrinsic dysfunction of glycoprotein IIb/IIIa

4. Deficiency in von Willebrand factor levels

Answer: Deficiency in von Willebrand factor levels

The deficiency in von Willebrand factor levels is not seen in uremic patients.

Q. Which of the following is considered a platelet toxic agent contributing to platelet dysfunction in uremia:

1. Urea
2. Guanidinoacetic acid
3. Creatinine
4. Methylguanidine

Answer: Guanidinosuccinic acid and methylguanidine

Note that urea and creatinine are not considered major platelet toxins.

Q. The drug of choice for bleeding due to uremia is:

1. Desmopressin
2. Factor VIIa
3. Estrogen
4. Cryoprecipitate

Answer: desmopressin

It is certainly the best drug for acute control of bleeding in uremic patients and it's also the least toxic.

Q. The major source of thrombopoietin is:

1. Liver
2. Kidney
3. Bone marrow
4. Lungs

Answer: liver

Q. The gene for thrombopoietin is found on:

1. Chromosome 3q
2. Chromosome 3p
3. Chromosome 5q
4. Chromosome 3p

Answer: Chromosome 3q

Note that there is only one copy for this gene in humans.

Q. In humans, thrombopoietin acts through which receptor:

1. c-Mpl
2. v-Mpl
3. p-Mpl
4. n-Mpl

Answer: c-Mpl

Q. Hepatic thrombopoietin production is usually constitutive:

1. True
2. False

Answer: true

Although levels may be affected by circulating platelet mass.

Q. Familial thrombocythemia occurs most commonly due to:

1. Activating mutations in the genes for TPO of c-Mpl transmitted in autosomal dominant pattern
2. Inactivating mutations in the genes for TPO of c-Mpl transmitted in autosomal dominant pattern
3. Activating mutations in the genes for TPO of c-Mpl transmitted in autosomal recessive pattern
4. Inactivating mutations in the genes for TPO of c-Mpl transmitted in autosomal recessive pattern

Answer: Activating mutations in the genes for TPO of c-Mpl transmitted in autosomal dominant pattern

Q. Which of the following statement is not true:

1. Thrombopoietin levels are done by ELISA assays
2. TPO concentrations are increased in bone marrow failure states
3. TPO levels are markedly elevated in immune thrombocytopenia (ITP)
4. TPO levels are usually normal in essential thrombocythemia

Answer: TPO levels are markedly elevated in immune thrombocytopenia (ITP)

It is an interesting point. In ITP the platelet count may be very low but still the levels of thrombopoietin are not proportionately elevated. Compare this with bone marrow failure states such as aplastic anemia, where the same levels of reduction in platelets will lead to markedly elevated thrombopoietin levels. One hypothesis for the explanation of the unexpectedly low rise of TPO in ITP is the enhanced clearance of TPO by megakaryocytes.

Q. In humans, megakaryocytes normally account for:

1. 0.05 to 0.1 percent of all nucleated bone marrow cells
2. 0.5 to 1 percent of all nucleated bone marrow cells
3. 1 to 5 percent of all nucleated bone marrow cells
4. 5 to 10 percent of all nucleated bone marrow cells

Answer: 0.05 to 0.1 percent of all nucleated bone marrow cells

Q. Megakaryocytes have an average diameter of:

1. 5 to 10 microns
2. 10 to 15 microns
3. 15 to 20 microns
4. 20 to 25 microns

Answer: 20 to 25 microns

Q. Each megakaryocyte produces how many platelets:

1. 1000 to 3000
2. 10000 to 30000
3. 100000 to 300000
4. Unlimited number of platelets

Answer: 1000 to 3000

Q. Thrombocytopenia due to bortezomib occurs as a result of:

1. Reduced number of megakaryocytes
2. Ineffective thrombopoiesis
3. Reduced platelet shedding
4. Inhibition of NF-kB

Answer: options 3 and 4 are correct

This is an interesting question. In most of the instances, the primary mechanism of chemotherapy induced thrombocytopenia is reduced number of megakaryocytes, primarily due to cytotoxicity of chemo and enhanced rate of apoptosis. But in the case of bortezomib that's not the case. Bortezomib has only minimal effect on the number of megakaryocytes, and its primary effect is reduced platelet shedding by inhibition of NF-kB.

Q. Chronic immune thrombocytopenia (ITP) is characterized by:

1. An increase in the number of bone marrow megakaryocytes
2. An increase in the size of bone marrow megakaryocytes
3. An increase in the ploidy of bone marrow megakaryocytes
4. All of the above

Answer: all of the above

Q. JAK2 mutations are found in approximately what percent of essential thrombocythemia patients:

1. 10
2. 20
3. 30
4. 50

Answer: 50

Approximately 5 to 10 percent of patients with ET have mutations in the thrombopoietin receptor (MPL), and around 75 percent have mutations in calreticulin (CALR).

Q. Megakaryocytes with a "pawn ball" nucleus are seen in:

1. Myelodysplastic syndrome
2. Primary myelofibrosis
3. Polycythemia vera
4. Essential thrombocythemia

Answer: myelodysplastic syndrome

Q. Which is the most potent activator of platelets:

1. Thrombin
2. Subendothelial collagen
3. Glycoprotein VI
4. ADP

Answer: thrombin

The most important receptor for thrombin in humans in PAR-1. Vorapaxar is an orally active PAR-1 antagonist used for preventing thrombosis in patients undergoing percutaneous coronary intervention.

Q. Aspirin results in what:

1. Irreversible inactivation COX-1
2. Irreversible activation COX-1
3. Reversible inactivation COX-1
4. Reversible activation COX-1

Answer: Irreversible inactivation COX-1

Q. Which of the following drug inhibits the final common pathway of platelet aggregation:

1. Abciximab
2. Tirofiban
3. Eptifibatide
4. All of the above

Answer: all of the above

Q. Which of the following TPO receptor agonist has not yet been approved for the treatment of ITP:

1. Romiplostim
2. Eltrombopag
3. Avatrombopag
4. All of the above mentioned drugs have been approved for ITP

Answer: All of the above mentioned drugs have been approved for ITP

Notes on approval of these agents:
1. In ITP all of these three have been approved.
2. In hepatitis C induced thrombocytopenia, only eltrombopag is approved.
3. For treatment of aplastic anemia eltrombopag and romiplostim has been approved

    4. Avatrombopag and lusutrombopag have been approved in patients with liver diseases who are about to undergo some invasive procedure

Note that this is based on data from various national guidelines. Not all the agents have the same approval worldwide for the indications listed above.

Q. Which of the following is not true about romiplostim:
    1. It is composed of two IgG1 kappa heavy chain constant regions linked via polyglycine
    2. It is FDA-approved for the treatment of ITP in adults and in children age ten and above
    3. It is administered weekly as a subcutaneous injection
    4. The dose ranges from 1 to 10 mcg/kg

Answer: It is FDA-approved for the treatment of ITP in adults and in children age ten and above

In fact, it is FDA-approved for the treatment of ITP in adults and in children age **one and above**.

Q. Eltrombopag is FDA-approved for the treatment of all except:
    1. Adults with ITP
    2. Patients with hepatitis C-related thrombocytopenia who are being treated with interferon
    3. Patients with aplastic anemia who are unresponsive to immunosuppressive therapy
    4. Children with ITP aged 2 years and above

Answer: Children with ITP aged 2 years and above

Eltrombopag is not approved for treatment of ITP in children.

Q. The advantages of avatrombopag over eltrombopag are:
1. It is approximately threefold more potent than eltrombopag
2. It does not alter liver function tests
3. It doesn't require any dietary restrictions
4. All of the above

Answer: all of the above

Q. Which of the following drug is not available orally:
1. Avatrombopag
2. Lusutrombopag
3. Eltrombopag
4. Romiplostim

Answer: romiplostim

Lusutrombopag is only approved to increase the platelet count in adult patients with chronic liver disease who are scheduled to undergo a procedure.

Q. Oprelvekin stimulates megakaryocyte growth and increases platelet production. It is:
1. IL-11
2. IL-13
3. TNF-alpha
4. Recombinant IFN-gamma

Answer: IL-11

Q. In patients of aplastic anemia unable to undergo HCT, the use of eltrombopag and romiplostim have been shown to be effective in improving which of the following hematologic parameters:
1. Neutropenia
2. Anemia
3. Thrombocytopenia
4. All of the above

Answer: all of the above

Although these drugs are expected to increase only platelet counts, their use in aplastic anemia patients has resulted in improvement of anemia and neutropenia as well; which is quite surprising but not entirely unexpected if we understand their mechanism of action.

Q. Which of the following is not true about adverse effects of thrombopoietic growth factors:
1. Antibody formation against romiplostim is a rare but alarming consequence
2. Eltrombopag has been associated with a risk of thrombosis in the portal venous system in patients with advanced liver disease
3. Increased rate of thrombosis in patients with immune thrombocytopenia (ITP)
4. Increased risk of bone marrow fibrosis

Answer: Increased rate of thrombosis in patients with immune thrombocytopenia (ITP)

This is an interesting question, as the results of trial data will lead to a correct answer rather than logic. While in many situations the use of thrombopoietic growth factors have been associated with an increased risk of thrombosis but in ITP this association has not been seen in trials.

Q. With which of the following drug, hepatotoxicity has been reported:
    1. Eltrombopag
    2. Romiplostim
    3. Avatrombopag
    4. All of the above

Answer: eltrombopag

Note that hepatotoxicity has not been reported with romiplostim or avatrombopag.

Q. The 5q- syndrome, a subtype of myelodysplastic syndrome, is commonly associated with:
    1. Thrombocytopenia
    2. Thrombocytosis
    3. Normal platelet count
    4. Abnormal platelet function with normal counts

Answer: thrombocytosis

Q. The normal mean platelet volume (MPV) is:
    1. 9 to 10 fL

2. 9 to 10 pL
3. 9 to 10 microL
4. 9 to 10 nL

Answer: 9 to 10 fL

fL is "femto litre".

Q. Which of the following is a cause of spurious thrombocytosis:

1. Mixed cryoglobulinemia
2. Severe hemolysis
3. Burns
4. All of the above

Answer: all of the above

Severe hemolysis and burns may cause fragmentation of RBCs, which may be mistaken for platelets.

Q. Thrombocytosis may be associated with:

1. Pseudohyperkalemia
2. Pseudohypokalemia
3. Pseudohypercalcemia
4. Pseudohypocalcemia

Answer: Pseudohyperkalemia

Artifactual elevation of potassium in serum but not in plasma may be seen with thrombocytosis, which is known as pseudohyperkalemia.

Notes:
In some cases of thrombocytosis, myeloproliferative neoplasms may be suspected. Most often, a clinician suspects an MPN because of atypical presentations like vasomotor or constitutional symptoms, splenomegaly, and/or an unusual thrombotic presentations.
Following tests are done on peripheral blood in such situations:
1. JAK2
2. CALR
3. MPL
4. Some form of testing for t(9;22) or its products

Q. A typical apheresis platelet unit provides:
1. 3 to 6 x 1011 platelets
2. 3 to 6 x 1010 platelets
3. 3 to 6 x 1012 platelets
4. 3 to 6 x 109 platelets

Answer: 3 to 6 x 1011 platelets

Q. Platelets are routinely stored at room temperature and not at cold temperature, why:
1. Cold induces clustering of von Willebrand factor receptors on the platelet surface
2. Cold induces morphological changes of the platelets
3. The cold induced changes lead to enhanced clearance by hepatic macrophages
4. All of the above

Answer: all of the above

Q. The shelf life of platelets stored at room temperature is:
1. 5 days
2. 1 day
3. 2 days
4. 9 days

Answer: 5 days

Q. Which of the following statement is not true:
1. Patients with thrombocytopenia and non-CNS bleeding, should be transfused with platelets immediately to keep platelet counts above 50,000/microL
2. Actively bleeding patients with thrombocytopenia and DIC should be transfused with platelets immediately to keep platelet counts above 50,000/microL
3. Patients having CNS bleeding with thrombocytopenia should be transfused with platelets immediately to keep platelet counts above 100,000/microL
4. Actively bleeding patients with thrombocytopenia and DIC should be transfused with platelets immediately to keep platelet counts above 100,000/microL

Answer: Actively bleeding patients with thrombocytopenia and DIC should be transfused with platelets immediately to keep platelet counts above 100,000/microL

In thrombocytopenic patients, in most bleeding situations

including disseminated intravascular coagulation (DIC), the platelet count should be kept above 50,000/microL.

I must admit that this is a very confusing topic and in many situations, the guidelines that we read are institution based and may not be universally accepted. Typical platelet count thresholds that are used for some common procedures are as follows:

1. Neurosurgery or ocular surgery – 100,000/microL
2. Most other major surgery – 50,000/microL
3. Endoscopic procedures – 50,000/microL for therapeutic procedures; 20,000/microL for low risk diagnostic procedures
4. Bronchoscopy with bronchoalveolar lavage (BAL) – 20,000 to 30,000/microL
5. Central line placement – 20,000/microL
6. Lumbar puncture – 10,000 to 20,000/microL in patients with hematologic malignancies and greater than 40,000 to 50,000 in patients without hematologic malignancies, but lower in patients with immune thrombocytopenia (ITP)
7. Epidural anesthesia – 80,000/microL
8. Bone marrow aspiration/biopsy – 20,000/microL

Q. The typical threshold for prophylactic platelet transfusion to prevent spontaneous bleeding in afebrile patients is:

1. Platelet counts below 10,000/microL
2. Platelet counts below 20,000/microL
3. Platelet counts below 30,000/microL
4. Platelet counts below 50,000/microL

Answer: Platelet counts below 10,000/microL

In patients who are febrile, have sepsis or organ dysfunction the threshold is higher. In unique situations like acute promyelocytic leukemia, the threshold is even higher (although there is no fixed number and different trials have used a different threshold for transfusion of platelets, most experts agree that platelet count should be kept 50,000/microL or more).

Q. Which of the following statement is true:

1. Prophylactic transfusion for patients with hematologic malignancies and HCT are used, with the threshold being platelet count less than 10,000/microL, except in cases of acute promyelocytic leukemia (APL)
2. In ITP, generally platelet transfusion is done for bleeding rather than at a specific platelet count
3. Although patients with HIT are at increased risk of thrombosis despite having thrombocytopenia, platelet transfusion should not be withheld from a bleeding patient due to concerns that platelet transfusion will exacerbate thrombotic risk
4. All of the above

Answer: all of the above

Q. The standard dose of platelets for prophylactic therapy in adults is:

1. One random donor unit per 10 kg of body weight
2. Two random donor units per 10 kg of body weight
3. One random donor unit per 20 kg of body weight
4. 5-6 random donor unit per 35 kg of body weight

Answer: One random donor unit per 10 kg of body weight

This amount usually translates to four to six units of pooled platelets or one apheresis unit (SDP).

Based on trial data, platelet doses more than this are not more effective whereas lower (half) dose may be equally effective but the standard guidelines recommend using the above mentioned doses.

A standard pediatric dose is 5 to 10 mL/kg.

Q. One unit of single donor platelets (SDP) is expected to raise the platelet count by approximately:

1. 30,000/microL
2. 10,000/microL
3. 50,000/microL
4. 20,000/microL

Answer: 30,000/microL

Q. Which of the following is not true about pooled versus apheresis platelets:

1. When given in recommended doses, the platelet count increment and hemostatic effects of pooled and apheresis platelets are comparable
2. The possibility of infection and alloimmunization is lower with apheresis platelets
3. It is easier to perform testing for infectious agents on apheresis platelets than on pooled tablets

4. When HLA-induced thrombolysis is there, pooled donor platelets are a safer choice

Answer: When HLA-induced thrombolysis is there, pooled donor platelets are a safer choice

Q. Leukoreduction aims at removing the contaminating white blood cells from the platelet transfusion. Which of the following is an indication for leukoreduction of platelet transfusion products:

1. Reduction of HLA alloimmunization
2. Reduction of CMV transmission
3. Reduction of transfusion-associated immuno-modulation
4. Reduction of transfusion-associated graft-versus-host disease
5. All of the above

Answer: all of the above

Note that, leukoreduction alone is not sufficient for prevention of ta-GVHD because some leukocytes may pass through the filtration channels. To prevent ta-GVHD, irradiation of platelets has to be done.

But please note that irradiation alone is also **insufficient** for prevention of ta-GVHD because the irradiated leukocytes may still trigger GVHD. So to prevent ta-GVHD both leukoreduction and irradiation are needed.

Leukoreduction also reduces the incidence of non-hemolytic febrile reactions.

Q. Which of the following statement is not true:
1. Platelets express ABO antigens on their surface
2. Platelets express HLA class I antigens on their surface
3. Platelets express HLA class II antigens on their surface
4. Platelets express Rh antigens on their surface

Answer: both options 3 and 4

Platelets do not express HLA class II antigens or Rh antigens.

Q. Which of the following is incorrect:
1. The hemolytic disease of the fetus and newborn (HDFN) results from Rh antigen mismatched platelets
2. Anti-D immune globulin is recommended if an Rh negative pregnant woman gets an Rh positive platelet transfusion
3. If only Rh+ platelets are available for transfusion in an Rh negative woman, then anti-D immune globulin can be coadministered with platelet transfusions
4. Each dose of anti-D immune globulin is considered sufficient to prevent alloimmunization for up to 15 mL of RhD-positive RBCs

Answer: The hemolytic disease of the fetus and newborn (HDFN) results from Rh antigen mismatched platelets

As we have discussed in a previous question, platelets don't express Rh antigen. The HDFN occurs due to the Rh positive RBCs that contaminate the platelet unit being transfused.

Most units of platelets do not contain more than 0.5 mL of RBCs, and since one dose of anti-D immune globulin is sufficient to prevent alloimmunization for upto **15 mL** of Rh positive RBCs, in most of the situations one dose is considered sufficient for this purpose.

Q. For an average sized adult, six units of pooled platelets or one apheresis unit of platelets is generally transfused over:
    1. 20 to 30 minutes
    2. 30 to 60 minutes
    3. 10 to 20 minutes
    4. 60-120 minutes

Answer: 20 to 30 minutes

There are many modifications of this duration, depending on comorbidities and other risk factors.

Q. Post-transfusion purpura develops:
    1. Within 48 hours of platelet transfusion
    2. 5 to 10 days after platelet transfusion
    3. After 24 hours but before 96 hours
    4. After 2 weeks or more

Answer: 5 to 10 days after platelet transfusion

This is a very rare complication of platelet transfusion and develops in individuals who lack the platelet antigen PIA1, also known as human platelet antigen 1a (HPA-1a).

Note that while the root cause of this complication is an innate lack of HPA-1a but the patient must have become pre-

viously sensitized to HPA-1a (like from a previous transfusion).
IVIG is the drug of choice if this complication develops.

Q. HIT results from an autoantibody directed against:
    1. Endogenous platelet factor 4 (PF4)
    2. Exogenous platelet factor 4 (PF4)
    3. Endogenous platelet factor 3 (PF3)
    4. Exogenous platelet factor 3 (PF3)

Answer: Endogenous platelet factor 4 (PF4)

This antibody **activates** platelets. HIT occurs due to the formation of the PF4-heparin complex.

Q. Which of the following is not correct about HIT type I:
    1. HIT type I (HIT I) is a mild, transient drop in platelet count that typically occurs within the first two days of heparin exposure
    2. The mechanism behind development of HIT type I is direct effect of heparin on platelets, causing immune-mediated platelet aggregation
    3. HIT type I is not associated with thrombosis
    4. Patients with HIT type I can be conservatively managed and discontinuation of heparin is not required

Answer: The mechanism behind development of HIT type I is direct effect of heparin on platelets, causing immune-mediated platelet aggregation

While it is true that HIT type I results from the direct effect of heparin on platelets, the platelet aggregation is **non-im-**

mune mediated.

Q. Which of the following is not true about HIT type II:
1. HIT type II occurs due to antibodies to platelet factor 4 (PF4) complexed to heparin
2. In HIT type II thrombosis along with thrombocytopenia is seen
3. Elimination of heparin from the patient is a must for its treatment
4. If heparin is eliminated then initiation of a non-heparin anticoagulant is not required

Answer: If heparin is eliminated then initiation of a non-heparin anticoagulant is not required

It must be clearly understood that if HIT type II is not correctly treated then mortality rates are very high and there are two essentials for its management:
1. Elimination of heparin
2. Initiation of non-heparin anticoagulant

Q. Delayed-onset HIT is defined by:
1. Thrombocytopenia occurring five or more days after heparin has been withdrawn
2. Thrombosis occurring five or more days after heparin has been withdrawn
3. Thrombocytopenia occurring more than 48 hours but with in five days after heparin has been withdrawn
4. Thrombosis occurring more than 48 hours but with in five days after heparin has been withdrawn

Answer: both options 1 and 2 are correct

The main crux of this question is the time frame but it also be stressed here, once again, that HIT is a unique disorder because it is a combination of thrombocytopenia and thrombosis.

This disorder occurs due to excessive presence of PF4/heparin complexes that were initially formed when the patient was exposed to heparin.

Note that the term "refractory HIT" is different from delayed HIT and it refers to a situation where HIT persists for many weeks after stopping heparin. There is no explanation for this.

Q. Which of the following is not true about HIT pathophysiology:
1. The IgM antibodies are formed usually within days for clinically significant manifestations
2. Even if the antibodies disappear, heparin rechallenge is no longer safe
3. Rechallenge with heparin in a patient who had developed HIT, does not always cause an anamnestic response
4. The culprit antibodies usually only cause clinical symptoms when heparin is present

Answer: The IgM antibodies are formed usually within days for clinically significant manifestations

While it's true that antibodies that result in HIT are formed within days of heparin exposure but these antibodies are **IgG** antibodies, not IgM antibodies. This is a unique feature of HIT that IgM antibodies are not formed and directly IgG antibodies are formed and that too within days.

Q. HIT has been reported in up to what percent of patients exposed to heparin for more than four days:
    1. 1
    2. 5
    3. 10
    4. <2

Answer: 5%

Q. In the "4 Ts" system for HIT, which of the following scores will fall under the intermediate probability category:
    1. 3
    2. 5
    3. 6
    4. 8

Answer: 5

In this system a score of 0 to 3 points means low probability (risk of HIT <1 percent), 4 to 5 points means intermediate probability (risk of HIT approximately 10 percent) and a score of 6 to 8 points means high probability (risk of HIT approximately 50 percent).

Many experts recommend an immunoassay (ELISA) for PF4-heparin in all patients with an intermediate or high probability 4 Ts score. In patients with low probability scores, experts consensus is that ELISA should not be performed, but it depends on the clinical situation.

For any 4 Ts score, if the ELISA OD is <0.60, the diagnosis of

HIT is ruled out. Once again, the guidelines may be slightly different for different expert groups and in some clinical situations exceptions may be there, discussion of which is beyond the scope of this book. In some cases there may be an indeterminate reading of OD by ELISA, in such cases functional assays may help in clarification.

Q. In individuals with a presumptive diagnosis of HIT based on the 4 Ts score, the diagnosis is considered to be confirmed if:

1. There is a positive ELISA with an optical density (OD) ≥2.00 for intermediate risk 4 Ts score
2. There is a positive ELISA with an OD ≥1.50 for patients with a high probability 4 Ts score
3. If there is a positive functional assay in cases of indeterminate ELISA OD
4. All of the above

Answer: all of the above

Q. Which is the more common type of HIT:

1. Type I HIT
2. Type II HIT
3. Delayed HIT
4. Spontaneous HIT

Answer: type I HIT

The frequency of type I HIT is 10-20% and that of type II is 1-3%.

Notes on phases of HIT:

1. Suspected: platelets are low but PF4-heparin assay

not yet done
2. Acute HIT: platelets are low **and** PF4-heparin assay is positive (functional assays **and/or** immunoassays)
3. Subacute HIT A: platelet counts are normalized and PF4-heparin assay still positive
4. Subacute HIT B: platelet counts are normalized and functional assay is negative **but** immunoassay still positive
5. Remote HIT: platelet counts are normal and both the functional as well as immunoassays are negative

Q. Which of the following is not a component of the 4 Ts scoring for estimating the pretest probability of HIT:
1. Thrombocytopenia
2. Timing of onset after heparin exposure
3. Thrombotic manifestations
4. Treatment responsiveness

Answer: treatment responsiveness

The fourth "T" is o**T**her cause for thrombocytopenia

It is easy to misread this one.

Q. In the typical presentation of drug induced immune thrombocytopenia, the drop in platelet count occurs:
1. Within two weeks of exposure to the drug
2. After 2 weeks but within 4 weeks of exposure to the drug
3. Within 48 hours of exposure to the drug
4. After at least 4 weeks of exposure to the drug

Answer: within two weeks of exposure to the drug

Note that quinine is the prototype drug for drug induced immune thrombocytopenia. Drugs may also cause thrombocytopenia by non-immune mechanisms, like linezolid.

Immune thrombocytopenia (ITP)

In the following section, we will discuss ITP (also known as idiopathic/immune thrombocytopenic purpura). Today the most accepted terminology is "immune thrombocytopenia", because it was observed that in many patients there is no purpura and the previous terminology was causing unnecessary confusion.

ITP can also occur in children, especially in the first decade of life. The ITP in children has many differences from ITP in adults, eg:
1. There is a higher likelihood of spontaneous remission in children
2. There is a lower incidence of underlying diseases and comorbidities in children
3. The risk of bleeding is lower in children with ITP compared to adults

Q. If 14 months have elapsed since the diagnosis of ITP and it has still not resolved then it will be referred to as:
1. Newly diagnosed
2. Persistent
3. Chronic
4. There is no such classification

Answer: chronic

ITP is called newly diagnosed ITP up to three months since diagnosis, persistent ITP from three to 12 months since diagnosis and chronic ITP if more than 12 months have elapsed since diagnosis.

Q. Which of the following is a mechanism of pathogenesis of ITP:
1. Antibody-mediated destruction of platelets
2. Autoreactive cytotoxic T cells mediated platelet destruction
3. Humoral and cellular autoimmunity directed at megakaryocytes
4. All of the above

Answer: all of the above

First of all, there is no agreed upon theory for pathogenesis of ITP. The most accepted one is that IgG autoantibodies are produced by the patient's B cells which target platelet membrane glycoproteins, the most important of which is GPIIb/IIIa.

Q. Antiplatelet antibodies are demonstrable in approximately what percent of patients with ITP:
1. 50
2. 70
3. 30
4. <20

Answer: 50%

The sensitivity of antiplatelet antibody assay in diagnosis of ITP is low.

Q. Which of the following is not true about clinical manifestations of ITP:

1. The bleeding in ITP typically occurs in the skin or mucous membranes
2. The purpura due to ITP is nonpalpable
3. Intracerebral hemorrhage is seen in less than 2% of adults with ITP
4. In patients with ITP, who are not having active bleeding, smaller sized platelets are often noted on the peripheral blood smear

Answer: In patients with ITP, who are not having active bleeding, smaller sized platelets are often noted on the peripheral blood smear

In fact, in ITP the size of platelets on the peripheral smear is often small.

But it must be noted here that the size of platelets or other morphological features of platelets are not characteristic for ITP and any aberration should raise suspicion for a disorder other than ITP.

Q. Most of the experts agree that therapies to increase platelet count are generally not required in patients with ITP having a minimum platelet count of (per microL):

1. >20000
2. >30000
3. >50000
4. >100000

Answer: >20000

The risk of severe bleeding is low with platelet counts >20,000/microL.

Note that ITP is a diagnosis of exclusion.

Q. Which of the following is not generally considered as a "first-line" treatment option for treatment of ITP:
    1. Glucocorticoids
    2. Intravenous immune globulin
    3. Anti-D immune globulin
    4. Rituximab

Answer: rituximab

Thrombopoietin receptor agonists are also **not** used in the first-line.

Q. Which of the following infectious agents need not be studied in a case of ITP:
    1. HBV
    2. HCV
    3. HIV
    4. CMV

Answer: CMV

Helicobacter pylori studies are also recommended by many experts.

Q. Which of the following is an initial treatment options for patients with severe bleeding and a platelet count <30,000/microL:

1. Platelet transfusion
2. IVIG, 1g/kg, repeated the following day if the platelet count remains <50,000/microL
3. Methylprednisolone, 1 g intravenously, repeated daily for three doses
4. Dexamethasone, 40 mg orally or intravenously, repeated daily for four days

Answer: all of the above

Romiplostim is also sometimes used but the evidence is lacking.

Q. Which of the following statement is not true about ITP:
1. Glucocorticoids are the first-line ITP therapy
2. Complete long-term remissions with glucocorticoids have been reported in approximately 50 percent of patients
3. When dexamethasone is used in the treatment of ITP, it is administered as 40 mg orally per day for four days with no taper
4. When prednisone is used in the treatment of ITP, it is administered at 1 mg/kg daily for one to two weeks followed by a gradual taper

Answer: Complete long-term remissions with glucocorticoids have been reported in approximately 50 percent of patients

The complete long term remission rate with glucocorticoids is around 20%.

Dexamethasone is preferred over prednisone by many experts, because dexamethasone has higher overall response rate, better complete response rate, no difference in overall or complete response at six months and fewer toxicities, compared with prednisone.

Notes on second line therapy options for ITP:
1. If first line therapy options fail then second line options are used.
2. They include splenectomy, rituximab, thrombopoietin receptor agonists or immunosuppressive therapy.

Note that if a patient of ITP develops a malignancy (breast cancer, for example) then myelosuppressive chemotherapy **should not be withheld** for the fear of worsening of thrombocytopenia. So chemotherapy should be given in patients in full doses according to the protocol.

Q. For patients who require additional therapy beyond first-line glucocorticoids, the treatment of choice is:
1. Rituximab
2. Thrombopoietic agents
3. Danazol
4. Splenectomy

Answer: splenectomy

Note that in hematology, there are no absolute treatment strategies and everything depends on the clinical context. Hence, words like "treatment of choice" don't have much of an inherent meaning. The point of this question is to test the ability of the exam going student to select the best course of action in a broader sense.

Out of all the second line options, splenectomy has the greatest chance of altering the disease course and resulting in a sustained remission and the toxicity is also acceptable.

If a patient is unfit for surgery or is unwilling for surgery then rituximab is the best option.

Q. Which of the following is an indication for use of thrombopoietin mimetics:
1. Persistent thrombocytopenia despite splenectomy and rituximab
2. Lack of suitability for splenectomy or rituximab
3. Requirement for a temporary increase in platelet count
4. All of the above

Answer: all of the above

It should be noted that the counts start increasing after 7 to 14 days of injection.

Q. Which of the following drug is available as a pill:
1. Romiplostim
2. Eltrombopag
3. Avatrombopag
4. All of the above

Answer: options 2 and 3

Romiplostim is available as a subcutaneous injection.

Q. Fostamatinib received US Food and Drug Administration approval for:

1. The treatment of thrombocytopenia in adults with chronic ITP in the first line
2. The treatment of thrombocytopenia in adults with chronic ITP who have had an insufficient response to a previous treatment
3. The treatment of thrombocytopenia in adults with acute ITP in second or subsequent line
4. All of the above

Answer: The treatment of thrombocytopenia in adults with chronic ITP who have had an insufficient response to a previous treatment

It is approved for only this indication.

MISCELLANEOUS

Q. The most common cause of thrombocytopenia in pregnancy is:
1. Gestational thrombocytopenia
2. HELLP syndrome
3. Preeclampsia
4. Immune thrombocytopenia (ITP)

Answer: gestational thrombocytopenia

Gestational thrombocytopenia accounts for nearly 60% of thrombocytopenia cases in pregnancy.

The characteristic features of gestational thrombocytopenia are:

1. It is most common in the third trimester and especially around delivery
2. Thrombocytopenia is mild
3. The risk of bleeding is not increased
4. There is no fetal or neonatal thrombocytopenia
5. It resolves spontaneously

Q. Which of the following statement is not true about thrombotic thrombocytopenic purpura (TTP):
1. It is associated with moderately to severely elevated activity of ADAMTS13
2. There is absence of coagulation abnormalities
3. The clinical course of TTP is not affected by delivery
4. The most important treatment of TTP is urgent plasma exchange therapy

Answer: It is associated with moderately to severely elevated activity of ADAMTS13

In fact it is associated with severely **reduced** activity of ADAMTS13. Typically the activity of ADAMTS13 in TTP is <10%.

Q. Which of the following is not a cause of secondary thrombocytosis:
1. Iron deficiency
2. Hemolysis
3. Mycobacterial infection
4. Hypersplenism

Answer: hypersplenism

Splenectomy or functional asplenia is the cause of thrombocytosis. Hypersplenism is a cause of thrombocytopenia.

Secondary thrombocytosis is also known as reactive thrombocytosis.

Q. All of the following are true about gestational thrombocytopenia except:
1. It develops in approximately 5 to 10 percent of pregnancies
2. It is mild, asymptomatic, occurs during early gestation
3. There is no associated risk of bleeding
4. There is no associated risk of fetal thrombocytopenia

Answer: It is mild, asymptomatic, occurs during early gestation

While it is true that gestational thrombocytopenia is mild and asymptomatic but it occurs in **late** gestation and not in early gestation. No treatment is required for this condition and it spontaneously resolves after delivery.

Gestational thrombocytopenia is a diagnosis of exclusion and the clinician must not miss the more dangerous causes of thrombocytopenia like **h**emolysis, **e**levated **l**iver enzymes, **l**ow **p**latelet count (HELLP) syndrome, preeclampsia, or thrombotic thrombocytopenic purpura (TTP) or even ITP.

Q. Which of the following drug is more commonly associated with immune mediated DITMA than with non immune

mediated DITMA:
1. Quinine
2. Calcineurin inhibitors
3. Methamphetamine
4. All of the above

Answer: quinine

Quinine is the classical drug for immune mediated DITMA.

Q. Which of the following is not a part of the pentad of TTP:
1. Microangiopathic hemolytic anemia
2. Thrombocytopenia
3. Hepatic insufficiency
4. Fever

Answer: hepatic insufficiency

Apart from the three findings above the other two findings are neurologic findings and renal insufficiency.

HEMOSTASIS

PNH (Paroxysmal nocturnal hemoglobinuria)

Q. PNH is associated with mutation of *PIGA* gene. This gene is:

1. Located on the X chromosome and the mutation takes place in a somatic cell
2. Located on the X chromosome and the mutation takes place in a germ line cell
3. Located on the chromosome 14 and the mutation takes place in a somatic cell
4. Located on the chromosome 14 and the mutation takes place in a germ line cell

Answer: Located on the X chromosome and the mutation takes place in a somatic cell

It is important to note that the PIGA gene mutation is an acquired, somatic mutation.

Q. Which of the following patients of PNH usually have more hemolysis, if the PNH clone population is similar:

1. Patients with a large percentage of type II RBCs
2. Patients with a small percentage of type II RBCs
3. Patients with a large percentage of type III RBCs
4. Patients with a small percentage of type III RBCs

Answer: Patients with a large percentage of type III RBCs

Notes:
1. Type II RBCs have partial absence of glycosylphos-phatidylinositol [GPI] anchored proteins
2. Type III RBCs have complete absence of GPI anchored proteins

Type III RBCs have the greatest degree of hemolysis because there are no GPI anchored proteins.

Q. Which of the following is not frequently encountered in patients of PNH:
1. Nocturnal hemolysis leading to cola coloured urine in the morning
2. Day time hemolysis due to activity of alternate complement pathway
3. Skeletal muscle dystonia
4. Smooth muscle dystonia

Answer: skeletal muscle dystonia

Note that the name of the disorder contains the word "nocturnal", meaning "at night" but most of the patients have chronic hemolysis occurring throughout the day and night.

Smooth muscle dystonia is often seen in PNH patients.

Q. Which if the most common gastrointestinal manifestation in PNH patients:
1. Esophageal spasm
2. Constipation
3. Gastric outlet obstruction
4. Lower GI bleeding

Answer: esophageal spasm

Q. Which of the following is the leading cause of death in patients with PNH:
1. Hemorrhage
2. Thrombosis
3. Pulmonary hypertension
4. Myocardial infarction

Answer: thrombosis

Q. Which of the following statement is wrong:
1. The incidence of PNH is significantly increased in patients with inherited aplastic anemia
2. The lifetime risk of PNH progressing to acute leukemia is 5 percent or less
3. Pure erythroid leukemia is often the most common

form of AML when transformation of PNH to acute leukemia occurs

4. None of the above

Answer: The incidence of PNH is significantly increased in patients with inherited aplastic anemia

Remember that the incidence of PNH is significantly increased in patients with **acquired** aplastic anemia, not inherited aplastic anemia.

Q. The hemolysis in PNH is generally:
1. Direct Coombs positive
2. Indirect Coombs positive
3. Coombs negative
4. Coombs indeterminate

Answer: Coombs negative

The characteristic hemolysis in PNH is "Coombs negative intravascular" hemolysis.

Q. Which of the following is not true about bone marrow examination findings in PNH:
1. Bone marrow examination is not required for the diagnosis of PNH
2. Patients with classical PNH usually have a hypercellular bone marrow with erythroid hyperplasia

3. Stainable iron is often abundantly present
4. Erythroid dysplasia is often present

Answer: Stainable iron is often abundantly present

In fact, stainable iron is often **absent**.

Q. Which is the most accepted method to confirm the diagnosis of PNH:
1. Flow cytometry including FLARE
2. Flow cytometry including FLAIR
3. Flow cytometry including FLAER
4. Flow cytometry including FLEAR

Answer: Flow cytometry including FLAER

For the diagnosis of PNH, flow cytometry is done on patient's peripheral blood cells with monoclonal antibodies which are fluorescently-labeled and bind to glycosylphosphatidylinositol (GPI)-anchored proteins.

These GPI-anchored proteins are absent or reduced on the blood cells in PNH. The most commonly assayed GPI-linked proteins are CD59 and CD55. Although there are many others.
Most labs also include **FL**uorescent **AER**olysin (FLAER) reagent. This reagent directly binds to the GPI anchor.

Note that the diagnosis of PNH by using flow cytometry is not always straightforward, as there can be confounding findings present. To overcome such difficulties, it is recommended that at least two independent flow cytometry reagents should be used on at least two cell lineages (eg, RBCs and WBCs) to establish the diagnosis of PNH.

Q. Which of the following is an established therapy for patients with hemolytic (classical) PNH:
1. Allogeneic hematopoietic cell transplantation
2. Eculizumab
3. Ravulizumab
4. All of the above

Answer: all of the above

Q. Which of the following statement is wrong about treatment of PNH:
1. In patients of PNH having significant disease manifestations attributable to hemolysis, treatment with a complement inhibitor is recommended
2. All patients should be vaccinated against *Neisseria meningitidis* ideally two weeks prior to the first dose of anti-complement therapy
3. Iron supplementation is routinely used during eculizumab therapy
4. Daily oral antibiotic prophylaxis is recommended in patients of PNH receiving complement inhibitors

Answer: Iron supplementation is routinely used during eculizumab therapy

Iron supplementation is **not** routinely used during eculiz-umab therapy.

Q. For patients of PNH who have not had a thrombotic event, prophylactic anticoagulation is indicated because throm-botic events are the leading cause of mortality in these pa-tients:
1. True
2. False

Answer: false

If a patient of PNH develops thrombosis then anticoagulants are used and they can then be continued after the throm-botic event has been resolved. But in a patient who never had a thrombotic event, prophylactic anticoagulants are **not** recommended.

Q. Which of the following is a curative therapy for PNH:
1. Allogeneic hematopoietic cell transplantation
2. Eculizumab
3. Ravulizumab
4. All of the above

Answer: allogeneic hematopoietic cell transplantation

Q. In pregnant patients with PNH, eculizumab therapy is contraindicated:
1. True
2. False

Answer: false

There are data suggesting decreased maternal mortality and no increased risk of fatal malformation with eculizumab. So, its use is **not** contraindicated.

Antiphospholipid syndrome (APS)

Q. Approximately what percent of APS patients have concomitant underlying systemic autoimmune disease:
1. 10
2. 20
3. 50
4. 90

Answer: 50%

Around 50% of cases of APS are associated with underlying systemic autoimmune disorder while rest of the patients (50%) have primary APS (without any concomitant auto-immune disease).

SLE is the most common autoimmune disease associated with APS.

Q. Thrombotic events are hallmarks of APS. Venous thrombosis is more common than arterial thrombosis. The risk of recurrent thrombosis is increased with "triple positivity," which includes all of the following except:
1. Lupus anticoagulant
2. Anti-cardiolipin antibodies
3. Anti-beta-2-glycoprotein-I antibodies
4. Alpha-1-stromelysin directed antibodies

Answer: Alpha-1-stromelysin directed antibodies

If a patient shows positivity for the first three (options 1, 2 and 3), "triple positivity" is said to be present. It is associated with increased risk of recurrent thrombosis.

Q. Which of the following are the most common sites of thrombosis in APS:
1. Deep veins of the lower extremities
2. Superficial veins of lower extremities
3. Renal veins
4. Pulmonary veins

Answer: deep veins of lower extremities

Q. Which is the most common site of arterial thrombosis in APS:
1. Cerebral vasculature
2. Pulmonary vasculature
3. Lower limb vasculature
4. Renal vasculature

Answer: cerebral vasculature

Q. Which of the following is a feature of Sneddon syndrome:
1. Livedo reticularis
2. Stroke
3. Myocardial infarction
4. All of the above

Answer: option 1 and 2 are correct

Sneddon syndrome is seen in some patients of APS, it has two components: widespread livido reticularis and stroke.

Q. Which of the following valve is most commonly involved in APS:
1. Mitral
2. Aortic
3. Pulmonary
4. Tricuspid valve

Answer: mitral

Q. Which of the following is the most common cutaneous abnormality in APS:
1. Livedo reticularis
2. Racemosa
3. Splinter haemorrhages
4. Cutaneous infarction

Answer: livedo reticularis

Notes on diagnostic criteria for APS:

APS is diagnosed if at least one of the clinical criteria **and** one of the laboratory criteria are met:

Clinical criteria:
1. Vascular thrombosis: One or more clinical episodes of arterial, venous, or small vessel thrombosis, in any tissue or organ. For diagnosis of thrombosis imaging studies and/or histopathologic studies must be done.
2. Pregnancy morbidity:

One or more of the following should be present:
   a. One or more unexplained deaths of a morphologically normal fetus at or beyond the 10th week of gestation, with normal fetal morphology documented by ultrasound or by direct examination of the fetus; **or**
   b. One or more premature births of a morphologically normal neonate before the 34th week of gestation

because of: (i) eclampsia or severe preeclampsia defined according to standard definitions, or (ii) recognized features of placental insufficiency; **or**

c. Three or more unexplained consecutive spontaneous abortions before the 10th week of gestation, with maternal anatomic or hormonal abnormalities and paternal and maternal chromosomal causes excluded.

Laboratory criteria:

1. Lupus anticoagulant (LA) present in plasma, on two or more occasions at least 12 weeks apart

2. Anticardiolipin antibody (aCL) of IgG and/or IgM isotype in serum or plasma, present in medium or high titer (ie, >40 GPL or MPL, or >the 99th percentile), on two or more occasions, at least 12 weeks apart, measured by a standardized ELISA.

3. Anti-beta-2 glycoprotein-I antibody of IgG and/or IgM isotype in serum or plasma (in titer >the 99th percentile), present on two or more occasions, at least 12 weeks apart, measured by a standardized ELISA.

Q. For the diagnosis of catastrophic APS, at least how many organs must be involved:

1. 2
2. 3
3. 4
4. 5

Answer: 3

For the diagnosis of **definite** catastrophic APS, all of the following four criteria must be met:

1. Evidence of involvement of **three or more** organs, systems, and/or tissues
2. Development of manifestations simultaneously or in less than a week
3. Confirmation by histopathology of small vessel occlusion in at least one organ or tissue
4. Laboratory confirmation of the presence of antiphospholipid antibodies (lupus anticoagulant, anticardiolipin antibodies, and/or anti-beta2-glycoprotein I antibodies)

There is another diagnostic entity, known as "probable APS". It has a different set of diagnostic criteria.

Q. Based on the latest trial data, which of the following is the anticoagulant of choice in patients with APS:

1. Aspirin
2. Warfarin
3. Rivaroxaban
4. Apixaban

Answer: warfarin

Warfarin has been the gold standard anticoagulant for patients of APS, but it requires monitoring of PT-INR. Trials have compared it with new oral anticoagulants, which have different mechanisms of action and don't require monitoring. But these newer drugs have lower efficacy than warfarin. Thus, warfarin is still the drug of choice for APS.

Q. In non-pregnant patients of APS, who never had a thrombotic event, thromboprophylaxis is indicated:
1. True
2. False

Answer: false

Primary prophylaxis of thrombosis is not indicated in patients with APS.

But once a patient of APS develops thrombosis, which resolves on treatment; **secondary prophylaxis is indicated,** typically with warfarin.

Q. For patients of APS who develop VTE and are treated with warfarin, what is the recommended range in which INR should be maintained:
1. 1-2
2. 2-3
3. 2.5-3.5
4. 3.5-4.5

Answer: 2-3

Haemophilia

Q. Which of the following is an option for the treatment of chronic hemarthrosis resulting as a sequelae of hemophilia:
   1. Short-term factor prophylaxis
   2. Synovectomy
   3. Total joint replacement
   4. All of the above

Answer: all of the above

Q. Hemophilia C occurs due to inherited deficiency of which coagulation factor:
   1. Factor VIII
   2. Factor IX
   3. Factor X
   4. Factor XI

Answer: factor XI

Notes:
   1. Haemophilia A: deficiency of factor VIII
   2. Haemophilia B (Christmas disease): deficiency of factor IX
   3. Haemophilia C (Rosenthal syndrome): deficiency of factor XI

Haemophilia A and B are X linked recessive disorders whereas haemophilia C is an autosomal recessive disorder. Some patients of haemophilia C may have other types of inheritance too.

Rarely, you may come across the term "acquired hemophilia", which most often means an acquired deficiency of factor VIII (as opposed to congenital deficiency).

Q. In moderate haemophilia, the factor activity level and factor concentration, respectively, are:
1. >1 to <5% and >0.01 to <0.05 IU/mL
2. <1% and >0.01 to <0.05 IU/mL
3. <5% and >0.03 to <0.05 IU/mL
4. None of the above

Answer: >1 to <5% and >0.01 to <0.05 IU/mL

Memorise the definition of severity of hemophilia:
1. Severe hemophilia: factor activity level <1 percent of normal, which corresponds to <0.01 IU/mL
2. Moderate hemophilia: factor activity level ≥1 percent of normal and ≤5 percent of normal, corresponding to ≥0.01 and ≤0.05 IU/mL
3. Mild hemophilia: factor activity level >5 percent of normal and <40 percent of normal, corresponding to ≥0.05 and <0.40 IU/mL

Q. Which of the following haemophilia is more likely to be

severe:
1. Hemophilia A
2. Hemophilia B
3. Hemophilia C
4. All of the above are equally severe

Answer: hemophilia A

Hemophilia A is the most common hemophilia and it is also the most severe one.

Q. All of the following is true about hemophilia B Leyden except:
1. There is mild hemophilia is childhood that becomes severe after puberty
2. Mutations in this disease occur in the factor IX promoter
3. Testosterone plays a role in alteration of disease course once the patient reaches puberty
4. None of the above

Answer: There is mild hemophilia is childhood that becomes severe after puberty

In this disease, there is **severe hemophilia is childhood which becomes mild after puberty.**

Some other diseases may be coinherited with hemophilia. If haemophilia is inherited along with a thrombotic disease, then the bleeding disorder of hemophilia may be less severe. This is called "coinheritance of hemophilia".

Notes on diagnostic criteria of hemophilia:
1. The diagnosis of hemophilia A requires a factor VIII activity level below 40% of normal
2. In some cases the factor VIII activity level may be 40% or more; in them a pathogenic factor VIII gene mutation must be present to make a diagnosis of hemophilia A
3. The diagnosis of hemophilia B requires a factor IX activity level below 40% of normal
4. In some cases the factor IX activity level may be 40% or more; in them a pathogenic factor IX gene mutation must be present to make a diagnosis of hemophilia B
5. The diagnosis of hemophilia carrier status requires identification of a hemophilia gene mutation. The "factor activity levels" can not be used for the diagnosis of haemophilia carriers.

Q. Approximately what percent of patients with hemophilia have a negative family history:
1. 33
2. 10
3. 50
4. 75

Answer: 33%

These cases arise due to de novo mutation.

Q. Emicizumab is useful in:
1. Hemophilia A
2. Hemophilia B
3. Acquired von Willebrand disease
4. PNH

Answer: hemophilia A

Emicizumab is a monoclonal antibody that substitutes for the function of factor VIII.

Notes on types of prophylaxis for haemophilia patients:
1. Episodic (on demand) treatment: replacement factor given at the time of bleeding
2. Intermittent (periodic) prophylaxis: replacement factor given to prevent bleeding for short periods of time such as during and after surgery
3. Continuous (regular) prophylaxis: replacement factor given to prevent bleeding for at least 45 of 52 weeks (85%) of a year. Continuous prophylaxis is of three types:
a. Primary prophylaxis: continuous prophylaxis started before age three years and before the second large joint bleed
b. Secondary prophylaxis: continuous prophylaxis started after two or more large joint bleeds but before the onset of chronic arthropathy
c. Tertiary prophylaxis: continuous prophylaxis started after the onset of arthropathy to prevent further damage

Q. What should be the target factor activity level in hemophilia patients who have life threatening intracranial bleed:
1. 1-2%
2. 10-20%
3. 80-100%
4. 40-50%

Answer: 80-100%

Life threatening bleeds like ICH and head trauma are medical emergencies and factor replacement must be done as urgently as possible. For hemophilia A, the dose is 50 units/kg of factor VIII and for hemophilia B, the dose is 100 to 120 units/kg of factor IX.

Q. In case a patient of hemophilia develops joint bleeding, what should be the target factor activity level:
1. 1-2%
2. 10-20%
3. 80-100%
4. 40-50%

Answer: 40-50%

Factor replacement should be done as urgently as possible at the first sign of joint bleeding. The dose for hemophilia A is 25 units/kg of factor VIII and for hemophilia B is 50 to 60 units/kg of factor IX.

Q. If a patient of hemophilia has a high titer and high-responding inhibitor (eg, ≥5 Bethesda units) who has serious bleeding; what is the treatment of choice for treatment of this acute condition:
1. Recombinant factor VIIa
2. Recombinant factor VIII
3. Recombinant factor VIIb
4. Recombinant factor X

Answer: Recombinant factor VIIa

Q. DDAVP is used most effectively in which setting in haemophilia patients:
1. For elective procedures in patients with mild hemophilia A
2. For emergency procedures in patients with mild hemophilia A
3. For elective procedures in patients with moderate to severe hemophilia A
4. For emergency procedures in patients with moderate to severe hemophilia A

Answer: For elective procedures in patients with mild hemophilia A

VWD

Q. Which is the most common inherited bleeding disorder:
1. Inherited von Willebrand disease
2. Acquired von Willebrand syndrome
3. Haemophilia A
4. Haemophilia B

Answer: inherited von Willebrand disease

Q. Which of the following may lead to acquired von Willebrand syndrome:
1. Autoantibodies to VWF
2. High shear stress
3. Adsorption of VWF to cells
4. Decreased protein production

Answer: all of the above

These are the four mechanisms which may lead to von Willebrand syndrome (VWS).

Q. Which of the following is more common:
1. Acquired VWS
2. Congenital VWS

Answer: congenital VWS

Congenital (or inherited) VWS has a 100 fold higher incidence than acquired VWS.

Notes on treatment of acquired VWS:
1. Treatment of underlying condition is the most important part of management.
2. In patients with acute bleeding, VWF concentrates, DDAVP, IVIG and antifibrinolytics are the mainstays. Immunosuppressive therapy is especially beneficial in individuals with autoantibodies to VWF.
3. In some patients, prophylaxis against bleeding and perioperative management may involve DDAVP, VWF concentrates, and/or IVIG.
4. Some patients may have concomitant essential thrombocytosis, such patients may be given anti platelet therapy. This, obviously, is very challenging but VWS in itself is **not** a contraindication to anti platelet therapy.

Q. Which of the following type of VWD occurs due to dysfunctional VWF:
1. Type 1
2. Type 2
3. Type 3
4. Type 4

Answer: type 2

Notes on types of VWD:

There are three major types of VWD:

a. Type 1: due to a quantitative reduction in von Willebrand factor (VWF) protein
b. Type 2: due to dysfunctional VWF (it is further subdivided into 2A, 2B, 2M and 2N)
c. Type 3: due to absent or severely reduced VWF

Q. Which of the following is the most common type of VWD:
1. Type 1
2. Type 2
3. Type 3
4. Type 4

Answer: type 1

Q. Which of the following VWD has an autosomal recessive inheritance:
1. Type 1
2. Type 2B
3. Type 2M
4. Type 3

Answer: type 3

Notes:
1. Autosomal dominant inheritance: 1, 2B and most types 2A and 2M
2. Autosomal recessive inheritance: 2N and 3

Note that all VWD are **autosomal,** and thus affected both males and females.

Q. Which type of VWD is not associated with a mild disease course:
1. Type 1
2. Type 2A
3. Type 2N
4. Type 3

Answer: type 3

Type 3 has an aggressive course, it has severe bleeding manifestations including both mucocutaneous and joint bleeding.

Notes on diagnosis of VWD:
The diagnostic work up of VWD is complex and nuanced. I will request you to go thorough a standard textbook to understand it thoroughly. The most important points are summarised below:
1. The screening tests for VWD in suspected patients are: VWF protein levels (VWF antigen [VWF:Ag]), a VWF functional (activity [VWF:Act]) test, and a factor VIII activity level.
2. An individual is diagnosed as having VWD if he or she has a positive personal or family history of bleeding and <30 percent (<30 international units/dL) VWF:Ag or VWF:Act.
3. If the VWF:Ag or VWF:Act is 30 to 50% then retesting is done and if again it comes out to be 30 to 50%

then a diagnosis of "low VWD" is made.

4. Once the diagnosis of VWD is confirmed using the criteria mentioned above, specialised tests are done to determine the type of VWD. Once again, I will advice you to go through a standard text book. The summary is as follows:

a. If there is a concordant reduction in VWF:Act and VWF:Ag, the likely diagnosis is type 1 VWD.

b. Individuals with discordant reductions in VWF:Act and VWF:Ag are likely to have type 2A, 2B, or 2M VWD.

c. Type 3 VWD patients have undetectable or absent VWD.

Q. Which of the following is not true about treatment of von Willebrand disease (VWD):

1. DDAVP is only effective in some individuals
2. DDAVP has a later onset and shorter duration of action
3. Type 2N VWD patients require factor VIII concentrates before major surgery
4. For major bleeding, the initial dose of plasma-derived VWF concentrates is in the range of 100 to 600 units/kg

Answer: For major bleeding, the initial dose of plasma-derived VWF concentrates is in the range of 100 to 600 units/kg

In fact, the initial dose range is 40 to 60 units/kg.

Notes on treatment of VWD:

1. There are two main treatment options: desmopressin and VWF concentrates.

2. Desmopressin is used before minor surgery or for treatment of minor bleeding. The problems with desmopressin are that it is not reliably effective in all patients, it has a later onset of action and it acts only in short term.

3. VWF concentrates are the mainstay for treatment of major bleeding and for prophylaxis when elective major surgery is planned. The treatment is individualised and the target ranges of VWF activity are also flexible.

4. There are certain special types of VWF that require additional products:

a. Type 2N VWD requires recombinant factor VIII for serious bleeding or surgery

b. Type 2B VWD requires platelet transfusions in addition to VWF concentrates

INHERITED THROMBOPHILIA

Notes:

1. For patients of inherited thrombophilia, the diagnostic and treatment strategies are not well defined.

2. They are generally suspected when an unprovoked episode of venous or arterial thromboembolism occurs; especially at unusual sites.

3. In these patients anticoagulants are to be started once an unprovoked thromboembolic episode takes place. The minimum duration of anticoagulant therapy is generally at least 3 to 6 months in such cases but may be longer.

4. Warfarin or direct oral anticoagulants are the main-

stays of treatment.
5. The role of primary prophylaxis is not well defined and primary prophylaxis is generally not recommended.
6. Oral contraceptive pills are relatively contraindicated in most of such disorders but may be used with extreme caution in certain situations.

Q. Antithrombin inhibits the function of which of the following:
1. Factor IIa
2. Factor Xa
3. Both of the above
4. All serine proteases

Answer: both of the above

Testing of antithrombin deficiency is best done by the functional assay for plasma AT activity, which is also known as the AT-heparin cofactor assay.

Q. What is the most common inheritance of antithrombin deficiency:
1. Autosomal dominant
2. Autosomal recessive
3. X linked dominant
4. X linked recessive

Answer: autosomal dominant

Q. Factor V Leiden is the most common inherited thrombophilia in individuals with venous thromboembolism:
    1. True
    2. False

Answer: true

It is the most common inherited thrombophilia in individuals with venous thromboembolism.

This disorder results from a point mutation.

Q. Protein C deficiency is inherited as:
    1. Autosomal dominant
    2. Autosomal recessive
    3. X linked dominant
    4. X linked recessive

Answer: autosomal dominant

Note that protein S deficiency is also an autosomal dominant condition.

Q. Which is the most common prothrombin point mutation resulting in inherited thrombophilia:

1. G20210A
2. G21210A
3. G20220A
4. G22010A

Answer: G20210A

MISCELLANEOUS TOPICS

Q. Which of the following statement is not true:
1. Patients with multiple myeloma treated with an immunomodulatory drug in combination with glucocorticoids have a rate of venous thromboembolism (VTE) greater than 20 percent
2. VTE prophylaxis is continued for as long as the patient of multiple myeloma is receiving treatment with thalidomide, lenalidomide, or pomalidomide
3. Ideally all patients of multiple myeloma being treated with immunomodulatory drugs should receive dual prophylaxis with aspirin plus warfarin or LMWH
4. Concurrent use of an H2-blocker or a proton pump inhibitor is recommended in multiple myeloma patients who are receiving immunomodulatory drugs and VTE prophylaxis

Answer: Ideally all patients of multiple myeloma being treated with immunomodulatory drugs should receive dual prophylaxis with aspirin plus warfarin or LMWH

Notes on VTE prophylaxis in multiple myeloma:
1. We must first assess the baseline risk of VTE. The risk factors are: previous VTE, inherited thrombophilia, central venous catheter or pacemaker, cardiac disease, diabetes, acute infection, immobilization, use of erythropoietin, chronic renal disease, and obesity. Based on these risk factors patients are classified in three risk groups.

2. Higher risk for VTE: patients being treated with immuno-modulatory drugs (thalidomide, lenalidomide or pomal-idomide) who have two or more risk factors or are receiving concomitant high dose dexamethasone (≥ 480 mg per month), doxorubicin, or multiagent chemotherapy. In these patients, LMWH or warfarin are used for VTE prophylaxis (aspirin is not used).

3. Standard risk for VTE: patients with no or one risk factor who are not receiving high dose dexamethasone, doxorubicin, or multiagent chemotherapy. In these patients, aspirin is used for VTE prophylaxis (LMWH or warfarin are not used.)

4. The prophylaxis is continued as long as immunomodulatory drugs are given.

Q. Modified Caprini risk assessment model is used for predicting risk of VTE in general surgical patients. Which of the following is not given "5" points in this model:
1. Age 75 years or more
2. Elective arthroplasty surgery
3. Hip fracture surgery
4. Less than one month old spinal injury

Answer: age 75 years or more

The modified Caprini model is very exhaustive, to read in its full extent please go to: Gould MK, Garcia DA, Wren SM, et al. Prevention of VTE in nonorthopedic surgical patients: antithrombotic therapy and prevention of thrombosis, 9th ed: American College of Chest Physicians evidence-based clinical practical guidelines. Chest 2012; 141:e227S.

There are only four factors which are given 5 points (all other factors are given 1, 2 or 3 points):
1. Stroke (<1 month)
2. Elective arthroplasty
3. Hip, pelvis, or leg fracture
4. Acute spinal cord injury (<1 month)

It is very important to note here that this model **does not apply to cancer surgeries.**

Q. Which of the following is not a factor in estimating the risk of venous thromboembolism is patients with cancer using the Khorana score:
1. Site of cancer
2. Pre-chemotherapy platelet count
3. Pre-chemotherapy hemoglobin level
4. Age

Answer: age

Please memorise the Khorana score, many times questions are asked about it. The risk factors are:

1. Site of primary tumor:
    1. Very high risk (stomach, pancreas): 2 points
    2. High risk (lung, lymphoma, gynecologic, bladder, testicular): 1 point
    3. All other sites: 0 points
2. Pre-chemotherapy platelet count ≥350,000/microL: 1 point
3. Hemoglobin level <10 g/dL or use of ESAs: 1 point
4. Pre-chemotherapy WBC >11,000/microL: 1 point
5. BMI ≥35 kg/m2: 1 point

These points are finally added and the sum is "Khorana score":

1. Low risk: 0 points
2. Intermediate risk: 1-2 points
3. High risk: 3 or more points

Q. Which of the following statement is false about treatment of DIC:

1. For patients who are not bleeding, prophylactic transfusion of platelets is indicated to maintain platelet count above 50,000/microL
2. Antifibrinolytic agents are contraindicated
3. Patients with purpura fulminans benefit from the

administration of protein C concentrate
4. All of the above

Answer: For patients who are not bleeding, prophylactic transfusion of platelets is indicated to maintain platelet count above 50,000/microL

Different societies and guidelines make different recommendations, but they all agree that prophylactic transfusion of platelets is not indicated if the platelet count is >10000 (>20000 according to some) and the patient is not bleeding. If the patient is bleeding or if a major surgical procedure is planned then the threshold may be high.

Caution must be taken as DIC has a unique biology and depending on the ongoing cascade, sometimes transfusion of platelets may lead to exacerbation of the problem.

Q. Typically what is the level of activity of ADAMTS13 in patients with acquired thrombotic thrombocytopenic purpura (TTP):
1. <10%
2. 10-20%
3. 20-30%
4. >30%

Answer: <10%

Acquired TTP usually presents as severe microangiopathic hemolytic anemia (MAHA) and thrombocytopenia.

TTP is characterised by ADAMTS13 deficiency.

Q. Treatment should be initiated promptly, even if only a presumptive diagnosis of acquired TTP is made:
1. True
2. False

Answer: true

It is considered a medical emergency.

Treatment options are:
1. Plasma exchange (preferred and most effective, may prove to be life saving in urgent situations)
2. Glucocorticoids (usually the regimen is high dose methylprednisolone followed by oral prednisone)
3. Rituximab
4. Caplacizumab

Q. How long should plasma exchange be continued in patients with TTP:
1. Indefinitely

2. Once the platelet count is ≥150,000/microL for at least two days
3. When a stable plateau in the normal or supranormal range of platelet count is approached for three days
4. In weekly pulses every 2 months, frequency may be guided by ADAMTS13 activity levels

Answer: options 2 and 3 are correct

If this question was not about the duration of plasma exchange but about the duration of glucocorticoids or caplacizuamb then the answer would have been: "tapering of these drugs is based on ADAMTS13 activity recovery to above 20 to 30 percent."

Q. Which of the following statement is false:
1. For acute lower limb DVT, anticoagulation is administered for a minimum of three months and extended for 6 to 12 months in some cases
2. For most patients with acute symptomatic proximal DVT, anticoagulation is recommended rather than no anticoagulation
3. An IVC filter is used for patients with acute proximal DVT who have recurrent embolism despite adequate anticoagulation
4. Low molecular weight heparin is relatively contraindicated in pregnant females having DVT

Answer: low molecular weight heparin is relatively contraindicated in pregnant females having DVT.

WHITE BLOOD CELL DISORDERS

BIOLOGY

Q. All of the following are true except:
1. Stem cell factor is also known as Steel factor
2. G-CSF is essential for the amplification and terminal differentiation of neutrophil progenitors and precursors
3. M-CSF/CSF1 is a monocyte lineage specific factor
4. IL-12 is an eosinophil lineage specific factor

Answer: IL-12 is an eosinophil lineage specific factor

In fact, **IL-5** is an eosinophil lineage specific factor.

Q. Which of the following point is wrong regarding development of myeloid lineage cells:
1. Myeloblasts are the earliest myeloid precursors recognizable by light microscopy
2. Promyelocytes are larger than myeloblasts with their size being > 20 microns
3. Myelocytes are the last precursor capable of undergoing cell division
4. Promyelocytes are characterized by secondary or azurophilic granules

Answer: Promyelocytes are characterized by secondary or

azurophilic granules

In fact, promyelocytes are characterized by primary or azurophilic granules.

Q. Which of the following is not a feature of bands:
    1. They have elongated, horseshoe-shaped nuclei
    2. The ratio of azurophilic primary granules to specific secondary granules is approximately 1:2 in these cells
    3. Tertiary (gelatinase) granules are not present
    4. These are fully functional phagocytes

Answer: Tertiary (gelatinase) granules are not present

In fact, tertiary granules are present.

To clarify the fourth option, the bands are fully functional and they are included in the absolute neutrophil count (ANC).

Q. Which of the following is not a feature of PMNs:
    1. They are of variable size with average diameter being 20 microns
    2. Their nucleus has three lobes on average
    3. Approximately 3 percent of PMNs from females have a visible Barr body which is an inactivated X chromosome
    4. They show peroxidase-positive primary granules and peroxidase-negative secondary granules

Answer: They are of variable size with average diameter being 20 microns

The fact is that PMNs are of consistently similar size and the average diameter is 13 microns.

Q. The maturation time for neutrophils from the myeloblast stage is:
    1. 1 day
    2. 8 days
    3. 14 days
    4. 28 days

Answer: 8 days

Q. What is the mean lifespan of neutrophils:
    1. 5-8 days
    2. 1-2 days
    3. 10-14 days
    4. More than a month

Answer: 5-8 days

Notes on fate of monocytes:
Monocytes differentiate further into fixed-tissue macrophages, including:
    1. Alveolar macrophages
    2. Hepatic Kupffer cells
    3. Dermal Langerhans' cells
    4. Osteoclasts
    5. Peritoneal and pleural macrophages
    6. Brain microglial cells (controversial)

Q. Human pulmonary alveolar proteinosis (PAP) is caused by:
1. Autoantibodies to GM-CSF
2. Autoantibodies to G-CSF
3. Autoantibodies to erythropoietin
4. Autoantibodies to stem cell factor

Answer: Autoantibodies to GM-CSF

LAB HEMATOLOGY

Notes on some formulas:
1. Mean corpuscular volume (MCV; in femtoliters [fL]) = 10 x HCT (percent) ÷ RBC (millions/microL)
2. Mean corpuscular hemoglobin (MCH; in picograms [pg]/red cell) = HGB (g/dL) x 10 ÷ RBC (millions/microL)
3. Mean corpuscular hemoglobin concentration (MCHC), in grams per deciliter (g/dL) = HGB (g/dL) X 100 ÷ HCT (percent)
4. Hematocrit = (RBC x MCV)/10

Q. In which of the following condition, RDW is only slightly elevated:
1. Iron deficiency
2. Transfused anemia
3. Myelodysplastic syndrome
4. Thalassemia trait

Answer: thalassemia trait

In the other three conditions, RDW is **very** elevated.

In anemia of chronic disease, RDW is slightly elevated.

Q. Use of which of the following agents during collection of peripheral blood is most commonly associated with pseudothrombocytopenia:
1. EDTA
2. Heparin
3. Sodium citrate
4. Dimethyl sulfoxide

Answer: EDTA

Q. Which of the following statement is correct:
1. Blood samples should be kept at room temperature if analysis is to occur within eight hours of collection
2. Blood samples should be refrigerated if the analysis is to occur up to 24 hours after collection
3. Samples more than 36 hours old should not be used for CBC testing
4. All of the above

Answer: all of the above

Q. In Coulter instruments, when taking readings about RBCs, a left "shoulder" extension to the curve indicates presence of what:
1. Schistocytes
2. Sideroblasts
3. Reticulocytes
4. RBC agglutinins

Answer: schistocytes

Notes on abnormalities of RBC distribution on Coulter instruments:
1. A left "shoulder" extension to the curve, or failure of the curve to reach baseline on the left side is due to RBCs with smaller volumes. It can be seen when microspherocytes or schistocytes are present. It may also be seen when platelet clumps or macrothrombocytes are present.
2. A separate RBC population to the left can indicate the presence of two populations of red cells, as seen in X-linked sideroblastic anemia.
3. A right-sided shoulder usually corresponds to a population of extremely large RBCs (macrocytes) or reticulocytes.
4. A trailing erythrocyte population to the extreme right can indicate the presence of RBC agglutinins.

Q. Platelets with a higher MPV are expected to be seen in:
1. Destructive thrombocytopenia
2. Marrow hypoplasia
3. Marrow aplasia
4. All of the above

Answer: Destructive thrombocytopenia

Higher MPV is seen when destruction of platelets is there but marrow is active as in immune thrombocytopenia [ITP]. It is also seen in some congenital thrombocytopenias like gray platelet syndrome, May-Hegglin anomaly, and Bernard-Soulier syndrome.

Low MPV is seen when marrow is not active enough, like

in aplastic anemia. It is also seen in Wiskott-Aldrich syndrome.

In hypersplenism platelets with low MPV are seen whereas in hyposplenic states platelets with higher MPV are seen.

Q. In instruments of hematology using scattered light for cell counting, the light is measured at low and high forward angles. How much is the low forward angle in these machines:
1. 0 to 3 degrees
2. 5 to 15 degrees
3. 15 to 30 degrees
4. 30 to 45 degrees

Answer: 0 to 3 degrees

Q. Which is the proposed international reference method for enumeration of platelets:
1. Immunologic method
2. Coulter method
3. Light scattering method
4. There is no consensus in this regard

Answer: immunologic method

CD61 monoclonal antibody is used for this. Another antibody is CD41a.

Q. While performing the differential leukocyte count by suspension method, the smallest size group of cells is:
1. Lymphocytes
2. Eosinophils

3. Band neutrophils
4. Monocytes

Answer: lymphocytes

These values are slightly different than the ones we usually memorize. In the "three-part differential" there are three groups of cells:
1. Lymphocytes and basophils are the smallest size group (35 to 90 fL)
2. Segmented and band neutrophils and eosinophils ("granulocytes") are the largest size group (>160 fL)
3. Monocytes and other mononuclear cells, including immature granulocytes and a portion of the eosinophils, are found in a smaller intermediate size peak between 90 and 160 fL

There are also five-part differential machines that report the basic five leukocyte subsets (neutrophils, eosinophils, basophils, lymphocytes, and monocytes) and also, seven part differential machines that add quantification of immature granulocytes and nucleated red blood cells to the five-part differential.

The current generation of instruments use the following techniques to produce a final DLC report:
1. Impedance volume with direct current (DC)
2. Radiofrequency (RF) conductivity (with impedance aperture)
3. Laser light scattering
4. Peroxidase staining
5. Propidium iodide fluorescence (for nucleated RBC and non-viable cells)
6. Cell-specific lysing reagents
7. Polymethine RNA/DNA histone dye
8. Digital imaging

Q. Which of the following is not a cause of spurious increase in MCHC:
1. A spuriously elevated HGB
2. A spuriously high RBC count
3. Lipemia
4. A very high WBC count

Answer: A spuriously high RBC count

In fact, it is the spuriously low RBC count that leads to spurious increases in MCHC. Apart from the three situations listed above, other causes of a spuriously high MCHC are presence of a precipitating monoclonal protein and presence of a cold agglutinin.

On the other hand, causes of spuriously decreased MCHC are:
1. Iron deficiency anemia
2. Hyperglycemia (it leads to temporary changes in readings)

Q. Peripheral smear examination offers many insights and is a cheap method. Which of the following is not true about a peripheral smear examination:
1. The thick of the slide may be useful in searching for the presence of malarial parasites
2. The thin end of the slide may be useful for identifying Auer rods
3. The thick end of the slide is more useful in identification of circulating tumor cells
4. None of the above

Answer: The thick end of the slide is more useful in identification of circulating tumor cells

In fact, CTCs are better visualized in the thin end.

Q. RBC rouleaux formation is seen in all except:
1. Multiple myeloma
2. Decreased levels of fibrinogen
3. Polyclonal gammopathy
4. Monoclonal gammopathy

Answer: decreased level of fibrinogen

In fact, increased levels of fibrinogen are associated with rouleaux formation.

Q. Which of the following is not true about the normal red cells:
1. They are the second most abundant cells in the peripheral smear
2. They are approximate the size of the lymphocyte nucleus
3. Their diameter is 7 to 8 microns
4. Their mean corpuscular volume (MCV) of approximately 90 femtoliters

Answer: They are the second most abundant cells in the peripheral smear

In fact, they are **the most** abundant cells in the peripheral smear.

Q. RBCs are generally round and have a smooth surface. Changes in their shape are known as poikilocytosis. Which of the following is not a correct statement in this regard:

1. Macroovalocytes suggest deficiency of vitamin B12 or folic acid
2. Schistocytes or helmet shaped cells are seen in idiopathic thrombocytopenic purpura
3. Teardrop-shaped red cells are seen in primary myelofibrosis
4. Teardrop shaped cells may be seen in thalassemia

Answer: Schistocytes or helmet shaped cells are seen in idiopathic thrombocytopenic purpura

In fact, schistocytes are seen in thrombotic thrombocytopenic purpura

Q. Approximately what fraction of area of red cell should appear clear on light microscopy:

1. 0%
2. 33%
3. 50%
4. 66%

Answer: 33%

This clear area is in the form of central pallor and occupies one-third of the red cell.

When hemoglobin concentration is low, this area is increased in size and in conditions like hereditary spherocytosis and autoimmune hemolytic anemia, this area is lost.

Q. Metamyelocytes and myelocytes may be seen in peripheral circulation during:
    1. Infections
    2. Pregnancy
    3. Leukemoid reactions
    4. They are never seen in nonmalignant conditions

Answer: first three options are correct

That being said, it's not usual for them to appear in the peripheral circulation in the above mentioned conditions but they may be seen. On the other hand, cells like promyelocytes and myeloblasts are almost exclusively seen in hematologic malignancies.

Q. Leuko-erythroblastic blood picture is defined as the combined presence of all of the following except:
    1. Early neutrophil forms
    2. Nucleated red blood cells
    3. Megakaryocytes
    4. Teardrop-shaped red blood cells

Answer: megakaryocytes

This picture is suggestive of bone marrow invasion and/or fibrosis.

Q. A leukemic hiatus is frequently seen in CML patients, which means:
    1. There is a greater percent of myelocytes than metamyelocytes in the peripheral blood

2. There is a lesser percent of myelocytes than meta-myelocytes in the peripheral blood
3. There is a greater percent of metamyelocytes than myelocytes in the bone marrow
4. There is a lesser percent of metamyelocytes than myelocytes in the bone marrow

Answer: There is a greater percent of myelocytes than meta-myelocytes in the peripheral blood

Q. Increased lobulation of neutrophils, known as hyperlobu-lation, is seen in all except:
1. Vitamin B12 deficiency
2. Iron deficiency anemia
3. Heat stroke
4. Myelodysplastic syndrome

Answer: myelodysplastic syndrome

In MDS, there is reduced lobulation of matured neutrophils known as the pseudo-Pelger-Huet anomaly. In the Pelger-Huet anomaly too, hypolobulation is seen. The abnormal cells in these two disorders have bilobed nucleus connected by a thin strand, giving a "pince-nez" appearance.

Q. In Chediak-Higashi syndrome, which abnormality of neu-trophils is seen:
1. Increased lobulation
2. Giant cytoplasmic granules
3. Reduced or absent toxic granules in cases of infec-tion
4. Recurrent pyogenic infection with neutrophil ab-normalities

Answer: Reduced or absent toxic granules in cases of infection

This syndrome is characterized by giant cytoplasmic granules within neutrophils.

Dohle bodies are light blue colored, situated near the periphery and seen in neutrophils of patients with infection.

Q. Which of the following is the least common circulating white blood cell:
    1. Eosinophil
    2. Basophil
    3. Monocyte
    4. Neutrophil

Answer: basophils.

They constitute less than 1% of total circulating white cell population.

Basophilia is seen in myeloproliferative disorders, hypersensitivity or inflammatory reactions, hypothyroidism (myxedema), and certain infections.

Q. Which are the largest normal cells seen on a peripheral blood smear:
    1. Monocytes
    2. Basophils
    3. Reticulocytes
    4. Lymphocytes

Answer: monocytes

Q. Large platelets may be seen in:
    1. Disseminated intravascular coagulation
    2. Thrombotic thrombocytopenic purpura
    3. Hemolytic uremic syndrome (HUS)
    4. All of the above

Answer: all of the above

Drug-induced thrombotic microangiopathy (DITMA) is also a cause.

Q. Microcytosis (of RBCs) in an adult may be seen in all except:
    1. Iron deficiency
    2. Thalassemia
    3. Sideroblastic anemias
    4. Chronic copper toxicity

Answer: chronic copper toxicity

The first three are recognized causes of microcytosis.

Chronic lead poisoning is another known cause of microcytosis.

Q. Polychromatophilia is typical of:
    1. Basophils

2. Eosinophils
3. Reticulocytes
4. Band forms

Answer: reticulocytes

Notes on shapes of RBCs:
1. Bite cells are seen in hemolytic anemia, especially G6PD. The rigid precipitates of denatured hemoglobin are known as Heinz bodies
2. In sickle cell anemia, the RBCs (obviously) look like sickles; other words are "canoe-like" or "pita bread-like".
3. Target cells have a "bull's eye" extra drop of hemoglobin in their center. They are seen in obstructive liver disease, postsplenectomy states, and hemoglobinopathies such as thalassemia and Hb C.
4. Echinocytes/burr cells/crenated cells are seen most commonly in uremia.
5. Acanthocytes or spur cells are seen in liver disease.
6. Teardrop-shaped red cells are are seen in primary myelofibrosis and thalassemic disorders.

Q. Nucleated red blood cells are seen in the peripheral blood in all of the following conditions except:
1. Severe hemolysis
2. Myelofibrosis
3. Profound stress
4. Severe iron deficiency anemia

Answer: Severe iron deficiency anemia

Q. Which of the following is not true:
1. Howell-Jolly bodies are nuclear remnants within

      red cells seen in hypersplenism
2. Heinz bodies are aggregates of denatured hemoglobin, found in G6PD deficient subjects
3. Basophilic stippling occurs due to ribosome precipitates and seen in thalassemias and lead poisoning
4. Pappenheimer bodies are iron-containing dark blue granules found in red cells in patients with sideroblastic anemia

Answer: Howell-Jolly bodies are nuclear remnants within red cells seen in hypersplenism

Howell-Jolly bodies are seen in patients with either absence of spleen or reduced function of spleen (like in cases of surgical removal of the spleen and in sickle cell anemia, when the crisis leads to infarction of spleen.

Q. The infectious agent most commonly leading to "red cell ghosts" is:
1. Clostridium perfringens
2. Staphylococcus aureus
3. Haemophilus influenzae
4. Neisseria meningitidis

Answer: Clostridium perfringens

Q. The formula for calculation of absolute neutrophil count is:
1. ANC = WBC (cells/microL) x percent (PMNs + bands) ÷ 100
2. ANC = WBC (cells/microL) x percent (PMNs + multinucleated cells) ÷ 100
3. ANC = WBC (cells/microL) x percent (PMNs +

bands)
4. ANC = WBC (cells/microL) x percent (PMNs) ÷ 100

Answer: ANC = WBC (cells/microL) x percent (PMNs + bands) ÷ 100

The point to remember here is that bands are considered functional neutrophils.

Q. In which of the following condition will the production of neutrophils will not be decreased:
1. Severe congenital neutropenia
2. Shwachman-Diamond syndrome
3. Chediak Higashi syndrome
4. None of the above

Answer: none of the above

In all of the above mentioned conditions the production of neutrophils will be decreased.

Other causes of decreased neutrophil production are aplastic anemia, paroxysmal nocturnal hemoglobinuria (PNH) etc.

Q. Chronic granulomatous disease is due to defects in:
1. NADPH oxidase
2. NADPH reductase
3. NADPH transcriptase
4. NADPH reuptake

Answer: NADPH oxidase

Defects in NADPH oxidase result in an inability of neutrophils to make superoxide.

This disease is most of the times X-linked and affects only males. In rare cases females may suffer from a mild form of CGD.

The diagnosis of CGD is established by showing absence of the ability to make superoxide in response to stimulation with phorbol myristate acetate (PMA). Superoxide production is indirectly assayed as an inability to reduce dihydrorhodamine (DHR) to its fluorescent form (which can be assayed using flow cytometry) or to reduce nitroblue tetrazolium (NBT), which is assayed using the NBT slide test.

Q. Leukocyte adhesion deficiency I is caused by:
1. Absence of the transmembrane protein CD18
2. Absence of the transmembrane protein CD28
3. Increased levels of the transmembrane protein CD18
4. Increased levels of the transmembrane protein CD18

Answer: Absence of the transmembrane protein CD18

On the other hand LAD-II is caused by decreased sialyl-Lewis-X on the neutrophil surface.

Q. Which of the following is not a feature of Chediak-Higashi syndrome:

1. Partial albinism
2. Nystagmus
3. Defects in chemotaxis
4. Absence of granules visible in the peripheral blood smear

Answer: Absence of granules visible in the peripheral blood smear

In fact, a feature of this syndrome is the presence of huge granules in the peripheral blood smear.

Q. Hyperimmunoglobulin E syndrome results in defects in neutrophil function due to mutations in:
1. STAT3
2. JAK1
3. BRAF
4. NADPH oxidase

Answer: STAT3

This syndrome is also known as Job syndrome.

Q. The definition of lymphocytosis in an adult is:
1. >4000 lymphocytes/microL in the peripheral blood
2. >8000 lymphocytes/microL in the peripheral blood
3. >2000 lymphocytes/microL in the peripheral blood
4. >1000 lymphocytes/microL in the peripheral blood

Answer: >4000 lymphocytes/microL in the peripheral blood

Q. The definition of lymphocytopenia in an adult is:
  1. <4000 lymphocytes/microL in the peripheral blood
  2. <8000 lymphocytes/microL in the peripheral blood
  3. <1500 lymphocytes/microL in the peripheral blood
  4. <1000 lymphocytes/microL in the peripheral blood

Answer: <1000 lymphocytes/microL in the peripheral blood

It should be noted that these values are not absolute and some
flexibility is allowed in interpretation.

Formula for calculation of absolute lymphocyte count (ALC) (cells/microL) = WBC (cells/microL) x percent lymphocytes ÷ 100

Q. In the peripheral blood, the most abundant lymphocyte population is of:
  1. T cells
  2. B cells
  3. NK cells
  4. All of the above are found in almost equal numbers

Answer: T cells

T cells are 60 to 80 percent, B cells are 10 to 20 percent and NK cells are 5 to 10 percent of total peripheral blood lymphocytes. Around 66% of T cells are CD4+ cells and 33% are CD8+ cells.

Q. Lymphocytosis is associated with:
1. *B. pertussis* infection
2. *B. parapertussis* infection
3. Both of the above
4. None of the above

Answer: *B. pertussis* infection

Q. All of the following are associated with lymphocytopenia except:
1. Wiskott-Aldrich syndrome
2. HIV infection
3. Protein energy malnutrition
4. EBV infection

Answer: EBV infection

In fact, EBV infection is **characterized** by lymphocytosis.

Drugs frequently associated with drug reaction with eosinophilia and systemic symptoms (DRESS):
1. Allopurinol
2. Carbamazepine, lamotrigine, phenytoin
3. Vancomycin, minocycline, dapsone, sulfamethoxazole

Notes on congenital causes of pancytopenia:
1. Wiskott Aldrich syndrome
2. Fanconi anemia
3. Dyskeratosis congenita/telomere biology disorders
4. Shwachman-Diamond syndrome
5. GATA2 deficiency
6. Hemophagocytic lymphohistiocytosis (HLH)

Q. The most accepted definition of neutropenia in adults is a neutrophil count in the peripheral blood of:
1. <1500 cells/microL
2. <2000 cells/microL
3. <1000 cells/microL
4. <500 cells/microL

Answer: <1500 cells/microL

It should be remembered that this value, and other such values, are not absolute and different institutes and organizations have different definitions; like the World Health Organization uses ANC of ≤1800 cells/microL to define neutropenia.

Notes on categories of neutropenia:
1. Mild: ANC ≥1000 and <1500 cells/microL
2. Moderate: ANC ≥500 and <1000 cells/microL
3. Severe: ANC <500 cells/microL
4. Agranulocytosis: ANC <200 cells/microL

Q. The most common cause of neutropenia is:
1. Infections
2. Medications

3. Nutritional
4. Familial

Answer: medications

Rheumatologic disorders are also common and important causes of neutropenia.

Q. In immunocompromised patients, the chest radiograph appearance of Pneumocystis jirovecii infection is:
1. Nodular infiltrates
2. Diffuse interstitial infiltrates
3. Basal infiltrates
4. Pleural effusion with patchy consolidation

Answer: Diffuse interstitial infiltrates

In viral infections, ARDS etc. too, there are diffuse interstitial infiltrates.

Q. Which of the following is not true about benign ethnic neutropenia:
1. It is an inherited cause of mild/moderate neutropenia
2. It is associated with increased risk for infections
3. It is more prevalent in people of African descent
4. It has been described in up to 25 to 40 percent of individuals of African origin

Answer: It is associated with increased risk for infections

Note the word "benign" in it. The risk of infections is not increased.

It is associated with a single nucleotide polymorphism (SNP) of the *ACKR1* gene.

Q. Patients with benign ethnic neutropenia are usually:
  1. Duffy null
  2. O negative and Rh negative
  3. Of Bombay blood group
  4. Of unclassifiable blood group type

Answer: Duffy null

HEMOPHAGOCYTIC LYMPHOHISTIOCYTOSIS

Q. Hemophagocytic lymphohistiocytosis most frequently affects which population:
  1. Infants
  2. Early adolescence
  3. Late adulthood
  4. Elderly

Answer: infants

HLH is a life-threatening syndrome of excessive immune activation. It most frequently affects infants from birth to 18 months of age.

The highest incidence is in infants of <3 months.

HLH is broadly of two types: primary and secondary. Primary HLH is caused by a gene mutation, either at one of the FHL loci or in a gene responsible for one of several immunodeficiency syndromes. Secondary HLH cases have **no** known familial mutation.

Macrophage activation syndrome is a form of HLH, which is often associated with juvenile rheumatologic diseases.

Q. Which of the following is true about pathogenesis and prognostic factors in HLH:
1. In HLH, macrophages become activated and secrete excessive amounts of cytokines
2. In HLH, NK cells fail to eliminate activated macrophages
3. In HLH, increased CD8 numbers and decreased CD4/CD8 ratios is associated with worse survival
4. Decreased total CD3 numbers is associated with a bad outcome

Answer: In HLH, increased CD8 numbers and decreased CD4/CD8 ratios is associated with worse survival

In fact, in HLH, increased CD8 numbers and decreased CD4/CD8 ratios is associated with **better** survival outcomes.

Q. Hemophagocytosis is frequently observed in HLH. Macrophage cytoplasm should show which kinds of cells or their fragments, to be categorized as hemophagocytosis:

1. Red blood cells
2. Platelets
3. White blood cells
4. Any of the above

Answer: any of the above

Q. Unbound (free) IL-18 levels are higher in:
1. Macrophage activation syndrome
2. Familial HLH
3. The levels are not elevated in either MAS or HLH
4. The levels are elevated to the same degree in both MAS and HLH

Answer: MAS

Unbound IL-18 level >24,000 pg/mL could distinguish MAS from familial HLH.

Q. Which is the most common infectious trigger for development of HLH:
1. EBV
2. HSV
3. HIV
4. CMV

Answer: EBV

Patients with X-linked lymphoproliferative disease (XLP) are at particularly high risk.

Interestingly, immune checkpoint inhibitors **may be** linked to the development of HLH.

Q. The genes for which cellular mechanisms are most commonly affected in HLH:
1. Perforin-dependent cytotoxicity
2. Antibody dependent cytotoxicity
3. Complement cascade
4. Cell energetics and anaerobic metabolism

Answer: Perforin-dependent cytotoxicity

Many HLH gene mutations map to loci that code for elements of the cytotoxic granule formation and release pathway, and have been labeled familial hemophagocytic lymphohistiocytosis (FHL) loci. The most important of these are:
1. PRF1/Perforin (FHL2)
2. UNC13D/Munc13-4 (FHL3)
3. STX11/Syntaxin 11 (FHL4)
4. STXBP2/Munc18-2 (FHL5)

Q. Which of the following immunodeficiency syndrome is least likely to be associated with increased incidence of HLH:
1. Griscelli syndrome
2. Chediak-Higashi syndrome
3. Severe combined immunodeficiency
4. X-linked immunoproliferative disease

Answer: severe combined immunodeficiency

Notes on immunodeficiency syndromes associated with

HLH:

1. Griscelli syndrome is caused by mutations of *RAB27A*
2. Chediak-Higashi syndrome is caused by mutations of *CHS1/LYST*. It is characterized by partial oculocutaneous albinism, neutrophil defects, neutropenia, and neurologic abnormalities.
3. X-linked lymphoproliferative disease is caused by mutations in SH2 domain protein 1A (*SH2D1A*).
4. XMEN disease: **X**-linked immunodeficiency with **m**agnesium defect, **E**BV infection, and **n**eoplasia (XMEN) disease
5. Hermansky-Pudlak syndrome is characterized by oculocutaneous albinism and platelet storage pool deficiency.

Q. Which of the following is not a usual clinical feature of HLH:

1. Splenomegaly
2. Hypertriglyceridemia
3. Increased ferritin levels
4. Decreased soluble CD25 levels

Answer: Decreased soluble CD25 levels

In fact, the soluble CD25 levels are elevated in HLH.

HLH patients have a constellation of symptoms and signs and that's why diagnosis is often delayed or missed, because these symptoms are present in many other conditions, both common and rare.

Hemophagocytosis is present in 82 percent of patients. Markers of macrophage activity are increased and NK cell activity is low or absent (as we have already discussed in the question about pathogenesis).

Q. Which of the following laboratory abnormality is not typical for HLH:
1. Anemia
2. Thrombocytopenia
3. Leukopenia
4. All of the above are characteristic for HLH

Answer: leukopenia

HLH characteristically has bicytopenia: anemia and thrombocytopenia.

Q. The most common malignancy related to HLH is:
1. Lymphoma
2. Leukemia
3. Plasma cell disorders
4. Solid childhood cancers

Answer: lymphoma

Q. The most common rheumatologic disorder associated with HLH is:
1. Systemic juvenile idiopathic arthritis
2. Adult onset rheumatoid arthritis
3. Polyarteritis nodosa
4. Juvenile Sjogren syndrome

Answer: Systemic juvenile idiopathic arthritis

It is also known as Still's disease.

HLH may develop any time during the course of a rheumato-logic disorder.

Q. Apart from complete blood count, liver function tests, serum ferritin and triglyceride levels; bone marrow evaluation should be done in which patients with HLH:
1. Patients having cytopenias
2. Patients having normal ferritin levels
3. In cases of diagnostic dilemma
4. In all patients regardless of other test results

Answer: In all patients regardless of other test results

All patients should have a bone marrow aspirate and biopsy to evaluate the cause of cytopenias and/or detect hemo-phagocytosis.

Bone marrow is infiltrated with macrophages in HLH and in majority of cases hemophagocytosis may also be seen but it must be noted that hemophagocytosis is **not** pathogno-monic for HLH.

Q. Which of the following finding is not consistent with HLH:
1. Elevated soluble IL-2R
2. Reduced NK function
3. Increased cell surface expression of CD107 alpha
4. Reduced perforin

Answer: Increased cell surface expression of CD107 alpha

In fact, the level of cell surface expression of CD107 alpha is reduced, which reflect reduced NK function.

Level of sIL-2R correlate most closely with disease activity.

Q. Genetic testing for HLH is indicated in which patients:
1. In all patients who meet the diagnostic criteria for HLH
2. In all patients with a high likelihood of HLH based on the initial evaluation
3. Both of the above
4. It is not indicated except as a part of a clinical trial

Answer: both of the above

For genetic testing of HLH, next generation sequencing or whole exome sequencing are preferred. Sometimes intronic sequencing may be needed.

Q. The currently accepted diagnostic criteria for HLH are based on which trial:
1. HLH-2014
2. HLH-2004
3. HLH-1994
4. HLH-2018

Answer: HLH-2004

These criteria are:
1. In children and adults presence of HLH mutations like *PRF1, UNC13D, STX11, STXBP2, Rab27A, SH2D1A, BIRC4, LYST, ITK, SLC7A7, XMEN, HPS* or

other genes related to immune regulation is diagnostic. In adults, an added condition is that along with heterozygosity of one of these genes, some clinical feature should also be present.

OR

Five of the following eight:

   a. Fever ≥38.5°C

   b. Splenomegaly

   c. Peripheral blood cytopenia, with at least two of the following: hemoglobin <9 g/dL (for infants <4 weeks, hemoglobin <10 g/dL); platelets <100,000/microL; absolute neutrophil count <1000/microL

   d. Hypertriglyceridemia (fasting triglycerides >265 mg/dL) and/or hypofibrinogenemia (fibrinogen <150 mg/dL)

   e. Hemophagocytosis in bone marrow, spleen, lymph node, or liver

   f. Low or absent NK cell activity

   g. Ferritin >500 ng/mL

   h. Elevated soluble CD25 (soluble IL-2 receptor alpha [sIL-2R]) two standard deviations above age-adjusted laboratory-specific norms

It should be noted here that the above mentioned criteria are not exhaustive and in a rare disease such as HLH, institutional practices and personal clinical experience play a big role in diagnosis. You may come across different sets of diagnostic criteria and to follow them would not be wrong.

Q. Which of the following is incorrect about HLH management:

   1. A period of observation is justified in most pediatric patients, as the disease runs a self-limiting course

   2. The HLH-94 consists induction chemo with etoposide and dexamethasone. Intrathecal methotrexate and hydrocortisone are given to those with central nervous system disease

3. After induction, patients who are recovering are weaned off therapy
4. After induction if the patient is not responding then allogeneic hematopoietic cell transplantation is performed

Answer: A period of observation is justified as in most pediatric patients, the disease runs a self-limiting course

HLH is a fulminant disease and treatment should be promptly initiated in most of the patients. That being said, if a patient is clinically stable and the ferritin is consistently below 10,000 ng/mL or rises from 1000 to 3000 ng/mL with only slightly elevated D-dimer and liver enzymes, many hematologists don't start treatment.

It goes without saying that if another disease is suspected underlying HLH (secondary HLH), then treatment of that disease should be initiated and in such cases HLH-94 protocol may not necessarily be followed.

The above mentioned treatment protocol is based on the HLH-94 trial, and another trial came later, known as the HLH-2004 trial which modified previous protocol by adding cyclosporine to the induction phase.

Q. Which of the following marker is not used for monitoring disease activity and/or response to treatment in cases of HLH:
1. Soluble IL-2 receptor alpha [sCD25]
2. Soluble hemoglobin-haptoglobin scavenger receptor [sCD163]
3. Ferritin
4. Bone marrow hemophagocytic count and ratio

Answer: Bone marrow hemophagocytic count and ratio

Q. The drug of choice for EBV induced HLH is:
1. Entecavir
2. Ritonavir
3. Rituximab
4. Ribavirin plus interferon-alpha

Answer: rituximab

IVIG is recommended as the drug of choice by some experts but the overall consensus is that rituximab is a more effective option.

Q. Which of the following is not an indication of allogeneic HCT in HLH:
1. Homozygous or compound heterozygous HLH gene mutations
2. Lack of response to initial HLH therapy
3. Central nervous system (CNS) involvement
4. Severe rheumatologic disorder

Answer: Severe rheumatologic disorder

The fourth indication of allo-HCT is hematologic malignancy.

Q. In patients of HLH who fail on initial HLH directed therapy as well as allo-HCT, the drug of choice is:
1. Alemtuzumab
2. Emapalumab

3. Etanercept
4. Abatacept

Answer: emapalumab

Emapalumab is an interferon gamma blocking antibody and it is used in combination with dexamethasone.

Alemtuzumab plus etoposide is also an option but is not preferred.

LANGERHANS CELL HISTIOCYTOSIS (LCH)

Q. LCH is derived from:
1. Myeloid progenitor cells from the bone marrow
2. Langerhans cells of the skin
3. Both of the above
4. None of the above

Answer: Myeloid progenitor cells from the bone marrow

LCH is a clonal myeloid malignancy.

There were many historical "names" for this disorder, like histiocytosis-X, Letterer-Siwe disease, Hand-Schüller-Christian disease etc.

The name eosinophilic granuloma is sometimes still used to describe an individual lesion.

Q. Erdheim-Chester disease comes under which category of disorders, as per the Histiocyte society:
1. C
2. L
3. R
4. M

Answer: L

The 5 categories of disorders in the Histiocyte society classification are:
1. L (Langerhans) group: LCH, indeterminate cell histiocytosis, Erdheim-Chester Disease (ECD), mixed LCH/ECD, and extracutaneous juvenile xanthogranuloma.
2. C (cutaneous and mucocutaneous) group: juvenile xanthogranuloma, adult xanthogranuloma, and cutaneous Rosai-Dorfman disease.
3. R (Rosai-Dorfman disease) group: Rosai-Dorfman disease and miscellaneous non-cutaneous histiocytosis.
4. M (malignant histiocytosis) group: includes histiocytosis secondary to malignant disorders.
5. H (hemophagocytic lymphohistiocytosis) group: primary and secondary hemophagocytic lymphohistiocytosis (HLH) and macrophage activation syndromes.

Q. LCH occurs most commonly in which age group:
1. 1-3 years
2. 3-6 years
3. 6-18 years
4. 18-24 years

Answer: 1-3 years

BRAF V600E mutation is commonly found in LCH cases.

Q. Acute disseminated, multisystem LCH is most commonly seen in:
1. Children less than three years old
2. Children more than three years old
3. Late adolescence and adults
4. Elderly population

Answer: children less than three years old

A more indolent disease involving a single organ is more common in older children and adults.

Q. Involvement of which of the following organ by LCH imparts the least risk compared to other organs mentioned below:
1. Liver
2. Hematopoietic system
3. Spleen
4. Lung

Answer: lung

In LCH, if certain organs are involved by the disease, prognosis will be worse. These organs are known as "risk organs" and include the hematopoietic system, liver, and/or spleen and denote a worse prognosis. Although the lung has been considered a "risk organ," more recent studies have suggested that it has less of an effect on prognosis.

Q. In adults, the most commonly affected bones by LCH are:
1. Jaws
2. Skull
3. Femur
4. Vertebra

Answer: jaws

The most frequent bony site of involvement in children is skull and in adults it is jaws, followed by the skull.

Q. Congenital self-healing reticulohistiocytosis is characteristically seen in:
1. LCH
2. MAS
3. Fabry's disease
4. Juvenile rheumatoid arthritis

Answer: LCH

It is the most common cutaneous manifestation of LCH along with an eczematous rash.

Q. Which is the most common endocrine abnormality encountered in LCH:
1. Diabetes insipidus
2. Diabetes mellitus
3. Acromegaly
4. Cushing's syndrome

Answer: diabetes insipidus

Q. The nucleus in the abnormal cells in LCH characteristically resemble which shape:
    1. Twisted towel
    2. Pillared hall
    3. Raindrop
    4. Blurred glass

Answer: twisted towel

The nucleus is sometimes may also be described as having a coffee bean appearance.

It should not be confused with the shape of the Birbeck granules, also seen in LCH, which is described as a tennis racket.

Note that identification of Birbeck granules is done by electron microscopy.

Q. LCH cells express all of the following markers except:
    1. CD1a
    2. S100
    3. CD207
    4. CD107

Answer: CD107

CD207 is also known as langerin.

Q. Which of the following is not true about LCH:

1. Diagnosis is often established by biopsy of an osteolytic bone lesion or skin lesion and at the time of biopsy, a wide excision should be performed
2. Biopsy of the pituitary gland is required in cases with isolated pituitary involvement and in challenging cases identification of *BRAF* V600E in the peripheral blood or cerebrospinal fluid can support the diagnosis
3. In patients with isolated pituitary disease in whom biopsy in not possible, empiric chemotherapy may be started based on MRI findings
4. A light microscopy exam showing Langerhans cells is not sufficient and their identity must be confirmed either by positive immunohistochemical staining for CD1a and CD207 or by the identification of Birbeck granules by electron microscopy

Answer: Diagnosis is often established by biopsy of an osteolytic bone lesion or skin lesion and at the time of biopsy, a wide excision should be performed

While it's true that diagnosis is often established by biopsy of an osteolytic bone lesion or skin lesion and but at the time of biopsy, a wide excision should **NOT** be performed as LCH bone lesions will have complete or near complete healing with curettage alone or chemotherapy.

Q. In which patient population of LCH is pulmonary involvement more common:

1. Male infants
2. Adult males
3. Female infants
4. Adult females

Answer: adult males

Lung involvement occurs in approximately 10 percent of cases. It is less frequent in children than in adults, in whom smoking is a key etiologic factor. So lung involvement is more common in smoker adult population. In the affected patients high-resolution computed tomography (CT) scan reveals cysts and nodules characteristic of LCH.

Q. Involvement of which of the following bones by LCH will not come under "CNS-risk" lesions category:
   1. Facial bones
   2. Bones of anterior cranial fossa
   3. Bones of middle cranial fossa
   4. Bones of posterior cranial fossa

Answer: bones of posterior cranial fossa

Q. Which of the following is not a part of the triad of Hand-Schüller-Christian disease:
   1. Exophthalmos
   2. Diabetes insipidus
   3. Skull lesions
   4. Hepatosplenomegaly

Answer: hepatosplenomegaly

Another disease of the same group as HSCD is Letterer-Siwe disease in which the findings are: lymphadenopathy, skin rash, hepatosplenomegaly, fever, anemia, and thrombo-cytopenia.

LCH of the bone (also known as eosinophilic granuloma of bone or histiocytosis X) is the third disease of this group.

Q. All of the following are correct about LCH of the bone except:
1. The most common age of presentation is 5 to 10 years
2. Monostotic bone lesion is more common than polyostotic bone lesions
3. Skull is the most commonly involved site in children and parietal bone is the most commonly affected bone
4. In adults the most common primary site of bone involvement is jaw

Answer: Skull is the most commonly involved site in children and parietal bone is the most commonly affected bone

While it's true that skull is the most common site in children but the most commonly involved bone of the skull is the frontal bone.

Q. The lesions of LCH are the least common in which part of the bone:
1. Diaphysis
2. Metaphysis
3. Epiphysis
4. The lesions are almost equally distributed throughout the bone

Answer: epiphysis

The lesions are mostly found in the diaphysis or metaphysis.

When LCH involves the vertebrae, in extreme cases there may be flattening of vertebra, that has a "coin on edge" appearance, also known as vertebra plana.

Q. On radionuclide bone scans, LCH typically is:
  1. Hot
  2. Cold
  3. Normal
  4. Not identified

Answer: hot

Q. Which of the following is not true about treatment of LCH:
  1. Almost all patients with osseous LCH are ultimately cured of their disease
  2. LCH of bone is most commonly treated with curettage and a clean margin is not required for treatment
  3. LCH lesions of the spine often involve the endochondral ossification centers, therefore reconstruction is a must
  4. High risk LCH patients should be treated with 12 months of vinblastine and prednisone as per the LCH-III protocol

Answer: LCH lesions of the spine often involve the endochondral ossification centers, therefore reconstruction is a must

In fact, LCH lesions of the spine **do not** involve the endochondral ossification centers.

To clarify the first option, we must understand that while almost all of the patients with LCH of the bone will be cured but that doesn't mean that there are no recurrences; in fact, recurrences are frequent.

If a question is asked about the role of radiation in LCH, then it will obviously depend on the clinical context. But to give a generalized view, radiation is not an initial or preferred approach and it is used in patients who recur despite repeated surgeries and/or chemo and in whom further surgery or chemo will not be of any benefit, as decided by the tumor board.

ERDHEIM-CHESTER DISEASE (ECD)

Q. Erdheim-Chester disease (ECD) is a:
    1. Langerhans histiocytic disorder
    2. Non-Langerhans histiocytic disorder
    3. It's a mixed Langerhans and non-Langerhans histiocytic disorder
    4. None of the above

Answer: non-Langerhans histiocytic disorder

This disorder arises from monocyte-macrophage lineage.

Q. ECD is characterized by:
    1. Multifocal osteosclerotic lesions of the long bones
    2. Multifocal osteosclerotic lesions of the short bones
    3. Multifocal osteolytic lesions of the long bones
    4. Multifocal osteolytic lesions of the short bones

Answer: Multifocal osteosclerotic lesions of the long bones

Q. The most common age of presentation of ECD is:
1. Children upto 4 years
2. Early adolescence
3. 50-60 years
4. More than 80 years

Answer: 50-60 years

Q. Touton cells are seen in which disorder:
1. Erdheim-Chester disease
2. Hemophagocytic lymphohistiocytosis
3. Langerhans cell histiocytosis
4. None of the above

Answer: Erdheim-Chester disease

Touton cells are multinucleated giant cells

Q. ECD cells express all of the following markers except:
1. CD68
2. CD163
3. Factor XIIIa
4. S100

Answer: S100

ECD cells don't express CD1a or S100, which are markers of LCH.

BRAF V600E mutation is found in about half of the patients with ECD.

Notes:
Treatment of ECD is not always indicated, the usual indications for beginning treatment are:
1. Symptomatic disease
2. Evidence of organ dysfunction
3. CNS involvement, either symptomatic or asymptomatic
4. Evidence of organ dysfunction, or impending organ dysfunction

Q. Which of the following is not an initial treatment option for ECD:
1. Vemurafenib
2. Interferon alfa
3. Cladribine
4. Glucocorticoids

Answer: cladribine

In patients with BRAF V600E mutation, vemurafenib is the preferred initial treatment option, whereas in patients lacking this mutation interferon is the drug of choice. Some patients can't tolerate either of these therapies, in such patients glucocorticoids alone may be used.

Cladribine and cyclophosphamide are second line options.

MEK inhibitors, cobimetinib and trametinib are also options for the second line or later line of therapy.

It should be noted here that there is no known cure for ECD and with currently available therapies, the 5 year OS is about 70%.

Q. Enlargement of which of the following lymph nodes is always pathological:
    1. Inguinal
    2. Left supraclavicular
    3. Epitrochlear
    4. Suboccipital

Answer: epitrochlear

CONGENITAL NEUTROPENIA

Notes on clues obtained by physical examination that point to the underlying disorder leading to congenital neutropenia (note that the final diagnosis is dependent on the genetic testing, as many of the physical examination findings overlap):
    1. Oculocutaneous albinism, peripheral neuropathy, and large granules in leukocytes – Chediak-Higashi syndrome
    2. Metaphyseal dysplasia, pancreatic insufficiency – Shwachman-Diamond syndrome
    3. Oculocutaneous albinism – Griscelli syndrome, Hermansky-Pudlak syndrome, p14 deficiency
    4. Warts – WHIM syndrome (warts, hypogammaglobulinemia, infections, myelokathexis syndrome)
    5. Hypoglycemia, growth retardation, hepatomegaly – Glycogen storage disease IB

6. Short-limbed short stature, hypoplastic hair – Cartilage hair hypoplasia
7. Skeletal myopathy, dilated cardiomyopathy – Barth's syndrome
8. Hypotonia, microcephaly, intellectual disability – Cohen syndrome

Q. Which of the following is not true about severe congenital neutropenia:
1. The most common mutation leading to SCN occurs in the *ELANE* gene and is transmitted as an autosomal dominant condition
2. In Kostmann syndrome, patients have mutations in *HAX1* with X-linked inheritance
3. In the Wiskott-Aldrich syndrome mutations is the WASP gene are seen
4. None of the above

Answer: In Kostmann syndrome, patients have mutations in *HAX1* with X-linked inheritance

While it's true that in Kostmann syndrome, patients have mutations in *HAX1* but the inheritance is autosomal recessive.

Q. Which of the following is not a part of the triad of Shwachman-Diamond syndrome:
1. Neutropenia
2. Metaphyseal dysplasia
3. Pancreatic insufficiency
4. Hyperglycemia

Answer: hyperglycemia

Q. Leukocyte adhesion deficiency is a cause of leukocytosis. Which of the following is responsible for LAD II:
    1. Defects of CD18
    2. Lack of sialyl Lewis X
    3. Excess of sialyl Lewis X
    4. None of the above

Answer: lack of sialyl Lewis X

There are three types of LAD. Type I is associated with defects of CD18, type II is associated with lack of sialyl Lewis X.

Q. Chronic neutrophilic leukemia (CNL) is associated with
    1. Activating germline mutation in *CSF3R*
    2. Deactivating germline mutation in *CSF3R*
    3. Activating somatic mutation in *CSF3R*
    4. Deactivating somatic mutation in *CSF3R*

Answer: Activating germline mutation in *CSF3R*

Notes: Infants with Down syndrome (trisomy of chromosome 21) may have a transient abnormal myelopoiesis (also called transient myeloproliferative disorder [TMD] of Down syndrome) that resembles congenital acute leukemia or chronic myeloid leukemia. TMD may resolve spontaneously, but evolves into overt acute myeloid leukemia in a subset of patients.

DRUG-INDUCED NEUTROPENIA

AND IMMUNE NEUTROPENIA

Q. Which of the following is not a risk factor for agranulocytosis:
1. Increasing age
2. Male gender
3. Renal failure
4. Underlying autoimmune disease

Answer: male gender

Agranulocytosis is more common in females.

An interesting risk factor is the combined use of ACE inhibitors and interferon.

Notes:
The list of drugs causing agranulocytosis is very long. The most important drugs that we should remember are: methimazole, carbimazole, sulfasalazine, trimethoprim-sulfamethoxazole, dipyrone combined with analgesics, clomipramine, and clozapine.

Q. Neonatal isoimmune neutropenia is more commonly caused by:
1. IgG antibodies to neutrophil-specific antigens inherited from the father
2. IgG antibodies to neutrophil-specific antigens inherited from the mother
3. IgM antibodies to neutrophil-specific antigens inherited from the father
4. IgM antibodies to neutrophil-specific antigens inherited from the mother

Answer: IgG antibodies to neutrophil-specific antigens inherited from the father

The prognosis of this disorder is good and apart from prophylactic antibiotics to prevent neonatal sepsis, nothing much needs to be done.

Q. Pure white cell aplasia is most often associated with:
1. Thymoma
2. Lymphoma
3. Small cell lung cancer
4. Non-small cell lung cancer

Answer: thymoma

Thymectomy and immunosuppressive therapy are used in this disorder.

Note that thymoma is also associated with pure red cell aplasia.

Q. Which of the following is not true about infections and neutropenia:
1. Leukopenia with neutropenia is seen in approximately 25 to 50 percent of adults with typhoid fever
2. Neutropenia occurs in 20 to 30 percent of adults and children with brucellosis
3. Lymphopenia is seen in up to 87 percent patients of tuberculosis with varying degrees of neutropenia
4. Leukopenia occurs in approximately 25 percent of patients with rickettsial pox

Answer: Leukopenia occurs in approximately 25 percent of patients with rickettsial pox

In fact, leukopenia is seen in almost 75% of the patients.

Clonal hematopoiesis of indeterminate potential (CHIP), Idiopathic and clonal cytopenias of uncertain significance (ICUS and CCUS)

Q. An individual hematopoietic stem cell would be expected to contribute to approximately what percent of blood cell production:
1. 0.001
2. 0.01
3. 0.1
4. 1.0

Answer: 0.001%

Q. Which is the least commonly involved single gene mutation in CHIP:
1. DNMT3A
2. TET2
3. ASXL1
4. TP53

Answer: TP53

Q. In which of the following situation, testing to exclude a germline mutation in a case of CHIP is not warranted:

1. Variant allele frequency 40 to 60 percent for mutations of *RUNX1*
2. Variant allele frequency 40 to 60 percent for mutations of *GATA2*
3. Variant allele frequency 20 percent or more for mutations of *DDX41*
4. Variant allele frequency 20 percent or more for mutations of *TP53*

Answer: Variant allele frequency 20 percent or more for mutations of *DDX41*

For DDX41 too, the variant allele frequency should be 40-60% to warrant germline mutation testing.

Genes like *DNMT3A, TET2, ASXL1* are not known to be inherited, and it is not necessary to exclude germline transmission if these mutations are identified with any frequency.

Q. Which of the following does not come under the definition of CHIP:

1. Variant allele frequency (VAF) ≥2 percent of an acquired mutation of a leukemia-associated gene
2. The most common mutations affect *DNMT3A, TET2*, and/or *ASXL1*
3. Abnormal peripheral blood counts
4. No clinical or pathologic evidence for a World Health Organization defined hematologic malignancy neoplasm

Answer: Abnormal peripheral blood counts

In fact, the peripheral blood counts should be normal.

If peripheral blood counts are not normal then the diagnosis in such cases will be clonal cytopenia of uncertain significance (CCUS).

It should be noted that modest levels of bone marrow dysplasia don't exclude the diagnosis of CHIP but if ≥10 percent of peripheral blood cells or bone marrow nucleated cells exhibit dysplasia, the condition should be classified as myelodysplastic syndrome (MDS).

Another related disorder is ARCH (aging related clonal hematopoiesis).

Q. The preferred method of testing for clonal hematopoiesis is:
    1. Next-generation sequencing (NGS)
    2. Flow cytometry
    3. Karyotype combined with FISH
    4. Proteomics analysis

Answer: next-generation sequencing (NGS)

A panel of leukemia-associated genes on peripheral blood or bone marrow are used for NGS.

Notes on diagnostic criteria for ICUS:
    1. Cytopenia in one or more blood lineages that remain unexplained despite appropriate evaluation
    2. No evidence of clonal hematopoiesis (CH); if

a leukemia-associated mutation is detected, the variant allele frequency (VAF) should be <2 percent
3. No other evidence of a hematologic malignancy, according to World Health Organization (WHO) criteria. Note that there should be no dysplasia and if dysplasia is there in either peripheral blood or bone marrow, it should be less than 10%

Notes on diagnostic criteria for CCUS:
1. Unexplained, clinically meaningful cytopenias
2. CH is detected with ≥2 percent VAF of a leukemia-associated gene
3. No other evidence of a hematologic malignancy, as described above

Q. The risk of progression to MDS or leukemias is more in:
1. ICUS
2. CCUS
3. The risk is similar in these two conditions
4. There is no risk of progression in either ICUS or CCUS

Answer: CCUS

It is so because CCUS is associated with more mutations than ICUS (read the diagnostic criteria for these conditions carefully).

RECOMBINANT HEMATOPOIETIC GROWTH FACTORS

Notes, clinical uses of HGFs:
1. Transient bone marrow failure following chemo-therapy
2. Hematopoietic stem cell and progenitor cell mobil-

ization
3. Recovery from hematopoietic cell transplantation
4. Myelodysplastic syndromes
5. Aplastic anemia
6. Some forms of neutropenia
7. Inherited bone marrow failure syndromes
8. Human immunodeficiency virus (HIV) infection-associated neutropenia
9. Chronic anemias (eg, renal failure, prematurity, chronic disease/inflammation, HIV infection)
10. ITP and chemotherapy induced thrombocytopenia

Q. Which of the following is not true about myeloid growth factors:
1. The recommended dose of G-CSF is 5 mcg/kg per day for most clinical situations and 10 mcg/kg per day for peripheral blood stem cell mobilization
2. The recommended dose of GM-CSF is 250 mcg/m2 per day
3. G-CSF is usually started within 24 hours after administration of chemotherapy
4. Following intravenous bolus injection, both GM-CSF and G-CSF induce a transient leukopenia in the first 30 minutes after administration

Answer: G-CSF is usually started within 24 hours after administration of chemotherapy

It must be understood that G-CSF is usually started **AFTER** at least 24 hours of chemotherapy.

Toxicities of myeloid growth factors:
1. Transient leukopenia
2. Flu-like symptoms
3. Bone pain, coincident with or shortly after administration

4. Increased risk of a therapy-related myeloid neoplasm
5. Pathogenic neutrophil infiltration (acute febrile neutrophilic dermatosis or Sweet syndrome) and cutaneous necrotizing vasculitis (leukocytoclastic vasculitis)
6. Capillary leak syndrome

Q. The most common side effect of erythropoietin is:
1. Hypertension
2. Flu-like syndrome
3. Deep venous thrombosis
4. Nephrotoxicity

Answer: hypertension

The drugs of choice for erythropoietin induced hypertension are beta-adrenergic blockers.

PROPHYLAXIS AND MANAGEMENT OF NEUTROPENIA

Q. The gold standard for determining the adequacy of the bone marrow's ability to produce neutrophils is:
1. Neutrophil stress test
2. Examination of a bone marrow
3. Flow cytometry
4. Functional oxidative stress assays

Answer: examination of the bone marrow

Q. Lymphocytopenia can occur in:
1. HIV-AIDS
2. Sepsis
3. Postoperative period
4. All of the above

Answer: all of the above

Indications for use of G-CSF in non-chemotherapy induced neutropenia:
1. Severe congenital neutropenia
2. Cyclic neutropenia
3. Neutropenia associated with early myeloid arrest
4. Acquired immune deficiency syndrome (AIDS)
5. Acquired bone marrow defects with severe neutropenia (ie, ANC <500 cells/microL)
6. Chronic idiopathic neutropenia with severe neutropenia
7. Drug-induced neutropenia/agranulocytosis with severe neutropenia

Q. Granulocyte transfusions are more useful in patients with sepsis who have not shown a clinical response to antibiotics within 24 to 48 hours and the pathogens are:
1. Gram negative bacteria
2. Gram positive bacteria
3. Invasive infections
4. Mycobacterial infections (disseminated)

Answer: Gram positive bacteria

Notes on diseases of immune function that can be treated by hematopoietic stem cell transplant:
1. Severe combined immunodeficiency

2. Wiskott-Aldrich syndrome
3. CD40 ligand deficiency (X-linked hyper IgM syndrome)
4. CD40 deficiency (autosomal recessive hyper IgM syndrome
5. X-linked lymphoproliferative disease
6. Interferon gamma receptor defects
7. NF kappa B essential modifier (NEMO) deficiency
8. Hemophagocytic lymphohistiocytosis
9. Chronic granulomatous disease
10. Leukocyte adhesion deficiency type 1
11. Griscelli syndrome type 2
12. Chediak-Higashi syndrome

Notes on CTCAE for hematologic toxicity:

NCI CTCAE (National Cancer Institute Common Terminology Criteria for Adverse Events) divides the categories of adverse effects in five grades, but note that it's not necessary for a toxicity to have 5 categories, sometimes it goes only up to grade 3.

1. Febrile neutropenia:
    a. There is no specified grade 1
    b. There is no specified grade 2
    c. Grade 3: ANC <1000/microL with a single temperature >38.3°C (100.4°F) or a sustained temperature ≥38°C (100°F) for more than one hour
    d. Grade 4: Life-threatening consequences; urgent intervention indicated
    e. Grade 5: death
2. Hemoglobin:
    a. Grade 1: <LLN to 10 g/dL
    b. Grade 2: 8 to 10 g/dL
    c. Grade 3: <8 g/dL
    d. Grade 4: Life-threatening consequences; urgent intervention indicated
    e. Grade 5: death
3. Neutrophils:
    a. Grade 1: <LLN to 1500/microL
    b. Grade 2: 1000 to 1500/microL

    c. Grade 3: 500 to 1000/microL
    d. Grade 4: <500/microL
    e. There is no specified grade 5
4. lymphocytes:
    a. Grade 1: <LLN to 800/microL
    b. Grade 2: 500 to 800/microL
    c. Grade 3: 200 to 500/microL
    d. Grade 4: <200/microL
    e. There is no specified grade 5
5. CD4 count:
    a. Grade 1: <LLN to 500/microL
    b. Grade 2: 200 to 500/microL
    c. Grade 3: 50 to 200/microL
    d. Grade 4: <50/microL
    e. There is no specified grade 5
6. Platelets:
    a. Grade 1: <LLN to 75,000/microL
    b. Grade 2: 50000 to 75000/microL
    c. Grade 3: 25000 to 50000/microL
    d. Grade 4: <25000/microL
    e. There is no specified grade 5

Q. Antimicrobial prophylaxis is generally not indicated in which patients of chemotherapy induced neutropenia:
1. Patients who are expected to be neutropenic with ANC <1500/microL for >7 days
2. Patients with neutropenia and ongoing comorbidities
3. Patients with neutropenia with significant hepatic or renal dysfunction regardless of duration of neutropenia
4. Antimicrobial prophylaxis is indicated in all of the above mentioned situations

Answer: Patients who are expected to be neutropenic with ANC <1500/microL for >7 days

Antimicrobial prophylaxis is indicated in patients of chemotherapy induced neutropenia who are at high risk of infectious complications, e.g.
1. Those who are expected to be neutropenic (ANC < 500 cells/microL) for > 7 days
2. Patients with neutropenic fever who have ongoing comorbidities regardless of the duration of neutropenia
3. Those having evidence of significant hepatic or renal dysfunction regardless of the duration of neutropenia
4. Those undergoing allogeneic HCT
5. Neutropenic patients receiving induction chemotherapy for acute leukemia

By contrast, low-risk patients are those in whom the duration of neutropenia (ANC < 500 cells/microL) is expected to be less than seven days and who have no comorbidities and no evidence of significant hepatic or renal dysfunction and in these patients antimicrobial prophylaxis is not indicated regardless of ANC.

Q. The preferred drug for antimicrobial prophylaxis in chemotherapy induced neutropenic patients at high-risk of infectious complications is:
1. Levofloxacin
2. Azithromycin
3. Carbapenems
4. Aztreonam

Answer: levofloxacin

The timing for initiating levofloxacin is not very clear but most of the times it's started on the day or the day after administration of chemotherapy and continued till neutropenia has resolved or if the patient becomes febrile, because if the patient becomes febrile then empiric antibacterial regimen should be initiated and levofloxacin should be discontinued.

Another drug still in use and extensively studied is ciprofloxacin. It has greater in vitro activity than levofloxacin against *P. aeruginosa*, but levofloxacin has greater in vitro activity against gram-positive bacteria (eg, alpha-hemolytic streptococci) and is given only once daily compared with twice daily dosing of ciprofloxacin. So these factors make levofloxacin a better drug.

Prolongation of the QT interval is a problematic side effect of quinolones and should be watched out for, especially if the patient is also receiving another drug that causes QT prolongation.

TMP-SMX was used in the past but it's no longer used due to its lack of activity against P. aeruginosa.

Q. The IDSA guidelines recommend that the prophylactic use of colony stimulating factors should be considered for afebrile patients in whom the anticipated risk of fever and neutropenia is:

    1. ≥10%
    2. ≥20%
    3. ≥30%
    4. In all patients regardless of the risk of fever and neutropenia

Answer: ≥20%

Please remember this number.

Notes on patients with chemotherapy-induced neutropenic fever who are at high risk for serious complications:

If a patient has any of the following characteristics then he will be considered at high risk:

1. Receipt of cytotoxic therapy sufficiently myelosuppressive to result in anticipated severe neutropenia (ANC <500 cells/mcL) for >7 days
2. MASCC risk index score <21
3. CISNE score of ≥3
4. Alemtuzumab use within the past two months
5. Uncontrolled or progressive cancer
6. Hepatic or renal insufficiency
7. Presence of uncontrolled comorbid conditions

Q. The term neutrophilia refers to what:

1. ANC >7700/microL
2. Total leukocyte count >11000/microL
3. ANC >4500/microL
4. ANC >10000/microL

Answer: ANC >7700/microL

Glucocorticoids lead to release of granulocytes from the bone marrow and are associated with neutrophilia.

Q. Fever in neutropenic patients is defined as:

1. A single oral temperature of ≥38.3°C
2. A temperature of ≥38.0°C sustained over a one-hour period
3. A temperature of ≥100.4°F sustained over a one-hour period
4. All of the above

Answer: all of the above

Q. Fever in a neutropenic patient should be considered a medical emergency and broad-spectrum antibacterials should be given:
    1. Within 60 minutes of triage
    2. Within 90 minutes of triage
    3. After receiving blood culture reports
    4. Not until the patient is hemodynamically stable

Answer: within 60 minutes of triage

Q. The most frequent pathogens identified during neutropenic fever episodes are:
    1. Gram-positive bacteria
    2. Gram-negative bacteria
    3. Fungi
    4. Viruses

Answer: Gram-positive bacteria

But it should be noted that the antibiotic coverage must be given for Gram-negative bacteria also because of their virulence and association with sepsis.

Q. Which of the following is not correct about the treatment of neutropenic fever:
    1. Ceftazidime monotherapy should not be used when there is concern for a gram-negative infection
    2. Antipseudomonal beta-lactam agent should be a part of the initial regimen
    3. Vancomycin may be added to the initial regimen if hypotension, mental status changes, pneumonia or cellulitis are there
    4. Anaerobic coverage should be added to the regimen

if there is suspicion of neutropenic enterocolitis

Answer: Ceftazidime monotherapy should not be used when there is concern for a gram-negative infection

The fact is that ceftazidime monotherapy should not be used when there is concern for a gram-**positive** infection because ceftazidime is not active against Gram-positive bacteria induced sepsis.

Antipseudomonal beta-lactam agents are: cefepime, meropenem, imipenem-cilastatin and piperacillin-tazobactam. As mentioned above ceftazidime monotherapy should not be used.

Notes about some key points in the management of neutropenic fever:
1. Monotherapy with the above mentioned beta-lactam agents generally demonstrated equivalent outcomes compared with two-drug regimens in clinical trials.
2. In a scenario where there is a high prevalence of multidrug-resistant gram-negative bacilli, initial empirical antibacterial therapy with piperacillin-tazobactam plus tigecycline may have some advantages over monotherapy.
3. Patients with a history of an immediate-type hypersensitivity reaction to penicillin should not receive beta-lactams or carbapenems.
4. Gram-positive bacteria targeting agents like vancomycin, are **not** recommended as a standard part of the initial regimen.
5. Gram-positive coverage should be added in patients with any of the following findings:
    a. Hemodynamic instability or other signs of severe sepsis
    b. Pneumonia

    c. Positive blood cultures for gram-positive bacteria
    d. Suspected central venous catheter (CVC)-related infection
    e. Skin or soft tissue infection
    f. In patients with increased risk of *viridans* group streptococcal infections

Caution should be taken with certain combinations, e.g., the combination of vancomycin and piperacillin-tazobactam has been associated with acute kidney injury.

Prolonged use of vancomycin has been associated with vancomycin resistant enterococci.

Q. Empiric antifungal coverage should be considered in high-risk patients who have persistent fever after how many days of a broad-spectrum antibacterial regimen:
    1. 1-2
    2. 3-4
    3. 4-5
    4. More than 1 week

Answer: 4-5

The most correct answer is 4 days with the range being from 4 to 7 days.

Q. Which of the following drug should be used for pneumonia caused by MRSA:
    1. Vancomycin
    2. Linezolid
    3. Daptomycin

4. All of the above

Answer: either vancomycin or linezolid

For MRSA infections, three antibiotics are commonly used: vancomycin, linezolid and daptomycin. Out of these, daptomycin should not be used in patients with pneumonia because it does not achieve sufficiently high concentrations in the respiratory tract.

Q. What are the treatment options for vancomycin resistant enterococci:
    1. Linezolid
    2. Daptomycin
    3. Both of the above
    4. None of the above

Answer: both of the above

Q. The drug of choice for extended spectrum beta-lactamase producing Gram-negative bacilli is:
    1. Meropenem
    2. Vancomycin
    3. Linezolid
    4. Daptomycin

Answer: meropenem

Carbapenems, eg, imipenem, meropenem, are the drug of choice for ESBL producing Gram-negative bacilli.

Q. What are the treatment options for carbapenemase-pro-
ducing bacteria:
    1. Colistin
    2. Tigecycline
    3. Both of the above
    4. None of the above

Answer: both of the above

Q. In patients receiving fluconazole prophylaxis, which is
the most likely cause of fungal infection:
    1. *Candida glabrata*
    2. *Candida krusei*
    3. *Aspergillus*
    4. All of the above

Answer: all of the above

Note that most of the Candida species are sensitive to fluconazole but glabrata and krusei are not.

Q. The 2010 IDSA guidelines for empiric antifungal therapy
recommend all of the following as suitable empiric antifungal therapy except:
    1. Amphotericin B deoxycholate
    2. Caspofungin
    3. Itraconazole
    4. Fluconazole

Answer: fluconazole

Other options are lipid formulations of amphotericin and voriconazole.

Notes that echinocandins (caspofungin) are not active against *Cryptococcus* spp, *Trichosporon* spp, and filamentous molds other than *Aspergillus* spp, such as *Fusarium* spp. They are also not active against the endemic fungi (*Histoplasma, Blastomyces, Coccidioides* spp).

Q. In cases of central venous catheter (CVC)-related infections, in addition to prompt initiation of antibiotics, CVC removal is recommended for patients with catheter-related bloodstream infections with which all of the following organisms except:
1. S. aureus
2. *P. aeruginosa*
3. *Candida*
4. Enterobacter

Answer: enterobacter

Other organisms which warrant the removal of CVC are rapidly growing nontuberculous mycobacteria.

Antibiotics should be administered for a minimum of 14 days following catheter removal **and** clearance of blood cultures.

Other scenarios where removal of CVC is recommended are:
1. Tunnel infection
2. Port pocket infection
3. Septic thrombosis
4. Endocarditis
5. Sepsis with hemodynamic instability
6. Bloodstream infection that persists despite ≥72

hours of therapy with appropriate antibiotics

Note that for CVC -associated bacteremia caused by co-agulase-negative staphylococci, the CVC may be retained.

Q. Which of the following strategy should be promptly used in all patients with established neutropenic fever:
    1. Empiric antibiotics
    2. G-CSF
    3. Both of the above
    4. None of the above

Answer: empiric antibiotics

This point should be clearly understood. According to the IDSA and other such guidelines, the use of colony stimulating factors is **NOT** recommended in all patients with established neutropenia and fever. They are indicated only in those patients who are at **high risk** of infectious complications.

Q. Which of the following is not correct:
    1. Use of granulocyte-macrophage colony stimulating factor (GM-CSF) has been associated with a higher incidence of thrombocytopenia and other complications when given with concurrent chemoradiotherapy
    2. G-CSF should be used cautiously, if at all, during concomitant chemoradiotherapy for head and neck cancer because it has been associated with reduced loco-regional tumor control
    3. Most of the guidelines have recommended against the use of CSFs in afebrile patients who have already developed severe neutropenia after chemotherapy

4. Use of CSFs is generally associated with significantly improved overall mortality and infection-related mortality as compared with antibiotics alone

Answer: Use of CSFs is generally associated with significantly improved overall mortality and infection-related mortality as compared with antibiotics alone

In fact, the use of CSFs is generally **NOT** associated with significantly improved overall mortality and infection-related mortality as compared with antibiotics alone

Notes on dose and timing of G-CSF and GM-CSF:
1. The recommended dose of G-CSF (filgrastim, filgrastim-sndz, tbo-filgrastim) is 5 mcg/kg per day and for GM-CSF (sargramostim), 250 mcg/m2 per day.
2. Therapy is usually begun 24 to 72 hours after cessation of chemotherapy and is often continued with twice weekly monitoring of blood counts, until the ANC reaches 5000 to 10,000/microL.
3. Because of the potential sensitivity of rapidly dividing myeloid cells to cytotoxic chemotherapy, growth factors should be discontinued several days before the next chemotherapy treatment and they should not be given on the same day as chemotherapy.
4. Myelosuppression is more profound if the myeloid growth factors were given immediately prior to or on the same day as the chemotherapy.
5. The recommended dose of pegfilgrastim is 6 mg in adults and 100 mcg/kg [maximum 6 mg] in children and it is given 24 hours after chemotherapy.

MISCELLANEOUS

Lymphoma

Notes on Ann Arbor staging for lymphoma:
1. Stage I: Involvement of a single lymph node region (I) or single extranodal site (IE)
2. Stage II: Involvement of two or more lymph node regions or lymphatic structures on the same side of the diaphragm alone (II) or with involvement of limited, contiguous, extra-lymphatic organ or tissue (IIE)
3. Stage III: Involvement of lymph node regions on both sides of the diaphragm (III), which may include the spleen (IIIS), or limited, contiguous, extralymphatic organ or tissue (IIIE), or both (IIIES)
4. Stage IV: Diffuse or disseminated foci of involvement of one or more extralymphatic organs or tissues, with or without associated lymphatic involvement

Note: All stages are further subdivided according to the absence(A) or presence (B) of systemic B symptoms including fevers, night sweats, and/or weight loss (>10% of body weight over 6 months prior to diagnosis).

Q. Which of the following variants of mantle cell lymphoma is characterized by IGV-mutated cells and has a more indolent course:
1. Classical
2. Leukemic

3. Blastoid
4. None of the above

Answer: leukemic

There are two variants of MCL: classical MCL, characterized by unmutated or minimally mutated IGV genes and leukemic, non-nodal MCL, characterized by IGV-mutated cells and which has a more indolent disease course.

Q. The characteristic translocation in mantle cell lymphoma is:
1. t(11;14)
2. t(11;18)
3. t(14;18)
4. t(8;14)

Answer: t(11;14)

It juxtaposes the IGH gene at 14q32 to a region containing the CCND1 gene on chromosome 11q13.

Q. Burkitt lymphoma has which of the following chromosomal abnormality:
1. t(8;14)
2. t(2;8)
3. t(8;22)
4. All of the above

Answer: all of the above

The primary genetic lesion in BL involves the MYC gene on

region 8q24 and one of the IG loci on the partner chromosome. In 80% of cases, this is t(8;14) and in the rest t(2;8) and
t(8;22) are found. Sometimes other rare translocations may
be present.

The consequence of these translocations is the constitutive
overexpression of the MYC proto-oncogene.
Interestingly, infection with plasmodium is a risk factor for
development of BL in the endemic areas.

Q. The most common low grade NHL is:
      1. Diffuse large B cell lymphoma
      2. Follicular lymphoma
      3. MALToma
      4. Burkitt lymphoma

Answer: follicular lymphoma

The genetic hallmark of FL is represented by chromosomal translocations of the BCL2 gene on chromosome band
18q21.

Notes on DLBCL molecular biology:
      1. DLBCL is the most common form of B-NHL
      2. Genetic lesions specific to GCB-DLBCL include
        the t(14;18) and t(8;14) translocations, which
        deregulate the BCL2 and MYC oncogenes

Q. The most common chromosomal abnormality in CLL is:
      1. Deletion of 17p
      2. Deletion of 13q
      3. Deletion of 17q
      4. Trisomy 12

Answer: deletion of 13q

CLL has many genetic abnormalities, like:
  1. Deletion of chromosomal regions 17p
  2. Deletion of chromosomal regions 11q
  3. Deletion of chromosomal regions 13q: most common
  4. Trisomy 12

Q. The genetic hallmark of ALK-positive ALCL is a chromosomal translocation:
  1. t(2;5)
  2. t(2;2)
  3. t(3;5)
  4. t(1;5)

Answer: t(2;5)

Q. Nodular lymphocyte-predominant Hodgkin lymphoma constitutes around what percentage of total Hodgkin lymphoma cases:
  1. 5
  2. 10
  3. 15
  4. 20

Answer: 5%

Notes on HL:
  1. HL is classified into two major subgroups: nodular lymphocyte-predominant HL (NLPHL) (~5% of

cases) and classical HL. Classical HL is divided into four: nodular sclerosis, mixed cellularity, lymphocyte rich and lymphocyte depleted.
2. Reed-Sternberg (RS) are characteristic for HL. They lack many of the mature B-cell markers such as CD19 and CD20 surface proteins, but they almost always express the B-cell specific transcription factor PAX5.
3. RS cells account for less than 2% of the tumor mass.
4. In the world, nodular sclerosis is the most common histologic subtype of HL. In this type, RS cells often have "lacunar" morphology.
5. In India mixed cellularity HL is the most common

Q. Which type of Hodgkin lymphoma is most often associated with Epstein-Barr virus infection:
   1. Nodular sclerosis
   2. Lymphocyte depleted
   3. Nodular lymphocyte predominant
   4. Mixed cellularity

Answer: mixed cellularity

80% of cases of mixed cellularity HL are associated with Epstein-Barr virus (EBV) infection.

In the Western world, EBV infection is mostly detected in cases of MCCHL and LDCHL and is less frequently detected in NSCHL and LRCHL. Conversely, EBV is found in HRS cells in nearly all cases of CHL occurring in patients infected with HIV.

Q. Hodgkin lymphoma is characterized by "contiguous" involvement of lymph nodes. This has implication in management planning as well. Which of the following type of HL, doesn't follow the rule of contiguous involvement and may involve distant sites without intervening nodal involvement:

1. Mixed cellularity
2. Lymphocyte rich
3. Nodular lymphocyte predominant
4. Lymphocyte depleted

Answer: Nodular lymphocyte predominant

Notes:
There are several criteria in use for risk stratification of early stage Hodgkin lymphoma. Which one of these will be used, depends on the protocol being followed as different groups have slightly different guidelines on the management of early stage Hodgkin lymphoma. Below are summarized the major criteria proposed by major groups. If a question is asked, without mentioning a particular group then we must take into consideration all of these factors. The abbreviation "CS" used below means: clinical stage.

EORTC
Risk factors
1. Large mediastinal mass (>1/3)
2. Age 50 y and older
3. ESR ≥50 mm/h without B symptoms or ≥30 mm/h with B symptoms
4. ≥4 nodal areas

Favorable:
CS I–II (supradiaphragmatic) without risk factors
Unfavorable:
CS I–II (supradiaphragmatic) with ≥1 risk factors

GHSG

607

Risk factors:
1. Large mediastinal mass
2. Extranodal disease
3. ESR ≥50 mm/h without B symptoms or ≥30 mm/h with B symptoms
4. ≥3 nodal areas

Favorable:
CS I–II without risk factors
Unfavorable:
a. CS I or CS IIA with ≥1 risk factor
b. CS IIB with risk factor 3 or 4 but without risk factors 1 and 2

NCCN
Risk factors:
1. Large mediastinal mass (>1/3) or >10 cm
2. ESR ≥50 mm/h or any B symptoms
3. ≥3 nodal areas
4. >1 extranodal lesion

Favorable:
CS I–II without risk factors
Unfavorable:
CS I–II with ≥1 risk factor (differentiating between bulky disease and other risk factors for treatment guidelines)

NCIC/ECOG
Risk factors:
1. Histology other than LP/NS
2. Age 40 y and older
3. ESR ≥50mm/h
4. ≥4 nodal areas

Favorable:
CS I–II without risk factors
Unfavorable:
CS I–II with ≥1 risk factor

Q. The management of early stage, favourable Hodgkin lymphoma has been debated and many trials have been done in an attempt to study the feasibility of reduction in the chemotherapy drugs administered, in order to prevent late toxicities but without compromising results. But even in the most favorable subsets of early Hodgkin lymphoma chemotherapy can't be reduced below a certain threshold, as was found in the trials. Which of the following constitutes the bare minimum treatment option for early stage favorable Hodgkin lymphoma:
    1. 2 cycles of ABVD and 20 Gy of IFRT
    2. 3 cycles of ABVD and 20 Gy of IFRT
    3. 2 cycles of ABVD and 30 Gy of IFRT
    4. 3 cycles of ABVD and 30 Gy of IFRT

Answer: 2 cycles of ABVD and 20 Gy of IFRT

It is based on the results of the GHSG HD10 and GHSG HD13 studies.

On the other hand, in the early stage but unfavorable group of Hodgkin lymphoma, it may be hazardous to reduce treatment below a threshold of four cycles of ABVD and 30 Gy of IFRT, unless some means can be found to select patients for whom further deintensification can be attempted, such as the use of functional imaging. These recommendations are based on the European intergroup H9-U study and the GHSG HD11 study.

Q. FDG-PET may be used to modify treatment plan of Hodgkin lymphoma, known as response-adapted treatment:
    1. True
    2. False

Answer: true

The RAPID study randomized patients with non bulky early-stage disease who had an interim PET score of 1 or 2 after three cycles of ABVD to either 30 Gy of IFRT or no further therapy. The survival outcomes were not different in the two groups.

Q. At any site uptake moderately increased compared to liver on PET scan is given a Deauville score of:
1. 1
2. 2
3. 3
4. 4

Answer: 4

Following is the Deauville scoring system:

No uptake above background = 1

Uptake ≤ mediastinum = 2

Uptake > mediastinum but ≤ liver = 3

Uptake moderately increased compared to the liver at any site = 4

Uptake markedly increased compared to the liver at any site = 5

New areas of uptake unlikely to be related to lymphoma = X

It should be noted here that there is no "0" score in Deauville scoring system.

Q. Which of the following is not a factor used in the prognostication of advanced stage Hodgkin lymphoma by the international prognostic score (IPS):
1. Age 40 years and more
2. Stage IV
3. Male gender
4. WBC ≥15,000 cells/µL

Answer: age 40 years and more

In fact the age criteria used in IPS is 45 years or more.

Other factors that impart a high risk are lymphocytes <600 cells/µL or <8% of WBC count, or both, albumin <4.0 g/dL and hemoglobin <10.5 g/dL.

Q. Checkpoint inhibitors may be used in Hodgkin lymphoma in all of the following indication except:
1. In a patient of classical Hodgkin lymphoma that has relapsed after autologous HSCT
2. In a patient of classical Hodgkin lymphoma that has relapsed after brentuximab vedotin
3. In a patient of relapsed classical Hodgkin lymphoma who is ineligible for HSCT
4. In a patient of classical Hodgkin lymphoma post allogeneic stem cell transplant

Answer: In a patient of classical Hodgkin lymphoma that has relapsed after brentuximab vedotin

The checkpoint inhibitor nivolumab may be given after failure of auto or allo-HSCT or in transplant ineligible patients or in those who failed on second line chemo. But in patients who receive and relapse on brentuximab, transplant or further chemo is a more suitable option, rather than switching to nivolumab and not doing a transplant.

In all other indications nivolumab is used but in patients who progress after alloHSCT, pembrolizumab may also be given.

Notes:
Indications of brentuximab vedotin:

It's a CD30-directed antibody-drug conjugate (ADC) consisting of chimeric IgG1 antibody cAC10, specific for human CD30 and the microtubule disrupting agent, monomethyl auristatin E (MMAE, or vedotin)

It should be noted that brentuximab is never given with bleomycin. And it should also be kept in mind that brentuximab is not effective in nodular lymphocyte predominant Hodgkin lymphoma because it is CD30 negative.

1. As first-line therapy for previously untreated Stage III or IV classical HL in combination with doxorubicin, vinblastine, and dacarbazine (AVD)
2. As consolidation in classical HL at high risk of relapse or progression **after** autologous hematopoietic stem cell transplantation (auto-HSCT)
3. In classical HL after failure of auto-HSCT or after failure of at least 2 prior multi-agent chemotherapy regimens in patients who are not auto-HSCT candidates
4. In previously-untreated systemic anaplastic large cell lymphoma
5. In treatment of systemic anaplastic large cell lymphoma after failure of at least 1 prior multiagent chemotherapy regimen

6. In primary cutaneous anaplastic large cell lymphoma or CD30 expressing mycosis fungoides (MF) who have received prior systemic therapy
7. In CD30-expressing peripheral T-cell lymphomas

Notes:

Infectious agents associated with the development of lymphoma:

1. Epstein-Barr virus
2. HIV-1 infection
3. HTLV-1
4. HHV-8
5. *Helicobacter pylori*
6. *Campylobacter jejuni*
7. *Chlamydia psittaci*
8. *Borrelia afzelii*
9. HCV
10. MTB

Q. Which of the following is not a part of the international prognostic index (IPI) used for follicular lymphoma:

1. Age older than 60 y
2. LDH > upper limit normal
3. ECOG performance status ≥2
4. Hgb < 12 g/dL

Answer: ECOG performance status ≥2

It should be noted that there are many types of international prognostic index (IPI) depending on the lymphoma in question.

The IPI (without any mention of a specific lymphoma) has five factors:

1. Age older than 60 y

2. LDH > upper limit normal
3. ECOG performance status ≥2
4. Ann Arbor stage III or IV
5. Number of extranodal disease sites greater than one

But the IPI used for follicular lymphoma, also known as FLIPI has different set of factors:
1. Age older than 60 y
2. LDH > upper limit normal
3. Hgb < 12 g/dL
4. Ann Arbor stage III or IV
5. Number of involved nodal areas greater than four

Q. Lymphoblastic lymphomas are mostly of:
1. T-cell lineage
2. B-cell lineage
3. NK/T-cell lineage
4. Dendritic cell origin

Answer: T-cell lineage

Approximately 85% to 90% of lymphoblastic lymphomas are of the T-cell lineage,with the remainder being of the B-cell type.

Q. The malignant cells of follicular lymphoma typically show which immunophenotype:
1. CD19 positive, CD20 positive, CD10 negative, CD5 positive and CD23 negative
2. CD19 positive, CD20 positive, CD10 positive, CD5 positive and CD23 negative
3. CD19 positive, CD20 negative, CD10 positive, CD5 positive and CD23 negative
4. CD19 positive, CD20 positive, CD10 positive, CD5

negative and CD23 negative

Answer: CD19 positive, CD20 positive, CD10 positive, CD5 negative and CD23 negative

Q. The treatment of choice for limited stage (I/II) follicular lymphoma is:
  1. Rituximab based chemotherapy for 3 cycles
  2. Rituximab based chemotherapy for 6 cycles
  3. Radiation therapy
  4. Observation

Answer: radiation therapy

It must be clearly understood that follicular lymphoma is an indolent lymphoma. In stage I and II, radiation is the treatment of choice. But in stage III and IV, we have to decide if the patient can be observed or should he be treated. There are criteria to decide for that, known as GELF and FLIPI criteria.

To repeat once again: in limited stage follicular lymphoma we have to treat the patient and radiation is the treatment of choice but in advanced stages we can choose observation and not treat the patient if there are no indications of treatment.

GELF Criteria
☐ Any nodal or extranodal tumor mass ≥7 cm
☐ ≥3 nodal sites, each >3cm
☐ Presence of B symptoms
☐ Splenomegaly
☐ Compression or vital organs compromise
☐ Significant serous effusions
☐ Lymphocyte count >5.0 x 10^9/L
☐ Cytopenias (granulocytes <1.0 x 10^9/L and/or platelets <100 x 10^9/L)

Table: GELF criteria. If any criteria is present, we may consider treatment.

Q. Which of the following is not seen with maintenance rituximab (versus no maintenance rituximab) in patients with follicular lymphoma who respond to initial chemo-immunotherapy:
1. Increased toxicity
2. Overall survival improvement
3. Progression free survival benefit
4. Higher chances of being in complete response at 2 years

Answer: Overall survival improvement

The PRIMA phase III intergroup trial randomized patients with previously untreated FL that responded to chemo-immunotherapy to maintenance with rituximab (375 mg/m2 every 8 weeks for 24 months) or placebo. At a median follow-up of 36 months from randomization, patients assigned to rituximab maintenance had a higher rate of PFS and a higher percentage of patients in CR or CR-unconfirmed at 24 months was also seen 2 years post randomization in patients receiving maintenance rituximab. There also was a significantly higher percentage of patients with grade III/IV adverse events and infections in the rituximab maintenance group. But overall survival (OS) was not different, even after 10 years of follow-up in the study.

Notes on follicular lymphoma grade III:
1. FL grade III has been historically referred to as follicular large cell lymphoma.
2. It is histologically defined by the presence of >15 centroblasts per hpf
3. It is further subdivided into grade IIIa, where centrocytes are present, and grade IIIb, where there are sheets of centroblasts.
4. It may be confused with pediatric-type FL, which may occur in young adults and has "aggressive" histologic features, but is genetically distinct from FL grade IIIb, pursues an indolent course, and is associated with an excellent prognosis
5. Follicular lymphoma grade IIIb is treated as DLBCL

Q. CLL immunophenotype is characteristically:
1. CD5 positive, CD23 positive
2. CD5 positive, CD23 negative
3. CD5 negative, CD23 positive
4. CD5 negative, CD23 negative

Answer: CD5 positive, CD23 positive

Around 40% of CLL cases express CD38. Expression of the tyrosine kinase ZAP70 is also observed in a subset of cases and correlates with a more aggressive clinical course.

Mantle cell lymphoma, on the other hand, expresses CD5 and usually lack CD10 and CD23.

Q. Out of the most characteristic chromosomal abnormalities, which has the most favorable outcome:
    1. 13q deletions
    2. del(11q)
    3. del(17p)
    4. Trisomy 12

Answer: 13q deletions

Q. Patients with small lymphocytic leukemia (SLL) characteristically have:
    1. An absolute lymphocyte count of < 5,000/µL
    2. An absolute lymphocyte count of < 1,000/µL
    3. An absolute lymphocyte count of < 10,000/µL
    4. Diagnosis of SLL doesn't depend on the absolute lymphocyte count

Answer: An absolute lymphocyte count of < 5,000/µL

Q. Patient of CLL may transform to:
    1. DLBCL
    2. Hodgkin lymphoma
    3. Both of the above
    4. Neither 1 nor 2

Answer: both of the above

The transformation to DLBCL is known as Richter syndrome.

Q. MYD88 activating mutations are characteristic and specific for lymphoplasmacytic lymphoma:
1. True
2. False

Answer: false

While its true that MYD88 activating mutations are found in most of the patients of LPL, they are not specific to this disease.

Q. Gastric MALT lymphomas may be associated with Helicobacter pylori infection. Which of the following is true about these tumors:
1. H. pylori treatment may result in long term disease control in early stages
2. Patients with a t(11;18) translocation don't benefit with eradication of H. pylori
3. If the lymphoma of an early stage fails to respond to H. pylori then RT is the preferred treatment modality.
4. All of the above

Answer: all of the above

Chemotherapy, immunotherapy, or chemoimmunotherapy is active in this disease but is generally reserved for patients with disease that is relapsed or refractory to antibiotic therapy or RT or patients with more advanced-stage or aggressive disease. Interestingly, MALT lymphoma of the ocular adnexa is associated with C. psittaci infection.

Q. What is a "double-hit" diffuse large B cell lymphoma:
1. DLBCL with MYC rearrangement and concurrent BCL2 or BCL6 rearrangements
2. DLBCL with MYC rearrangement and concurrent BCL2 but not BCL6 rearrangements
3. DLBCL with MYC rearrangement and concurrent BCL6 but not BCL2 rearrangements
4. DLBCL without MYC rearrangement but with concurrent BCL2 and BCL6 rearrangements

Answer: DLBCL with MYC rearrangement and concurrent BCL2 or BCL6 rearrangements

Double hit lymphomas have a poorer prognosis and in the new WHO classification, they are classified as a new disease entity.

Q. Which of the following is not true about DLBCL management:
1. The current recommendation for the treatment of advanced-stage DLBCL is combination chemotherapy with RCHOP for patients both younger than 60 years and older than 60 years
2. GELA trial reported that eight cycles of RCHOP was superior to CHOP alone in terms of PFS, disease-free survival (DFS), and OS, with no added toxicity
3. In the U.S. Intergroup study comparing administering CHOP or RCHOP given on a different schedule in a similar population and randomizing responding patients to receive either rituximab maintenance therapy or no maintenance found PFS benefit of maintenance rituximab following RCHOP induction
4. The RICOVER-60 trial found no benefit of eight cycles of RCHOP over six cycles

Answer: In the U.S. Intergroup study comparing administering CHOP or RCHOP given on a different schedule in a similar population and randomizing responding patients to receive either rituximab maintenance therapy or no maintenance found PFS benefit of maintenance rituximab following RCHOP induction

In fact, maintenance rituximab failed to show benefit.

Notes:
1. Trials comparing RCHOP administered every 21 days (RCHOP-21) to RCHOP administered every 14 days (RCHOP-14) found no benefit of RCHOP-14 and toxicity were increased. Thus establishing RCHOP given every 21 days for 6 cycles as the standard of care.
2. A meta-analysis of patients treated on 15 randomized trials with either conventional therapy or ASCT in first CR showed no difference in EFS, OS, or treatment-related mortality.
3. The results to date do not support ASCT as a consolidation for first remission.

Q. In testicular DLBCL which of the following treatment strategies is used:
1. Orchiectomy of the involved testis
2. Systemic or intrathecal methotrexate
3. Prophylactic radiation of the contralateral testis
4. All of the above

Answer: all of the above

Testicular DLBCL is a unique entity as there are higher chances of involvement of CNS and contralateral testis. For this purpose its management involves all of the above mentioned options along with systemic chemo.

Notes on other sites and characteristics, lymphomas of which have high chances of having CNS spread:
1. Testis
2. Ovary
3. Bone marrow
4. Breast
5. Epidural space
6. Paranasal sinuses
7. High intermediate or high IPI score
8. Multiple extranodal sites

There is a CNS-IPI model available for assessing the risk to CNS. It has the same five parameters used in the standard IPI with the addition of involvement of the kidneys and/or adrenal glands to define three risk groups: low, intermediate, and high risk.

Q. Starry sky appearance on histology is seen in:
1. Burkitt lymphoma
2. DLBCL
3. Mantle cell lymphoma
4. Nodular lymphocyte predominant Hodgkin lymphoma

Answer: Burkitt lymphoma

Notes on Burkitt lymphoma:
1. It generally occurs in the pediatric population
2. It has three major forms:
   a. The endemic or African form presents as a jaw or facial bone tumor and spreads to extranodal sites, including the ovary, testis, kidney,

breast, and especially bone marrow and meninges.

b. The non endemic form usually has an abdominal presentation with massive disease, ascites, and renal, testis, and/or ovarian involvement and, like the endemic form, also spreads to the bone marrow and CNS.

c. Immunodeficiency-related cases more often involve lymph nodes and may present with peripheral blood involvement. BL has a male predominance and is typically seen in patients younger than 35 years of age.

Q. Hallmark cells are most commonly found in:
1. Burkitt lymphoma
2. Mixed cellularity Hodgkin lymphoma
3. Anaplastic large cell lymphoma
4. Peripheral cutaneous T cell lymphoma

Answer: Anaplastic large cell lymphoma

Notes on ALCL:
1. It has three distinct clinicopathologic entities: primary systemic ALCL, ALK positive; primary systemic ALCL, ALK negative; and primary cutaneous ALCL.
2. Virtually all cases are CD30+

Q. ATLL is associated with HTLV-1 in what percentage of cases:
1. 50
2. 10
3. 72
4. 100

Answer: 100%

The tumor cells of ATLL circulating in the blood have a sun-flower or starburst appearance.

Q. ATLL is a tumor of:
1. Pre T cells
2. NK/T cells
3. CD4+ T cells
4. CD8+ T cells

Answer: CD4+ T cells

Q. Which are the therapeutic strategies used in cases of post-transplant lymphoproliferative disorder:
1. Reduction in immunosuppression
2. Antiviral therapy
3. Single-agent rituximab
4. Chemoimmunotherapy

Answer: all of the above

If the examiner asks what is the "first" step in management of PTLD then its reduction in immunosuppression in form of a 25% to 50% reduction in cyclosporine and tacrolimus and discontinuation of azathioprine and mycopheno-late mofetil.

Q. Which of the following is not a diagnostic criteria re-quired for Sézary syndrome:

1. Absolute Sézary count of at least 1,000 cells/mm3 in the bone marrow
2. Expanded CD4+ populations and/or loss of antigens such as CD2, CD3, CD5, or CD4
3. Presence of a T-cell clone in the blood
4. None of the above

Answer: Absolute Sézary count of at least 1,000 cells/mm3 in the bone marrow

In fact the absolute Sézary count of at least 1,000 cells/mm3 is required in the blood and not in the bone marrow.

The criteria for the diagnosis of this syndrome are provided by the International Society for Cutaneous Lymphoma (ISCL), which include an absolute Sézary count of at least 1,000 cells/mm3 in the blood, immunophenotypic abnormalities (expanded CD4 + populations and/or loss of antigens such as CD2, CD3, CD5, or CD4), or presence of a T-cell clone in the blood.

Notes on mycosis fungoides;
1. Mycosis fungoides, also known as Alibert-Bazin syndrome or granuloma fungoides, is the most common form of cutaneous T-cell lymphoma.
2. The immunophenotypic profile of MF is one of clonal mature CD4+CD45RO+ T cells with a marked homing capacity for the papillary dermis and epidermis.
3. Antigen loss is characteristic of the disease, with loss of CD7, CD5, or CD2 and dim staining for CD3.
4. Sézary cells express a TH2 phenotype, with secretion of interleukin (IL)-4, IL-5, IL-6, IL-10, and IL-13.
5. The pruritus characteristic of the disease is related to secretion of IL-5 as well as other chemokines.
6. One of the most striking features of MF/SS is epider-

motropism, or infiltration of the epidermis by malignant T cells.

7. The pathognomic feature of MF is the Pautrier microabscess, a collection of clonal malignant cells **within the epidermis**.

8. Skin-directed modalities include those for localized disease (radiotherapy, bexarotene, carmustine) and those applicable to total skin therapy (topical chemotherapy with nitrogen mustard [NM], phototherapy, and total skin electron-beam therapy [TSEBT]).

9. Systemic therapy options Interferon-α, vorinostat, alemtuzumab, mogamulizumab (a humanized anti-CCR4 antibody) and brentuximab vedotin among others

Q. The most common type of primary CNS lymphoma is:
1. DLBCL
2. Follicular lymphoma
3. High grade lymphoma, NOS
4. Lymphoblastic lymphomas

Answer: DLBCL

Notes on PCNSL:
1. The common sites are the cerebral hemisphere (38%), basal ganglia and thalamus (16%), and corpus callosum (14%).
2. It is characterized o n T1-weighted, postcontrast images by homogeneous enhancement with well-defined borders. It is typically isointense to hypointense on T2-weighted MRI and has restricted diffusion on diffusion-weighted imaging (DWI).

Q. The staging system used for PCNSL is:
   1. Ann Arbor
   2. Lugano
   3. McDonalds
   4. None of the above

Answer: none of the above

There is no validated staging system for PCNSL.

Q. The most effective systemic therapy option for PCNSL is:
   1. High dose intravenous methotrexate
   2. Rituximab
   3. Thiotepa
   4. High dose cyclophosphamide +/- steroids

Answer: High dose intravenous methotrexate

The most effective treatment for PCNSL is intravenous, HD-MTX at variable doses (1 to 8 g/m2), typically utilized in combination with other chemotherapeutic agents and/or WBRT.
MATRix regimen addition of thiotepa and rituximab to the HD-MTX/cytarabine combination

Q. Which of the core binding factor targeting chromosomal translocation is not characteristically found in AML:
   1. t(8;21)
   2. inv(16)
   3. t(12;21)
   4. All of the above are characteristically found in AML

Answer: t(12;21)

The ETV6/RUNX1 (aka TEL/AML1) fusion that is expressed as a consequence of t(12;21) is more commonly found in pediatric B-ALL and not in AML.

Core binding factor targeting mutations confer good prognosis to acute leukemia patients.

Notes on APL (acute promyelocytic leukemia):
1. It is a result of t(15;17) fusion gene
2. The RARα gene on chromosome 17 is fused to promyelocytic leukemia (PML) gene on chromosome 15.
3. It is classified in low and high risk (based on the WBC count upto 10000/mm3 or more). Some groups use an intermediate risk classification as well, that takes into account platelet count as well.
4. The treatment of low risk APL may be done without chemo and by using a combination of all trans retinoic acid (ATRA) and arsenic. The most used of which is the Lococo regimen.
5. The treatment of high risk incorporates ATRA, arsenic and chemo
6. The cure rates in low risk APL are well above 90% where as they are lower in the high risk group.
7. There are some variant gene fusions as well like the PLZF/RARα fusion, resulting from t(11;17). In the patients harboring this mutation, ATRA is not effective.

Q. Which of the following is not true:
1. Approximately 1% to 2% of de novo AML are BCR/ABL1 rearranged
2. BCR/ABL1 rearrangement is present in 20% to 30% of pediatric ALL
3. Most patients with ALL express a 190-kDa protein

(p190) as a result of BCR/ABL1 rearrangement

4. In CML patients the BCR/ABL1 rearrangement results in expression of a 210-kDa oncoprotein (p210)

Answer: BCR/ABL1 rearrangement is present in 20% to 30% of pediatric ALL

In fact, this rearrangement is present in 20% to 30% of adult ALL and 2% to 3% of children with ALL.

Q. Activating mutations in FLT3 have been reported in what percentage of AML patients:
1. 30-35
2. <20
3. 60-70
4. They are not found in AML

Answer: 30-35%

They are most commonly internal tandem duplications (ITDs) within the JM domain that result in constitutive activation of FLT3.

This mutation confers high risk.

Q. A marrow or peripheral blood blast count ≥20% is absolutely necessary for the diagnosis of AML and if blast percentage is any lower a diagnosis of AML can't be made:
1. True
2. False

Answer: false

While its true that according to the WHO a marrow or peripheral blood blast count ≥20% is necessary for the diagnosis of AML, but it's not always required. For example, in cases with t(8;21), inv(16), t(16;16) (core-binding factor), or t(5;17) (APL), the diagnosis of AML can be made with lower blast percentage.

Notes on risk stratification of AML:
The revised European LeukemiaNet classification system:
Favorable risk
   1. t(8;21)(q22;q22.1); RUNX1-RUNX1T1
   2. inv(16)(p13.1q22) or t(16;16)(p13.1;q22); CBFB-MYH11
   3. Mutated NPM1 without FLT3-ITD or with FLT3-ITD low
   4. Biallelic mutated CEBPA
Intermediate
   1. Mutated NPM1 and FLT3-ITD high
   2. Wild-type NPM1 without FLT3-ITD or with FLT3-ITD low (without adverse-risk genetic lesions)
   3. t(9;11)(p21.3;q23.3); MLLT3-KMT2A
   4. Cytogenetic abnormalities not classified as favorable or adverse
Adverse
   1. t(6;9)(p23;q34.1); DEK-NUP214
   2. t(v;11q23.3); KMT2A rearranged
   3. t(9;22)(q34.1;q11.2); BCR-ABL1
   4. inv(3)(q21.3q26.2) or t(3;3)(q21.3;q26.2); GATA2,MECOM(EVI1)
   5. -5 or del(5q); -7; -17/abn(17p)
   6. Complex karyotype, monosomal karyotype
   7. Wild-type NPM1 and FLT3-ITD high
   8. Mutated RUNX1
   9. Mutated ASXL1
      10.   Mutated TP53

Q. The 7+3 regimen used in the treatment of AML is:
1. 7 days of cytarabine administered by continuous infusion for 7 days together with 3 days of an anthracycline
2. 7 days of an anthracycline administered by continuous infusion for 7 days together with 3 days of cytarabine
3. 7 days of cytarabine together with 3 days of an anthracycline administered by continuous infusion
4. 7 days of an anthracycline together with 3 days of cytarabine administered by continuous infusion

Answer: 7 days of cytarabine administered by continuous infusion for 7 days together with 3 days of an anthracycline

The dose of cytarabine is usually 100 mg/m2 daily continuous infusion for 7 days (total dose 700 mg/m2) along with three days of an anthracycline (daunorubicin or idarubicin). The dose of daunorubicin is generally 60 mg/m2 daily for 3 days.

Q. Gemtuzumab ozogamicin is an antibody directed to:
1. CD30
2. CD33
3. CD52
4. CD22

Answer: CD33

Notes on midostaurin:
1. The RATIFY trial randomized patients of AML to 3+7 plus or minus midostaurin in patients with

FLT3-mutated AML. Consolidation was with high-dose ara-C with or without midostaurin and allogeneic stem cell transplant was allowed in first CR. Those in remission continued their midostaurin or placebo for maintenance.

2. OS and event-free survival were significantly better for the patients randomized to receive midostaurin, even after censoring patients who underwent allogeneic stem cell transplant. This has led to the approval of midostaurin for the treatment of patients with newly diagnosed FLT3-mutated AML.

Q. Which of the following is not an adverse prognostic factor in adult acute lymphoblastic leukemia:
1. Age <35 years
2. Leukocytosis of >30000/mm3 for B cell lineage
3. Leukocytosis of >100000/mm3 for T cell lineage
4. Early T cell precursor immunophenotype

Answer: age <35 years

In fact, age >35 years is an adverse prognostic risk factor.

Notes on unfavorable prognostic features in adult acute lymphoblastic leukemia:
1. Age >35 y
2. Leukocytosis >30000/mm3 for B lineage and >100000/mm3 for T lineage
3. Early T-cell precursor immunophenotype
4. t(9;22)(q24;q11.2), t(4;11)(q21;q23), t(8;14)(q24.1;q32), complex, low hypodiploidy
5. Molecular profile: IKZF1, CRLF2, TP53, LYL1
6. Treatment Related:
    a. Therapy response Time to morphologic CR >4 wk
    b. Persistent MRD up to 10 to 12 wk postinduc-

tion

Q. Adults with ALL have lower chances of achieving long term disease free survival compared with pediatric ALL patients:
    1. True
    2. False

Answer: true

Only 25% to 50% of adults achieve long-term DFS.

Q. Starry sky appearance on microscopy is seen in which type of ALL:
    1. L1
    2. L2
    3. L3
    4. None of the above

Answer: L3

The FAB classification divided ALL based on cell morphology in to three subtypes:
    1. L1 lymphoblasts, which have small to intermediate in size (the most common type of ALL)
    2. L2, which has slightly larger sized blasts
    3. L3, which has large blasts, described as having a starry sky appearance, which were seen in Burkitt leukemia or lymphoma.

Q. The most common type of ALL, the precursor B ALL, shows all of the following features except:
    1. Surface immunoglobulin positivity

2. TdT positivity
3. CD10 (CALLA) positivity
4. Cytoplasmic CD79a positivity

Answer: Surface immunoglobulin positivity

Notes on ALL immunophenotypes:
1. Of all cases of ALL, 85% are of B-cell lineage, and the most common form is the precursor B phenotype (also called common precursor-B-ALL or early precursor-B-ALL); these cells express a B-cell immunophenotype (CD19, CD22), terminal deoxynucleotidyl transferase (TdT), cytoplasmic CD79A, CD34, CD10 (CALLA), and lack cytoplasmic μ and surface immunoglobulin (sIg).
2. Pro-B-ALL, lacks CD10 expression and may represent an earlier level of B-cell maturation.
3. Mature B-cell lineage ALL has the immunophenotype of mature B cells with sIg expression and is seen with Burkitt leukemia or lymphoma.
4. T-lineage ALL accounts for 15% to 20% of cases. This common thymocyte type expresses pan T-cell markers, CD2, cytoplasmic CD3 (cCD3), CD7, CD5, and distinctively shows co-expression of CD4 and CD8 and expression of CD1a.
5. A more primitive type called prothymocyte or immature thymocyte type has TdT, cCD3, and variable expression of CD5, CD2, and CD7, but lacks CD4, CD8, and CD1a. Notably, using molecular profiling, a distinct subset within the immature thymocyte group has been identified as early T-cell precursor with very poor prognosis.
6. Mature T-lineage phenotype expresses the pan T-cell markers, variable TdT, but lacks CD1a.

Q. All of the following are associated with poor prognosis in ALL except:

1. t(9;22)
2. t(4;11)
3. t(12;21)
4. Five or more chromosomal abnormalities

Answer: t(12;21)

Other poor prognostic features are t(8;14), low hypodiploidy or near triploidy.

Q. The term "Philadelphia chromosome" is used for which abnormal chromosome:
　　1. 9
　　2. 22
　　3. 11
　　4. The product of t(9;22) is called the philadelphia chromosome

Answer: 22

The Philadelphia chromosome was described by Nowell and Hungerford as a "minute" chromosome 22 in CML cells.

The genes juxtaposed by the translocation are ABL1 (Abelson) on 9q34 and breakpoint cluster region (BCR) on chromosome 22q11.

Q. In patients of CML the breakpoints within ABL1 (on chromosome 9q34)occur most frequently:
　　1. Upstream of exon 1b
　　2. Downstream of exon 1a
　　3. Between exon 1b and exon 1a
　　4. None of the above

Answer: between exon 1b and exon 1a

Q. CML is characterized by the Philadelphia chromosome. What is the minimum number of bone marrow metaphases required to be examined for classical cytogenetics analysis for the detection of the Ph chromosome:
1. 10
2. 20
3. 30
4. 40

Answer: 20

In up to 90% of the patients, a typical t(9;22)(q34;q11) translocation can be identified; in the remaining patients, variant translocations are present.

Q. Which of the following is not true about atypical CML patients:
1. They have clinical and cytological features, like basophilia, of CML but are negative for Ph chromosome or BCR-ABL1 rearrangement on cytogenetics, QRPCR, and FISH analysis
2. In 40% of these patients, mutations in the SETBP1 or ETNK1 genes are detected
3. Atypical CML has a poor prognosis with median survival being only 2 to 3 years
4. Nonspecific chromosomal alteration may be present in a few cases

Answer: They have clinical and cytological features, like basophilia, of CML but are negative for Ph chromosome or BCR-

ABL1 rearrangement on cytogenetics, QRPCR, and FISH analysis

The above mentioned statement is true except the word "basophilia". These cases don't have basophilia.

Q. Which of the following TKI is not approved by US-FDA for the treatment of CML in any phase:
1. Dasatinib
2. Radotinib
3. Bosutinib
4. Ponatinib

Answer: radotinib

Radotinib is approved in some Asian countries but not by US-FDA.

There are five TKIs are licensed for CML treatment: imatinib, dasatinib, nilotinib, bosutinib, and ponatinib.

Notes on adverse effects of imatinib:
1. The common one are related to the inhibition of PDGFR
2. The common adverse effects are edema with weight gain, conjunctival irritation and lacrimation, scleral and mucosal hemorrhage, muscle cramps, asthenia, and diarrhea. Skin rash is also possible, with nummular lesions in lower limbs, trunk, or forearms.
3. Less frequent AEs include skin hypopigmentation (due to KIT blockage) and fragility, liver function test (LFT) alterations, anemia, thrombocytopenia, and neutropenia.

4. Hematologic AEs are considered as such only when occurring in patients who have already obtained a cytogenetic remission (CyR).
5. Most of the adverse effects are not severe and are reversible.

Q. Which is not true about dasatinib:
1. DASISION was a major trial studying dasatinib in CML
2. It is more specific than imatinib
3. It is approved for treatment of CML both in the first line and in later lines
4. The most important adverse effect of dasatinib is development of pleural and pericardial effusions

Answer: It is more specific than imatinib

In fact it is **less** specific than imatinib as it inhibits more than 30 tyrosine kinases, but it is more potent.

Pleural and pericardial effusion are seen in 30% to 40% of patients and are treated with treatment interruption and supportive therapy with steroids and diuretics.

Q. Nilotinib is not associated with which of the following side effects:
1. Edema and muscle cramps
2. Cutaneous toxicity
3. Acute pancreatitis
4. Metabolic syndrome

Answer: edema and muscle cramps

Unlike imatinib, nilotinib is not associated with edema and muscle cramps.

The metabolic syndrome is characterized by hypergly-cemia, increased cholesterol and triglyceride levels, and progression of atherosclerotic lesions.

Nilotinib is approved in both the first line and later lines of therapy.

ENESTnd was a pivot trial of nilotinib in CML.

Q. Which of the following TKI inhibits T315I mutated cells in CML:
1. Bosutinib
2. Dasatinib
3. Ponatinib
4. Radotinib

Answer: ponatinib

Ponatinib is the only TKI that acts on the T315I mutation.

It is **not** approved in the first line therapy of CML patients. Its most troublesome toxicity is cardiovascular events that can include both arterial and venous events (deep vein thrombosis, pulmonary emboli) and which can develop after a few months of treatment, again at difference with nilotinib. These events are frequent as they involved 35% (arterial) and 6% (venous) of patients.

Notes on response monitoring of TKI therapy in CML:
There are three levels of response assessment:

1. The first level of response is represented by the normalization of cell blood count, and this is called hematologic response. In order to achieve a complete hematologic response (CHR), symptom disappearance (if present) and normalization of spleen size (if splenomegaly is present) must also be obtained.

2. A second level of response is achieved when a "cytogenetic response" (CyR) is obtained. Such a response is called partial when the number of Ph-positive metaphases are between 1% and 35% and complete (CCyR) when there is no Ph-positive cell out of a minimum of 20 evaluated metaphases. The term major cytogenetic response includes both partial CyR and CCyR.

3. A third level of response is the one produced by the availability of QRPCR for BCR/ABL1. With this assay, the results are expressed as the number of BCR-ABL1 molecules divided by the number of molecules amplified from a control gene (ABL1 or GUSB). Any ratio below 0.1% is called major molecular remission (MMR); we speak of MR4.0, MR4.5, or MR5 if the ratio falls below 1/10,000, 1/32,000 or 1/100,000, respectively. Results obtained in different labs can be made more comparable by using the International Standard (IS), although a variation by a factor of at least three to four cannot be eliminated even by this method. The term complete molecular remission (CMR) applies when the QRPCR results show no amplification for the BCR-ABL1 gene.

Q. Which of the following TKI is not approved for first line treatment of CML:
  1. Nilotinib
  2. Bosutinib

3. Ponatinib
4. Dasatinib

Answer: ponatinib

There are four TKIs presently approved for treatment of CML is the first line: imatinib, bosutinib, dasatinib and nilotinib.

The usual dosage is 400 mg per day for imatinib, 400 mg per day for bosutinib, 100 mg per day for nilotinib, and 300 mg twice a day (fasting) for nilotinib.

Q. In patients of CML treated with TKIs, who achieve a major molecular response, how often should QRPCR be performedIt is advisable to perform QRPCR:
1. Every 3 months in the initial 5 years and every 6 to 12 months thereafter
2. Every 6 months in the initial 5 years and every year thereafter
3. Every 3 months in the initial 5 years and then monitoring with PCR may be stopped
4. Every 3 months in the initial 2 years and every 6 thereafter

Answer: Every 3 months in the initial 5 years and every 6 to 12 months thereafter Monitoring by QRPCR must be continued indefinitely as CML relapses have been documented

This is the conventional view and also the most practised one but as we will see later that nowadays some patients may be candidates for stopping treatment with TKIs, in such patients the schedules of performing PCR are different.

Q. Which of the following is true about second generation TKIs used in the treatment of CML;

1. Second-generation TKIs uniformly produced a faster and deeper decrease in BCR-ABL1 messenger RNA values as detected by QRPCR compared with imatinib.
2. Some studies showed a significantly higher CCyR rates at or by 12 months in patients receiving second-generation TKIs compared with imatinib.
3. Some studies showed a significant difference in progression to AP or BC CML with the use of second generation TKIs as compared with imatinib.
4. No studies showed a significant difference in OS with second generation TKIs compared with imatinib.

Answer: Some studies showed a significant difference in progression to AP or BC CML with the use of second generation TKIs as compared with imatinib

In fact, **no studies showed** a significant difference in progression to AP or BC CML with the use of second generation TKIs as compared with imatinib (which essentially is another way of saying that there was no significant difference in progression free survival between second generation TKIs and imatinib).

Notes on monitoring patients of CML:
    A. Bone marrow cytogenetics is performed:
        1. At diagnosis
        2. Failure to reach response milestones
        3. Any sign of loss of response (defined as hematologic or cytogenetic relapse)
    B. qPCR using IS is performed:
        1. At diagnosis
        2. Every 3 months after initiating treatment.

    3. After BCR-ABL1 (IS) ≤1% (>0.1%–1%) has been achieved, every 3 months for 2 years and every 3–6 months thereafter.

    4. If there is 1-log increase in BCR-ABL1 transcript levels with MMR, qPCR should be repeated in 1–3 months.

BCR-ABL1 kinase domain mutation analysis is performed in cases of:
1. Failure to reach response milestones.
2. Any sign of loss of response (defined as hematologic or cytogenetic relapse).
3. 1-log increase in BCR-ABL1 transcript levels and loss of MMR.
4. Disease progression to accelerated or blast phase.

Notes on the definitions of CML blast phase and accelerated phase:
It should be noted here that different institutions follow different criteria and there are no agreed upon universal criteria. So minor variations are to be expected in questions being asked, depending on what the examiner has in mind while framing a particular question.

Definition of CML blast phase according to the International Bone Marrow Transplant Registry:
1. ≥30% blasts in the blood, marrow, or both
2. Extramedullary infiltration of leukemic cells

Definition of CML accelerated phase according to the Modified MD Anderson Cancer Center (MDACC) Criteria:
1. Peripheral blood myeloblasts ≥15% and <30%
2. Peripheral blood myeloblasts and promyelocytes combined ≥30%
3. Peripheral blood basophils ≥20%
4. Platelet count ≤100 x 109 /L unrelated to therapy
5. Additional clonal cytogenetic abnormalities in Ph

+ cells

Notes on criteria for different kinds of responses and relapse in CML:
1. Complete hematologic response (all of the following must be met):
    a. Complete normalization of peripheral blood counts with leukocyte count <10000/microL
    b. Platelet count <450 x 109 /L
    c. No immature cells, such as myelocytes, promyelocytes, or blasts in peripheral blood
    d. No signs and symptoms of disease with resolution of palpable splenomegaly
2. Molecular response:
    a. Early molecular response (EMR) - BCR-ABL1 (IS) ≤10% at 3 and 6 months
    b. Major molecular response (MMR) - BCR-ABL1 (IS) ≤0.1% or ≥3-log reduction in BCR-ABL1 mRNA from the standardized baseline, if qPCR (IS) is not available
    c. Complete molecular response (CMR) is variably described, and is best defined by the assay's level of sensitivity (eg, MR4.5)
3. Cytogenetic response:
    a. Complete cytogenetic response (CCyR) - No Ph-positive metaphases
    b. Major cytogenetic response (MCyR) - 0%–35% Ph-positive metaphases
    c. Partial cytogenetic response (PCyR) - 1%–35% Ph-positive metaphases
    d. Minor cytogenetic response - >35%–65% Ph-positive metaphases

Relapse is defined as:
1. Any sign of loss of response (defined as hematologic or cytogenetic relapse)
2. 1-log increase in BCR-ABL1 transcript levels with

loss of MMR should prompt bone marrow evaluation for loss of CCyR but is not itself defined as relapse (eg, hematologic or cytogenetic relapse)

Notes on criteria for TKI Discontinuation (if all three criteria are met then TKI therapy for CML may be discontinued):

1. Age ≥18 years
2. Chronic phase CML
3. No prior history of accelerated or blast phase CML
4. On approved TKI therapy for at least 3 years
5. Prior evidence of quantifiable BCR-ABL1 transcript
6. Stable molecular response (MR4; BCR-ABL1 ≤0.01% IS) for ≥2 years, as documented on at least 4 tests, performed at least 3 months apart
7. Access to a reliable qPCR test with a sensitivity of detection of at least MR4.5 (BCR-ABL1 ≤0.0032% IS) and that provides results within 2 weeks
8. Monthly molecular monitoring for one year, then every 2 months for the second year, and every 3 months thereafter (indefinitely) is recommended for patients who remain in MMR (MR3; BCR-ABL1 ≤0.1% IS) after discontinuation of TKI therapy
9. Prompt resumption of TKI within 4 weeks of a loss of MMR with monthly molecular monitoring until MMR is re-established, then every 3 months thereafter is recommended indefinitely for patients who have reinitiated TKI therapy after a loss of MMR.
10. For those who fail to achieve MMR after 3 months of TKI resumption, BCR-ABL1 kinase domain mutation testing should be performed, and monthly molecular monitoring should be continued for another 6 months.

Q. Which of the following is not a component of the EURO score used for risk stratification of patients with CML:

1. Age
2. Spleen size below costal margin
3. Blast percentage in the bone marrow

4. Eosinophil count

Answer: Blast percentage in the bone marrow

In fact, blast percentage in the peripheral blood is used (not in the bone marrow).

There are three scores for CML risk stratification which have been extensively used:
1. Sokal: age, spleen, platelet count, blasts in peripheral blood.
2. Hasford, also known as EURO: age, spleen size [cm below costal margin], percent blasts in peripheral blood, percent eosinophils, basophils, platelet count.
3. EUTOS (ELTS): age, spleen size cm below the costal margin, blasts in peripheral blood.

Sokal score, for instance, may be low <0.8, intermediate 0.8-1.2 or high >1.2.

The implications of this risk stratification are that they can impact treatment selection. In for example the score is low, then we may choose imatinib or any other second generation TKIs that have been approved for the treatment of CML in the first line but if the score is high then second generation TKIs become the preferred choice and imatinib is not preferred.

Q. The most common leukemia in western countries is:
1. CML
2. CLL
3. AML
4. ALL

Answer: CLL

Q. The characteristic immunophenotype of CLL cells is:
1. CD5+, CD20+, CD23+
2. CD5+, CD20-, CD23+
3. CD5+, CD20+, CD23-
4. CD5-, CD20+, CD23+

Answer: CD5+, CD20+, CD23+

There is sometimes confusion between CLL and MCL. We can remember this by using a trick that CLL has two "L" so it is positive for both CD5 and CD23 whereas MCL (mantle cell lymphoma) has only one "L" in it so it is positive for only one of these markers: CD5 positive and negative for CD23.
CD200 is expressed on CLL cells, but not on mantle cell lymphoma cells, and may be used as a distinguishing marker.

Notes on MBL (monoclonal B lymphocytosis):
1. Around 3.5% of otherwise normal individuals over the age of 40 years may harbor a population of clonal (by light chain analysis) CD5+/CD19+/CD23+ B cells.
2. These asymptomatic individuals **do not** have an absolute lymphocytosis, lymphadenopathy, or other clinical evidence of CLL.

Q. The most common chromosomal abnormality in CLL is:
1. Del(13q)
2. Del(11q)
3. Trisomy 12
4. Del(17p)

Answer: del(13q)

Deletion 13q [del(13q)] is the most common chromosome abnormality in CLL; it is found by FISH as a sole abnormality in 55% of cases, followed by 11q deletion (18%) [del(11q)], 12q trisomy (16%), and 17p deletion (7%) [del(17p)].

The prognosis is worst for del(17p).

The prognosis in best for del13q.

The survival times associated with these abnormalities are: 32, 79, 114, 111, and 133 months for del(17p), del(11q), 12q trisomy, no abnormalities, and del(13q), respectively.

Notes on diagnostic criteria of CLL:
These criteria are proposed by the International Workshop on Chronic Lymphocytic Leukemia (IWCLL)
1. A blood monoclonal B lymphocyte count >5000/ microL, with <55% of the cells being atypical (pro-lymphocytes)
2. B lymphocyte monoclonality should be demon-strated with cells expressing B-cell surface antigens (CD19, CD20, CD23), low density surface Ig (M or D), and CD5.

Q. The monoclonal B cell count specified to distinguish CLL from small lymphocytic lymphoma (SLL) in patients with palpable lymph nodes or splenomegaly is:
1. 5000/mm3
2. 10000/mm3
3. 3000/mm3
4. There is no such distinction and it depends on the immunophenotype

Answer: 5000/mm3

Q. Wells syndrome is frequently seen in:
1. CLL
2. CML
3. MDS
4. T-PLL

Answer: CLL

Exaggerated skin reaction to a bee sting or an insect bite (Wells syndrome) is frequently seen in CLL.

Notes on certain interesting features associated with CLL:
1. Smudge cells are commonly seen in the peripheral smear, reflecting fragility and distortion during preparation of the peripheral smear on a glass slide.
2. A positive direct antiglobulin (Coombs) test is seen in approximately 25% of cases, but autoimmune hemolytic anemia (AIHA) of clinical significance is not common.

Q. Which of the following belongs the Rai stage III of CLL:
1. Lymphocytosis with splenomegaly
2. Lymphocytosis with lymphadenopathy and hepatomegaly
3. Anemia with or without lymphocytosis
4. Thrombocytopenia with lymphocytosis

Answer: Anemia with or without lymphocytosis

Following are the Rai stages of CLL:

0 = Lymphocytosis only

I = Lymphocytosis and lymphadenopathy

II = Lymphocytosis and splenomegaly with/without lymphadenopathy

III = Lymphocytosis and anemia (hemoglobin, <11 g/dL)

IV = Lymphocytosis and thrombocytopenia (platelets, <100,000/mm3)

There is also Binet staging for CLL, which divides the patients in three stage groups: A, B and C.

Q. Which of the following patients of CLL will **not** require active treatment:
  1. A patient with extreme fatigue
  2. A patient with fever
  3. If a patient develops AIHA responsive to steroids
  4. A patient with lymphadenopathy of more than 10 cm longest diameter

Answer: If a patient develops AIHA responsive to steroids

Treatment may be indicated in patients with AIHA **unresponsive** to steroids.

It is an important point to note that not all patients of CLL require treatment and some may be observed without any treatment (as opposed to, for example AML or CML, where all patients have to be treated). For this, the IWCLL has proposed criteria for active disease as indications to initiate treatment:

1. Presence of constitutional symptoms attributable to CLL: weight loss (>10% of baseline weight within the preceding 6 months), extreme fatigue (Eastern Cooperative Oncology Group [ECOG] performance status 2 or higher), fever (temperature higher than 38°C or 100.5°F for at least 2 weeks), or night sweats without evidence of infection.
2. Evidence of progressive bone marrow failure characterized by the development of or worsening of anemia, thrombocytopenia, or both.
3. AIHA or autoimmune thrombocytopenia, or both, poorly responsive to corticosteroid therapy.
4. Massive (>6 cm below the left costal margin) or progressive splenomegaly.
5. Massive (>10 cm in longest diameter) or progressive lymphadenopathy.
6. Progressive lymphocytosis defined as an increase in the absolute lymphocyte count by >50% over a 2-month period, or a doubling time predicted to be <6 months.

The sixth point is especially confusing and should be read very carefully.

If **any** of these characteristics is present in a patient then we may initiate treatment.

Q. Which is preferred treatment for a patient aged 55 years, having IGHV-mutated status but without del(17p):
  1. Ibrutinib
  2. FCR
  3. BR
  4. Obinutuzumab plus venetoclax

Answer: FCR

Notes on first line therapy of CLL:
1. Tremendous progress has been made in the treatment of CLL, especially over the recent years.
2. The list of approved protocols is too long and one must read a thorough reference book for this purpose, like Devita's oncology (quarterly updates) or the NCCN guidelines. I will try to provide a brief overview of the treatment here.
3. In young (<65 years) patients who are fit, in young patients (<65 years) who are not fit, in old (65 years or more) patients; **so essentially in all patients having del(17p)**, the Bruton tyrosine kinase inhibitor "ibrutinib" is the drug of choice.
4. In young and fit patients not having del(17p) and having IGHV (immunoglobulin heavy chain) mutated status, FCR is the therapy of choice (combination of fludarabine, cyclophosphamide and rituximab).
5. In older patients and those young patients who are not fit to receive intensive combination FCR chemo, who don't have del(17p) and have IGHV-mutated status; some less intensive chemoimmunotherapy or ibrutinib should be used.
6. In young and fit patients not having del(17p) and having IGHV-**un**mutated status, treatment options are chemoimmunotherapy or ibrutinib. Same is true for old or unfit patients.
7. The term chemoimmunotherapy means use of an anti-CD20 molecule, like rituximab, obinutuzumab, ofatumumab and a chemo molecule like bendamustine, chlorambucil etc.
8. The main clinical implication of choosing ibrutinib over chemoimmunotherapy is that ibrutinib has to be taken lifelong but chemoimmunotherapy is given for a specific duration of time.

Q. Which of the following drug used in CLL works on Bcl-2:
   1. Ibrutinib

2. Idelalisib
3. Venetoclax
4. Selumetinib

Answer: venetoclax

Idelalisib is a PIK-3 inhibitor.

Selumetinib is not used in CLL.

Q. Which is the most common second neoplasm developing in CLL patients:
　　1. Skin cancer
　　2. Lung cancer
　　3. Myelodysplastic syndrome
　　4. PNH turning into MDS

Answer: skin cancer

Approximately 25% of patients with CLL develop second neoplasms, the most common being skin cancer.

Q. CLL may sometimes evolve into a high grade lymphoma, known as Richter transformation. This transformation occurs in what percentage of cases:
　　1. 1-5
　　2. 5-10
　　3. <2
　　4. 20

Answer: 1-5%

The exact mentioned percentages range from 2 to 6%.

The prognosis of Richter transformation is poor, with a median survival of only 6 months.

Q. In high risk patients of CLL, not having del(17p), rituximab maintenance is recommended:
    1. True
    2. False

Answer: false

A trial was done that randomized patients to receive rituximab every 3 months for up to 2 years versus observation. There was improved PFS with rituximab versus observation; there was no difference in OS. There was also a higher incidence of grade 3/4 neutropenia and infections for patients who received rituximab.

So in conclusion, CD20 monoclonal antibody maintenance therapy post-chemoimmunotherapy improved PFS, but not OS, and is associated with neutropenia and infection. It is **not** recommended.

Q. Which of the following is not true about hairy cell leukemia;
    1. Hairy cells may be seen in the peripheral blood which are twice as large as normal lymphocytes
    2. Bone marrow has a "fried egg" appearance
    3. Immunophenotypic analysis of cHCL cells shows the presence of CD11c, CD23, CD25, CD103, CD123, as well as CD19, CD20, and CD22
    4. BRAF V600E gain of function mutation is found in

the cells from patients with classical HCL

Answer: Immunophenotypic analysis of cHCL cells shows the presence of CD11c, CD23, CD25, CD103, CD123, as well as CD19, CD20, and CD22

It must be noted that in contrast to CLL, hairy cells are negative for CD5 and CD23 and negative for CD10, CD27, and CD79b. So, the immunophenotypic analysis of cHCL cells shows the presence of CD11c, CD25, CD103, CD123, as well as CD19, CD20, and CD22.

Notes:
1. HCL can be of two types: classical and variant.
2. The variant HCL cells are negative for CD25 and CD123.
3. In variant HCL, BRAF V600E mutations are not seen.

Q. Which of the following is curative in cases of HCL:
1. Cladribine
2. Pentostatin
3. Vemurafenib and dabrafenib
4. Vemurafenib plus auto-HSCT

Answer: none of the above

It was a trick question, it should be remembered that for HCL there is no curative therapy, except perhaps allo-HCT.

Pentostatin (2′ deoxycoformycin) and cladribine (2-CdA) are nucleoside analogs and are the mainstay of treatment of HCL.

Because cladribine is given only for one course and pentostatin for many cycles, cladribine is preferred.

Vemurafenib and other BRAF inhibitors are used in classical HCL, either as monotherapy or in combination with anti-CD20 drugs. It should be noted that variant HCL is devoid of these mutations and not responsive to BRAF inhibitors.

Moxetumomab pasudotox is a novel drug which is a CD22 MAb-drug conjugate.

Q. Which is the most common recurrent abnormality in myelodysplastic syndromes:
    1. del(5q)
    2. -7
    3. 7q-
    4. +8

Answer: del(5q)

The most common recurrent abnormalities were del(5q) (30%), -7 or 7q- (21%), and +8 (16%).

Notes on some features of MDS:
    1. Macrocytic anemia is the most common hematologic feature.
    2. One-third patients will undergo transformation into AML.
    3. The classification of MDS was recently updated by the WHO and the reader is advised to read it up from their website.
    4. There are many risk assessment (stratification) tools for MDS: IPSS, International Prognostic Scoring System; IPSS-R, revised IPSS; WPSS, WHO Prognostic Scoring System; MDAS, MD Anderson Scoring

System; LR-MDAS, Lower Risk MDAS etc.

5. The IPSS and IPSS-R are most commonly used systems. Their components are:

   a. IPSS: bone marrow blasts, karyotype, cytopenia

   b. IPSS-R: bone marrow blasts, karyotype, hemoglobin, ANC, platelet count

   c. The IPSS divides patients into Low, Int-1, Int-2 and High.

   d. The IPSS-R divides patients into very good, good, intermediate, poor and very poor risk

   e. The karyotype abnormalities in the IPSS-R are:

      1. Very good: –Y, del(11q)

      2. Good: normal karyotype, single del(5q), del(12p), del(20q), or double including del(5q).

      3. Intermediate: single del(7q), +8, I (17q), +19, or any double not including del(5q).

      4. Poor: der(3q), monosomy 7, double including –7/7q, or three abnormalities.

      5. Very poor: **more than three** abnormalities.

Q. What will be the optimal initial treatment of a patient with high risk MDS:

1. Azacitidine for 4 to 6 cycles followed by evaluation for allo-HCT

2. Azacitidine for 4 to 6 cycles with response evaluation after every two cycles and finally evaluation for allo-HCT

3. Azacitidine is continued indefinitely and patients showing progression on azacitidine are evaluated for allo- or auto-HCT

4. Either decitabine or azacitidine are used for 4 to 6 cycles and then patients are put on active surveillance

Answer: Azacitidine for 4 to 6 cycles followed by evaluation for allo-HCT

If the patient is not a candidate for allogeneic HCT due to any reason, then azacitidine should be continued indefinitely.

Another important point to note is that the response to azacitidine is evaluated after four to six cycles.

Decitabine is also an option and the principles are similar to azacitidine.

Q. In lower risk MDS, anemia is the most common indication for therapy. In patients with a low endogenous serum erythropoietin level (<500 mU/ml) and low transfusion burden, treatment is begun with an ESA, like epoetin-α or darbepoetin-α. If no response is seen at 12 weeks then what should be the ideal next step:
   1. Increasing the dose of ESA
   2. Adding G-CSF
   3. Lenalidomide for non-del(5q) lower risk MDS
   4. Switching to azacitidine

Answer: adding G-CSF

There is no perfect answer for this question and practice varies depending on the institute.

Lenalidomide and azacitidine have also been used in these patients. Another interesting treatment option for MDS patients **younger than 60 years of age with a short duration of transfusion dependence, a CD4:CD8 ratio <2.0, or those with trisomy 8**, is immunosuppressive therapy (IST).

In del(5q) lower risk MDS patients who have either failed on ESA or are not candidates for treatment with an ESA, lenalidomide is the treatment of choice.

Q. The preferred method for detecting bone disease in multiple myeloma is:
1. Whole-body low-dose CT
2. PET-CT
3. Skeletal survey
4. MRI survey of abdomen

Answer: whole body low dose CT

Other modalities may also be used, in fact, they are frequently used.

Notes on ideal initial treatment strategies for multiple myeloma:
1. If a patient is not a transplant candidate and is fit, then preferred regimens are Bortezomib/lenalidomide/dexamethasone, Bortezomib/cyclophosphamide/dexamethasone and other recommended regimens are Carfilzomib/lenalidomide/dexamethasone and Ixazomib/lenalidomide/dexamethasone.
2. If a patient is not a transplant candidate and is frail, then the preferred regimens are: Bortezomib/lenalidomide/dexamethasone, Daratumumab/lenalidomide/dexamethasone, Lenalidomide/low-dose dexamethasone, Bortezomib/cyclophosphamide/dexamethasone. Other recommended regimens are Carfilzomib/lenalidomide/dexamethasone, Ixazomib/lenalidomide/dexamethasone, Daratumumab/bortezomib/melphalan/prednisone.

3. If a patient is transplant eligible, then there are two strategies:
   a. Early transplant: a combination of bortezomib, lenalidomide and dexamethasone is given for 3-4 cycles and autologous HCT is done followed by bortezomib maintenance for high risk patients or lenalidomide maintenance for standard risk patients.
   b. Delayed transplant: a combination of bortezomib, lenalidomide and dexamethasone is given for many more cycles and transplant is done later.

In some cases a tandem transplant (auto-HCT followed by another planned auto-HCT) or an auto- followed by allo-HCT is done.

Some experts recommend treatment with a combination of **carfil**zomib, lenalidomide and dexamethasone in high risk patients to begin with.

Devita oncology has this wonderful table on management of relapsed myeloma, which everybody should go through.

Q. SLAM-F7 targeting molecule used in multiple myeloma treatment is:
   1. Elotuzumab
   2. Daratumumab
   3. Panobinostat
   4. Selinexor

Answer: elotuzumab

Daratumumab is an anti-CD38 MAb.

Panobinostat is an HDAC inhibitor.

Pomalidomide is an immunomodulator.

Q. In patients of multiple myeloma, to prevent skeletal events bisphosphonates are indicated. For how long should bisphosphonates are administered every month in them:
1. 1 to 2 years
2. 3 to 5 years
3. Indefinitely
4. Bisphosphonates should ideally be given every 3 months indefinitely

Answer: 1 to 2 years

The dose of zoledronic acid is 4 mg intravenously over 15 to 30 minutes every 4 weeks and dose of pamidronate is 90 mg intravenously over at least 2 hours every 4 weeks.

When bisphosphonates are used, monthly use should be limited to the first 1 to 2 years. Thereafter, the frequency should be reduced to once every 3 to 4 months.

Some trials suggest that a reduced frequency of administration, i.e., once every 3 months may be as effective as monthly administration.

Q. Extramedullary plasmacytoma is localized most commonly to:
1. Upper respiratory tract
2. Lower GI tract
3. Upper GI tract
4. Retroperitoneum and thigh

Answer: upper respiratory tract

They are found in the nasal cavity and sinuses, nasopharynx, and larynx in over 80% of cases.

Q. What is the treatment of choice for solitary plasmacytoma:
    1. 40 to 50 Gy of radiation
    2. Surgery followed by 40 to 50 Gy of radiation
    3. 40 to 50 Gy of radiation followed by surgery
    4. Surgery alone and radiation only in high risk patients

Answer: 40 to 50 Gy of radiation

Notes on POEMS syndrome:
    1. Polyneuropathy
    2. Organomegaly
    3. Endocrinopathy
    4. Monoclonal plasma cell disorder
    5. Skin changes

Almost all patients with POEMS syndrome have either osteosclerotic lesions or Castleman disease.

Q. The treatment of choice for patients of smoldering myeloma is:
    1. Observation
    2. Radiation to involved sites
    3. Low dose myeloma directed therapy
    4. Immunomodulators

Answer: observation

Observation is done every 3 to 6 months.

Q. Which of the following is not an additional entity present in the revised ISS criteria for multiple myeloma compared with the ISS criteria:
1. Serum LDH
2. Chromosomal abnormalities by FISH
3. PCR multiplex gene analysis
4. None of the above

Answer: PCR multiplex gene analysis

The ISS criteria are:
1. Stage I: Serum beta-2 microglobulin <3.5 mg/L, Serum albumin ≥3.5 g/dL
2. Stage II: Not ISS stage I or III
3. Stage III: Serum beta-2 microglobulin ≥5.5 mg/L

The R-ISS criteria are:
1. ISS stage I and standard-risk chromosomal abnormalities by FISH and Serum LDH ≤ the upper limit of normal
2. Stage II: Not R-ISS stage I or III
3. Stage III: ISS stage III and either high-risk chromosomal abnormalities by FISH or Serum LDH > the upper limit of normal

The high-risk chromosomal abnormalities by FISH are: presence of del(17p) and/or translocation t(4;14) and/or translocation t(14;16). It should be noted here that some centres use different sets of high-risk chromosomal markers. But the above mentioned ones are most commonly used.

Q. All of the following may be labelled as smoldering myeloma except:
1. Serum monoclonal protein ≥3 g/dL
2. Bence-Jones protein ≥500 mg/24 h
3. Clonal bone marrow plasma cells 10%–59%
4. 2 or less focal lesions on MRI studies ≥5 mm

Answer: 2 or less focal lesions on MRI studies ≥5 mm

Diagnostic criteria for smoldering myeloma:
Serum monoclonal protein ≥3 g/dL or Bence-Jones protein ≥500 mg/24 h and/or clonal bone marrow plasma cells 10%–59% and absence of myeloma-defining events or amyloidosis
Diagnostic criteria for multiple myeloma:

Clonal bone marrow plasma cells ≥10% or biopsy-proven bony or extramedullary plasmacytoma **and** Any one or more of the following:
1. Calcium >0.25 mmol/L (>1 mg/dL) higher than the upper limit of normal or >2.75 mmol/L (>11 mg/dL)
2. Renal insufficiency (creatinine >2 mg/dL) [>177 μmol/L] or creatinine clearance <40 mL/min
3. Anemia (hemoglobin <10 g/dL or hemoglobin >2 g/dL below the lower limit of normal)
4. One or more osteolytic bone lesions on skeletal radiography, CT, or FDG PET/CT
5. Clonal bone marrow plasma cells ≥60%
6. Involved:uninvolved serum FLC ratio ≥100 and involved FLC concentration 10 mg/dL or higher
7. >**1** focal lesions on MRI studies ≥5 mm

Notes on some response categories of multiple myeloma:

1. Stringent complete response: Complete response as defined below plus normal FLC ratio and absence of clonal cells in bone marrow biopsy by immunohistochemistry (κ/λ ratio ≤4:1 or ≥1:2 for κ and λ patients, respectively, after counting ≥100 plasma cells).

2. Complete response: Negative immunofixation on serum and urine and disappearance of any soft tissue plasmacytomas and <5% plasma cells in bone marrow aspirates.

3. Very good partial response: Serum and urine M-protein detectable by immunofixation but not on electrophoresis or ≥90% reduction in serum M-protein plus urine M-protein level <100 mg per 24 h.

4. Partial response: ≥50% reduction of serum M-protein plus reduction in 24-h urinary M-protein by ≥90% or to <200 mg per 24 h. If the serum and urine M-protein are unmeasurable, a ≥50% decrease in the difference between involved and uninvolved FLC levels is required in place of the M-protein criteria. If serum and urine M-protein are unmeasurable, and serum-free light assay is also unmeasurable, ≥50% reduction in plasma cells is required in place of M-protein, provided baseline bone marrow plasma-cell percentage was ≥30%. In addition to these criteria, if present at baseline, a ≥50% reduction in the size (sum of the products of the maximal perpendicular diameters [SPD] of measured lesions) of soft tissue plasmacytomas is also required.

Printed in Great Britain
by Amazon

28353634R00381